Drug Development for Malaria

Drug Development for Malaria

Novel Approaches for Prevention and Treatment

Edited by Pravin Kendrekar

WILEY-VCH

Editor

Dr. Pravin Kendrekar
University of Central Lancashire
Centre for Smart Materials
Preston PR1 2HE
United Kingdom

Cover Image: © Christoph Burgstedt/Shutterstock

Library of Congress Card No.: applied for

British Library Cataloguing-in-Publication Data
A catalogue record for this book is available from the British Library.

Bibliographic information published by the Deutsche Nationalbibliothek
The Deutsche Nationalbibliothek lists this publication in the Deutsche Nationalbibliografie; detailed bibliographic data are available on the Internet at <http://dnb.d-nb.de>.

Print ISBN: 978-3-527-34860-2
ePDF ISBN: 978-3-527-83060-2
ePub ISBN: 978-3-527-83059-6
oBook ISBN: 978-3-527-83058-9

Cover Design: Wiley
Typesetting Straive, Chennai, India
Printing and Binding CPI Group (UK) Ltd, Croydon, CR0 4YY

Printed on acid-free paper

C110176_030822

Contents

Part I

Introduction

1

Chronology of Drug Development for Malaria

Nalini Kurup and Nikhil Rajnani

Principal K. M. Kundnani College of Pharmacy, Department of Pharmaceutics, Mumbai 400005, India

1.1 Introduction

The deadly malaria parasite is transmitted by mosquitoes and has been documented since earlier times. Malaria still remains an important cause of illness and death in children and adults in countries in which it is endemic. World Health Organization defines malaria as a life-threatening disease caused by parasites that are transmitted to people through the bites of infected female *Anopheles* mosquitoes, and it is preventable and curable [1]. The name malaria comes from the Italian word *mal'aria*, meaning "bad air." This was due to the reason that people thought the disease was transmitted via contaminated air (miasmas). Human malaria is caused by four different species of *Plasmodium* namely *P. falciparum*, *P. malariae*, *P. ovale*, and *P. vivax*. Of the four, *P. falciparum* and *P. vivax* pose the greatest threat. Scientists succeeded in sequencing the *P. falciparum* genome in 2002, which has permitted researchers to make great progress in comprehending better ways to target it [2].

The history of malaria depicts many attempts to defeat it. Quinine, a substance derived from the bark of the cinchona tree, has been known to be effective against malaria since the 1600s [3]. After discovering the role of mosquitoes in malaria transmission, scientists focused on vector control. They presumed that by killing the vector, they could halt the cycle of infection. As a result, DDT and other insecticides came into vogue in the mid-1900s and have been used ever since. Bed nets to protect sleeping people from mosquito bites are another form of vector control that is not only effective, but also extremely cost-effective [4]. Subsequently, the development of different anti-malaria drugs has changed the way travelers view malaria-endemic countries and the risk associated with traveling. In fact, and likely due to all of the above measures, estimated deaths from malaria fell 13%, from 755 000 in 2000 to 655 000 in 2010 [5]. Cases of the disease fell as well, although less dramatically, from 223 million in 2000 to about 216 million in 2010.

With all of these developments, why does malaria remain a problem? The emergence of resistance to drugs and insecticides is a major concern. Research in recent decades has shed light on many aspects of *Plasmodium* biology, broadening

Drug Development for Malaria: Novel Approaches for Prevention and Treatment, First Edition.
Edited by Pravin Kendrekar.

understanding of how parasites interact with the human immune system, cause human disease, and are transmitted by mosquitoes [6]. The malaria parasite has survived for more than 50 000 years, and natural selection favors strains of the organism with mutations that help them evade threats. Today we are seeing more and more drug-resistant parasites and insecticide-resistant mosquitoes. Global efforts are underway in the next era of malaria prevention: the development of malaria vaccines that have the potential to save countless lives and that could ultimately help eradicate this historic plight.

The World Malaria Report 2019 by WHO pays attention to the burden of malaria in two high-risk groups – children and pregnant women. In 2018, an estimated 228 million cases occurred worldwide and 405 000 deaths were reported. Twenty-seven countries reported less than 100 cases of malaria in 2018 compared with 17 countries in 2010. Inadequate funding being a barrier to future progress renewed R&D agenda is one of the major priorities to achieve a malaria-free world.

The report details on regional and global trends in burden of malaria cases and deaths, maternal, infant, and child health consequences of malaria, high burden to high-impact approach, investments in malaria programs and research, preventing malaria, diagnostic testing and treatment, world malaria report 2019 malaria surveillance systems and responding to biological threats to the fight against malaria [7].

The global technical strategy for malaria 2016–2030 adopted by the World Health Assembly in May 2015 provides a comprehensive framework to guide countries in their efforts to accelerate progress toward malaria elimination. The strategic framework comprising of three major pillars and two supporting elements sets the target of reducing global malaria incidence and mortality rates by at least 90% by 2030. The three major pillars being: (i) ensure universal access to malaria prevention, diagnosis, and treatment; (ii) accelerate efforts toward elimination and attainment of malaria-free status; and (iii) transform malaria surveillance into a core intervention. The two supporting elements are (i) innovation and research and (ii) a strong enabling environment. The program aims at achieving the vision – a world free of malaria [8].

There are many review articles emphasizing on the approaches available for prevention and treatment of malaria. This chapter aims at summarizing the information available on the erstwhile, current, and promising future in the drug development for malaria (Figure 1.1).

1.1.1 Life Cycle of Malaria (Adapted from CDC)

The malaria parasite life cycle involves two hosts [9].

During a blood meal, a malaria-infected female *Anopheles* mosquito inoculates sporozoites into the human host. Sporozoites infect liver cells and mature into schizonts, which rupture and release merozoites. (Of note, in *P. vivax* and *P. ovale*, a dormant stage [hypnozoites] can persist in the liver [if untreated] and cause relapses by invading the bloodstream weeks or even years later.) After this initial replication in the liver (exo-erythrocytic schizogony), the parasites undergo asexual multiplication in the erythrocytes (erythrocytic schizogony). Merozoites infect

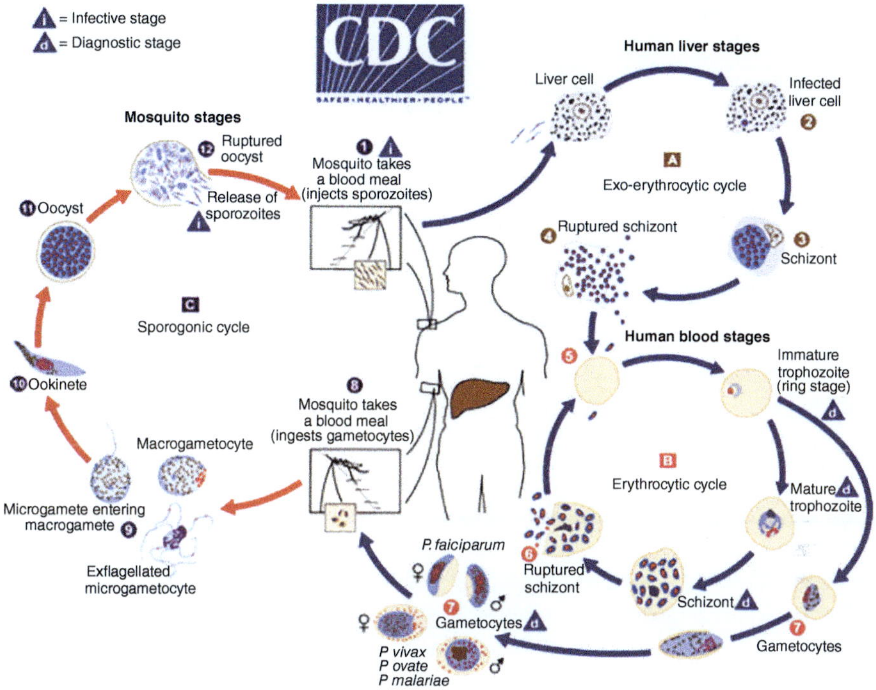

Figure 1.1 Life cycle of malaria adapted from CDC.

red blood cells. The ring stage trophozoites mature into schizonts, which rupture releasing merozoites. Some parasites differentiate into sexual erythrocytic stages (gametocytes). Blood stage parasites are responsible for the clinical manifestations of the disease. The gametocytes, male and female, are ingested by an *Anopheles* mosquito during a blood meal. The parasites' multiplication in the mosquito is known as the sporogonic cycle. While in the mosquito's stomach, the microgametes penetrate the macrogametes generating zygotes. The zygotes in turn become motile and elongated (ookinetes), which invade the midgut wall of the mosquito where they develop into oocysts. The oocysts grow, rupture, and release sporozoites, which make their way to the mosquito's salivary glands. Inoculation of the sporozoites into a new human host perpetuates the malaria life cycle.

1.2 Malaria – Erstwhile Memories

1.2.1 Progress Fighting Malaria

Since the dawn of modern microbiology research, beginning in the nineteenth century, scientists have known that the disease is actually caused by a microscopic parasite called Plasmodium, which is spread by mosquitoes common to wet, marshy places. Two of the earliest Nobel Prizes went to the scientists who made these basic discoveries, and at the dawn of the twentieth century, the situation had never seemed

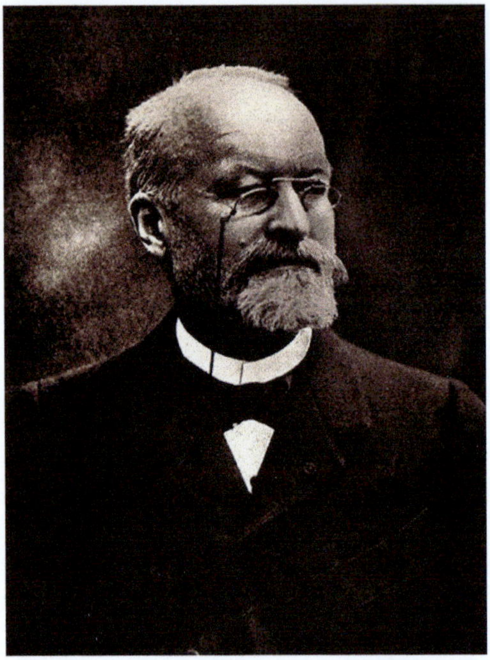

Figure 1.2 Charles Louis Alphonse Laveran first identifies the malaria parasite. Credit: Photo Researchers/ Science History Images/Alamy Stock Photo.

brighter. The possibility that malaria would be eliminated or eradicated was exciting and real then. History proved otherwise (Figures 1.2 and 1.3, Table 1.1).

Full malaria eradication was a major public health effort in the first half of the twentieth century and was intensively pursued after World War II. Since that effort was launched, 108 countries have eliminated malaria from within their borders, with another 39 countries en route to that goal. Despite those efforts, malaria remains a major cause of illness in many parts of the world. Today almost half the world's population lives in places where the disease is common.

According to the Centers for Disease Control and Prevention, about 1500 cases of malaria still occur in the United States each year, but most are imported when people travel abroad. The real problem exists in several Asian and sub-Saharan African countries, where malaria is both a major leading cause of death and a significant drain on the economy. The World Health Organization estimates that the disease eats up nearly half of all public health expenditures and measurably lowers the gross domestic product of countries where it is common.

Several new approaches to controlling malaria have become available in the last few decades, such as insecticide-treated bed nets, but there remains a dire need for new drugs and for effective vaccines to control it.

There are many references in early history indicating malaria afflicting mankind. In earlier times herbal remedies found importance in treatment of malaria [11]. The first efficacious treatment for malaria was quinine from the bark of the cinchona

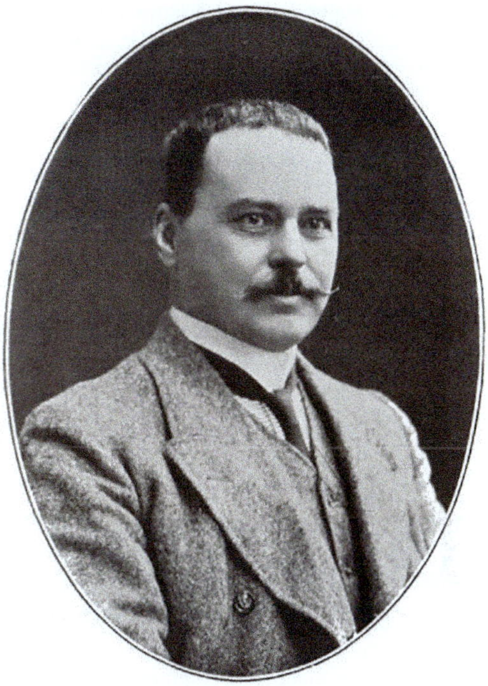

Figure 1.3 Sir Ronald Ross first demonstrates mosquitoes transmit malaria.

tree. With the association of spread of malaria to mosquitoes, many control measures such as spraying of insecticides, covering of open water surfaces, insecticide treated nets were initiated.

With the global increase in malaria cases, need was felt to develop stronger measures in prevention and treatment of malaria. Following the isolation of quinine from the bark of cinchona tree in 1820, a number of other natural and synthetic drugs have been developed as shown in the table below (Table 1.2):

1.3 Current Chemotherapy Used to Treat Malaria

Antimalarials mostly act by mechanisms that seek to inhibit one or two stages of the parasite's life cycle. The treatment aims to act on the parasite in two different ways. One of them is to interrupt the schizogenic blood stage responsible for the symptoms of the disease, that is, to kill the parasite during the evolutionary cycle. The other is to employ drugs that prevent the development of gametocytes parasites in the tissue cycle of the species *P. vivax* and *P. ovale*, interrupting the transmission of the parasite and avoiding relapses. Various drugs are available for achieving these goals, where each acts in a specific way to inhibit the development of the parasite in the host (Table 1.3).

Table 1.1 Major events in discovery of antimalarials.

1820	Quinine first purified from tree bark. For many years prior, the ground bark had been used to treat malaria
1880	Charles Louis Alphonse Laveran first identifies the malaria parasite. He was awarded the 1907 Nobel Prize for the discovery
1898	Sir Ronald Ross demonstrates that mosquitoes transmit malaria. He wins the 1902 Nobel Prize for this work
1934	Hans Andersag in Germany discovers the anti-malarial drug Chloroquine, which is not widely used until after World War II
1939	Paul Hermann Muller in Switzerland tests the insecticide DDT. He won the Nobel Prize for this work in 1948
1952	Malaria is eliminated in the United States
1957	First documented case of resistance to Chloroquine is reported
1976	William Trager and JB Jensen grow parasites in culture for the first time, opening the way for drug discovery and vaccine research
1989	The U.S. Food and Drug Administration approves the use of the anti-malaria drug Mefloquine hydrochloride, registered as Lariam® by Hoffman-LaRoche
1992	Malaria vaccine candidate RTS, -S, developed by GlaxoSmithKline and the Walter Reed Army Institute of Research, enters clinical trials
2000	The U.N. General Assembly adopts the Millennium Development Goals, setting a target to halt and begin reversing malaria incidence by 2015
2001	WHO prequalifies first fixed-dose Artemisinin combination therapy (ACT), sold by Novartis as Coartem® and recommends ACT as first-line malaria treatment
2002	Genome sequencing of *Anopheles gambiae* (mosquito) and *Plasmodium falciparum* (parasite) completed
2005	The World Health Assembly adopted a target of 80% worldwide coverage of insecticide nets and ACTs by 2010
2007	UCSF study shows combination malaria therapy effective in treating African children
2007	World Malaria Forum convenes in Seattle, hosted by Bill and Melinda Gates Foundation
2008	The Global Health Group at UCSF comes forward with the first high-level strategy for the eventual achievement of malaria eradication. This strategy has since been widely adopted
2008	The United Nations adopted April 25 as World Malaria Day

Source: Data from Ref. [10].

A great challenge for malaria treatment in recent decades has been to overcome the parasite's ability to acquire resistance to antimalarials, requiring the development of more effective drugs.

(1) **Aminoquinoline** [13, 14]

In general they are the derivatives, i.e. quinolines substituted in any position by one or more amino groups. Depending upon the substitution, they are further classified to 4-aminoquinoline and 8-aminoquinoline. Drugs that belong to this class are chloroquine (CQ), amodiaquine, primaquine, bulaquine, etc.

Table 1.2 Origin of antimalarial drugs.

Name of the drug	Structure	Origin	Year	Current status
Quinine	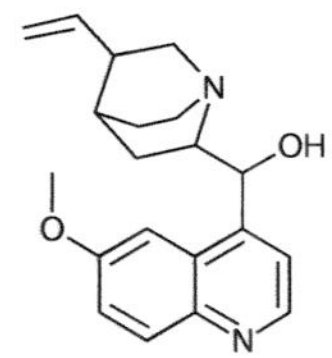	Natural Alkaloid from bark of cinchona tree	1820	Resistance was reported in 1980 but still used in severe malaria cases when artemisinin was not available. Appears on WHO's Model List of Essential Medicines (MLEM)
Mepacrine (Quinacrine)	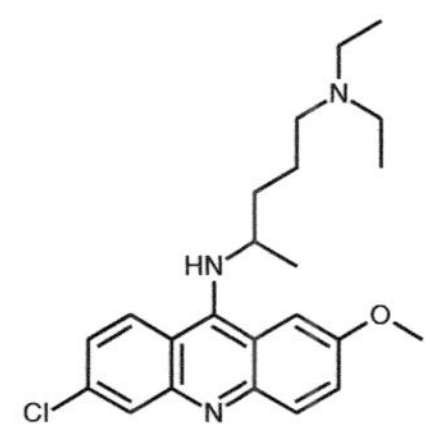	Synthetic Acridine derivative	1930	No longer used due to side effects of toxic psychosis
Chloroquine	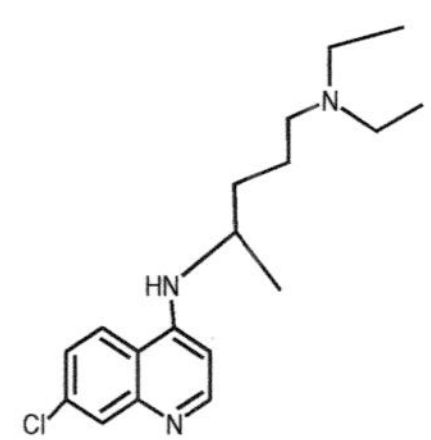	Synthetic Quinoline derivative	1934	Resistance reported in 1950. Appears on MLEM and used where resistance is not developed and for treatment of *P. vivax*

Table 1.2 (Continued)

Name of the drug	Structure	Origin	Year	Current status
Mefloquine	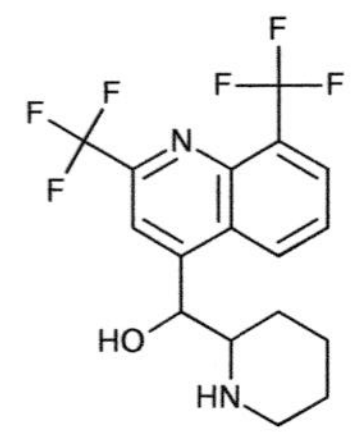	Synthetic	1970	No longer used due to CNS toxicity. Appears on MLEM to be used in combination with artesunate
Halofantrine	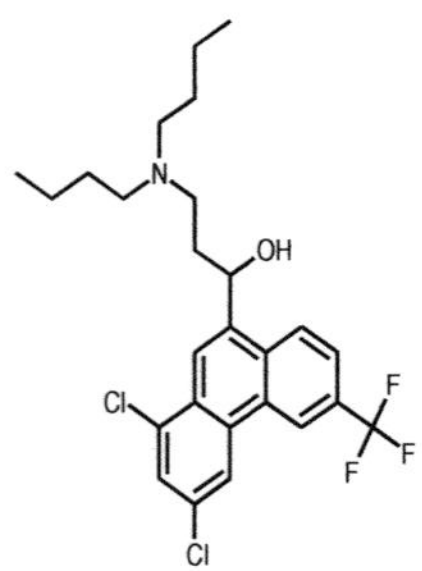	Synthetic	1980	Still used in patients free of heart diseases. Used in severe and resistant forms of malaria

Source: Based on Tse et al. [12].

Table 1.3 Classification of the antimalarial drugs.

Past drugs	A. Aminoquinolines	Chloroquine, Hydroxychloroquine, Amodiaquine
	B. 8-Aminoquinolines	Primaquine, Tafenoquine, Bulaquine
	C. Arylamino alcohols	Quinine
Present drugs	D. Methanols i. 4-Quinoline methanol ii. 9-Phenanthrene methanol	Mefloquine Halofantrine, Lumefantrine
	E. Biguanides	Proguanil
	F. Diaminopyrimidines	Pyrimethamine
	G. Antimalarial endoperoxides i. First generation endoperoxides (Artemisinin derivatives) ii. Second generation endoperoxides a. Trioxanes b. Tetroxanes	Artesunate, Artemether, Arteether
	H. Hydroxynaphthoquinone	Atovaquone
	I. Benzonaphthyridine derivative	Pyronaridine
	J. Antibiotics	Sulfonamides, Tetracycline, Doxycycline, Clindamycin, Azithromycin

Mechanism of action: Generally not known, but it believes that it accumulates in acidic pH Vescuoles, thus forming drug – heme complex thus preventing the free heme toxic to be available for the parasite.

(2) **Methanols/aryl amino alcohol** [15]

Drugs that belong to this class include quinine, lumefantrine, mefloquine, halofantrine

Mechanism of action: Interfere with the digestion of hemoglobin in blood stage of malaria life cycle by accumulating in the acidic vacuole of the parasite. Higher concentration of drug leads to polymerization of heme.

(3) **Biguanides** (https://go.drugbank.com/drugs/DB01131, [16])

Popularly known as proguanil (chloroguanide). It is a biguanide derivative, which is converted to an active metabolite called cycloguanil pamoate.

Mechanism of action: By inhibiting the enzyme parasitic dihydrofolate reductase (DHFR) thus inhibiting bacterial growth. It has both suppressive and prophylactic attack against *P. falciparum* and also effective against vivax malaria.

(4) **Diaminopyrimidines** [17]

Like biguanides, they also inhibit enzyme DHFR, which interfere in the synthesis of tetrahydro folic acid, a cofactor needed for bacteria to make the nucleotide bases thymine, guanine, uracil, and adenine.

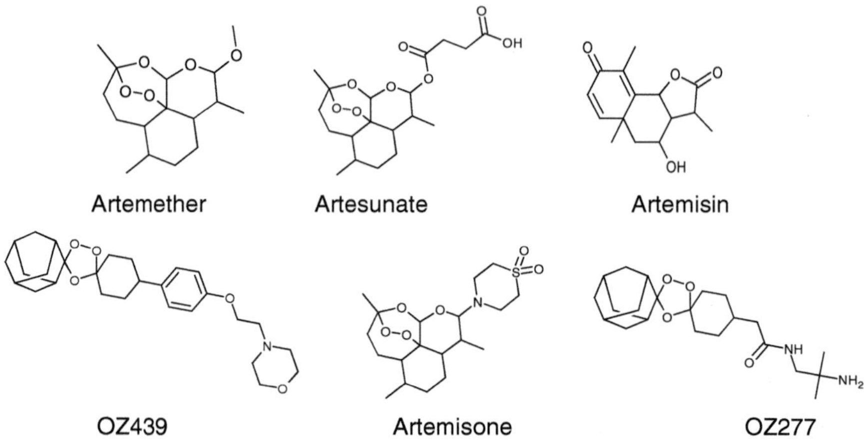

Figure 1.4 Structure of antimalarial drugs belonging to class endoperoxide.

(5) **Antimalarial endoperoxides** [18]

Drugs belonging to this class include artemisinin (ART) and its derivatives, first- and second-generation endoperoxides. This class of antimalarial drugs has several advantages over other antimalarial drugs

- Little or no cross resistance
- Clear the peripheral blood parasite
- Short half life
- Sustained effect

ART and its derivatives also act as gametocytocidal and effective against specific stages in the malaria life cycle. Trophozoites and parasites are more susceptible while the liver stage of *P. vivax* and *P. falciparum* is not affected.

Mechanism of action: It acts as free radical scavengers, thus high oxygen tension is increased and. Drugs in this class produce oxygen free radicals such as superoxide, which damage the malarial cell. Other effects can also be seen as hemolysis, decreased erythrocytes deformability.

It acts differently from other drugs; instead of reacting with oxygen, it produces large quantities of oxygen-free radicals such as superoxide and OH^-.

(6) **Hydroxynaphthoquinone** [19, 20]

Drugs belonging to this class, i.e. atovaquone, are used for both prevention and treatment of malaria. Usually atovaquone is given in a fixed-dose combination with proguanil. Its primary mode of action is it acts on mitochondrial functions. And with proguanil, it gives asynergistic effect and interferes with mitochondrial membrane potential.

Mechanism of action: It inhibits cytochrome c reductase activity in *P. falciparum* by binding with cytochrome bc1 complex of the parasite mitochondrial electron transport chain. Thus, disposes of electrons generated by dihydroorotate dehydrogenase during the synthesis of pyrimidines and inhibition of this process kills parasites (Figures 1.4–1.9).

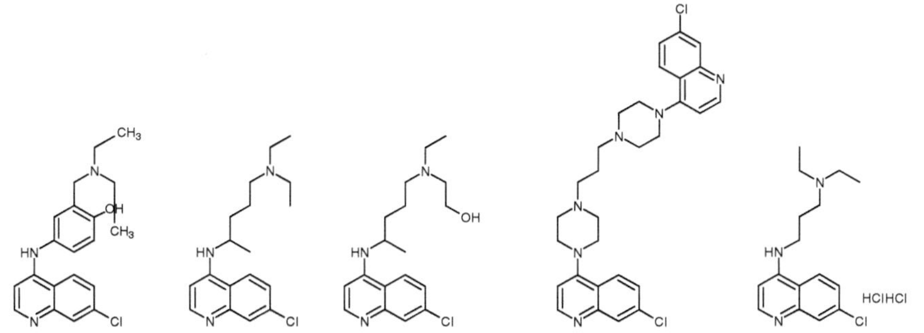

Amodiaquine Chloroquine Hydroxychloroquine Piperaquine AQ-13 Dihydrochloride

Figure 1.5 Structure of antimalarial drugs belonging to class 4-aminoquinolines.

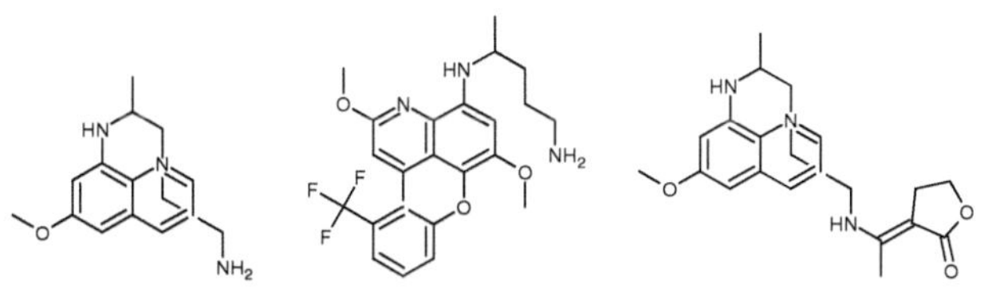

Primaquine Tafenoquine Bulaquine

Figure 1.6 Structure of antimalarial drugs belonging to class 8-aminoquinolines.

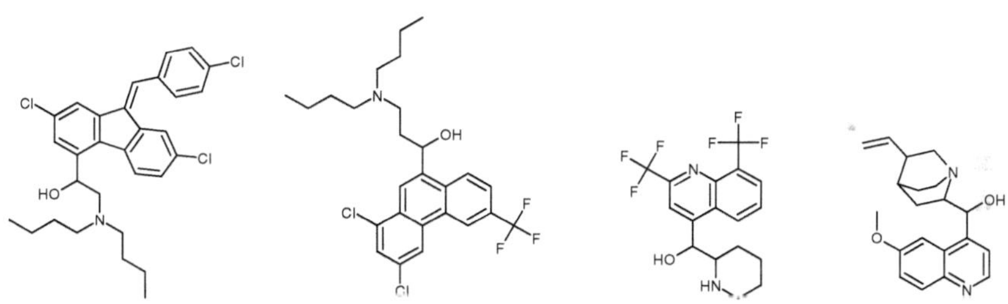

Lumefantrine Halofantrine Mefloquine Quinine

Figure 1.7 Structure of antimalarial drugs belonging to class quinoline derivatives.

1.3.1 Current Combination Therapy

The combination of a fast-acting ART derivative and a long-acting antimalarial with different mechanisms of action is called artemisinin-based combination therapy (ACT). The use of ACTs with at least two drugs is recommended by the WHO to prevent or reduce the development of antimalarial resistance. These combined therapies may act concomitantly through several mechanisms of action and in different biochemical targets of the parasite, achieving better results than monotherapy. Replacement of monotherapy by ACT has started in all countries where *P. falciparum* is endemic. ART derivatives are considered the basis for the treatment of *P. falciparum* malaria and are used to combat uncomplicated malaria.

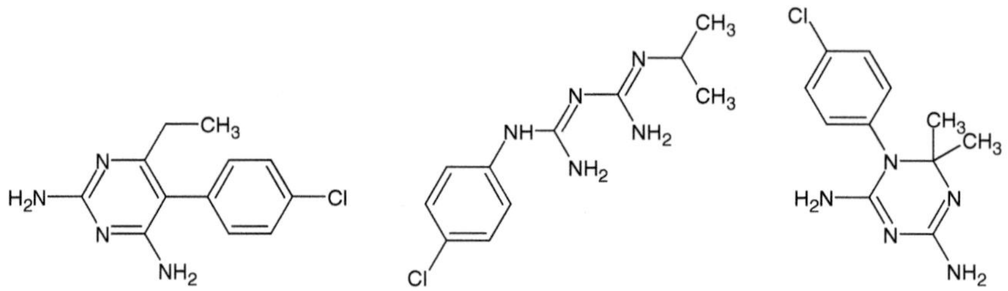

Pyrimethamine Proguanil Cycloguanil

Figure 1.8 Structure of antimalarial drugs belonging to class antifolates.

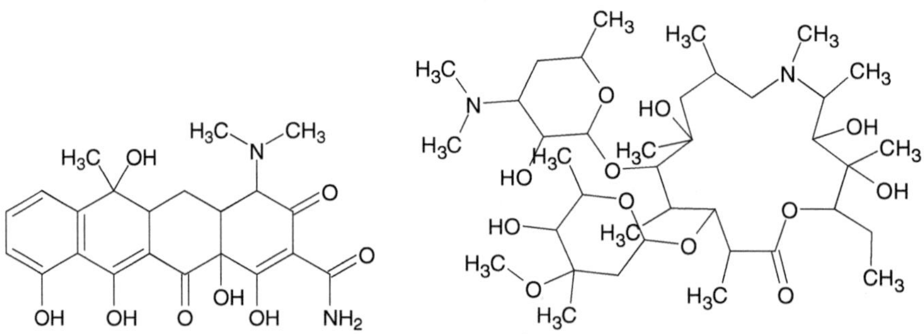

Tetracycline Azithromycin

Figure 1.9 Structure of antimalarial drugs belonging to class antibiotics.

The ACTs for the treatment of malaria are as follows:

- Dihydroartemisinin + piperaquine (Eurartesim®)
- Artemether + lumefantrine (Coartem®)
- Artesunate + mefloquine (ASMQ)
- Artesunate + amodiaquine (Winthrop® or Coarsucam™)
- Artesunate + sulfadoxine + pyrimethamine
- ARCO® (artemisinin + naphthoquine)

1.4 Drug Resistance of Antimalarial Drugs

Resistance to antimalarial drugs has been described for two of the four species of malaria parasites that naturally infect humans; *P. falciparum* and *P. vivax*. *P. falciparum* have developed resistance to nearly all antimalarials in current use.

Antimalarial drug resistance has been defined as the "ability of a parasite strain to survive and/or multiply despite the administration and absorption of a drug given in doses equal to or higher than those usually recommended but within tolerance of the subject." This definition was later modified to specify that the drug in question must "gain access to the parasite or the infected red blood cell for the duration of the time necessary for its normal action" [21].

Most researchers interpret this as referring only to persistence of parasites after treatment doses of an antimalarial rather than prophylaxis failure, although the latter is a useful tool for early warning of the presence of drug resistance [22].

This definition of resistance holds true if the patient has been administered the required treatment dose and also demonstrates adequate blood drug and metabolite concentrations using laboratory methods such as high-performance liquid chromatography or *in vitro* tests.

A differentiation must be made between a failure to clear malarial parasitemia and true antimalarial drug resistance. While drug resistance can cause treatment failure, not all treatment failures are due to drug resistance. Factors that contribute to treatment failure include incorrect dosing, noncompliance with duration of dosing regimen, poor drug quality, drug interactions, poor or erratic absorption, and misdiagnosis.

Mechanisms of antimalarial resistance – In general, resistance appears to occur through spontaneous mutations that confer reduced sensitivity to a given drug or class of drugs. For some drugs, only a single point mutation is required to confer resistance, while for other drugs, multiple mutations appear to be required. Provided the mutations are not deleterious to the survival or reproduction of the parasite, drug pressure will remove susceptible parasites while resistant parasites survive. Single malaria isolates have been found to be made up of heterogeneous populations of parasites that can have widely varying drug response characteristics, from highly resistant to completely sensitive [23].

The biochemical mechanism of resistance has been well described for chloroquine, the antifolate combination drugs, and atovaquone.

In chloroquine resistance, as the malaria parasite digests hemoglobin, large amounts of toxic by-product are formed. The parasite polymerizes this by-product in its food vacuole, producing nontoxic hemozoin (malaria pigment). It is believed that resistance of *P. falciparum* to chloroquine is related to an increased capacity for the parasite to expel chloroquine at a rate that does not allow chloroquine to reach levels required for inhibition of heme polymerization [15]. This chloroquine efflux occurs at a rate of 40–50 times faster among resistant parasites than sensitive ones [24]. Further evidence supporting this mechanism is provided by the fact that chloroquine resistance can be reversed by drugs, which interfere with this efflux system [25]. It is unclear whether parasite resistance to other quinoline antimalarials (amodiaquine, mefloquine, halofantrine, and quinine) occurs via similar mechanisms [15].

Combination drugs, such as sulfadoxine + pyrimethamine, act through sequential and synergistic blockade of two key enzymes involved with folate synthesis. Pyrimethamine and related compounds inhibit the step mediated by DHFR while sulfones and sulfonamides inhibit the step mediated by dihydropteroate synthase (DHPS) [21]. Specific gene mutations encoding for resistance to both DHPS and DHFR have been identified. Specific combinations of these mutations have been associated with varying degrees of resistance to antifolate combination drugs [26].

Atovaquone acts through inhibition of electron transport at the cytochrome bc1 complex [27]. Although resistance to atovaquone develops very rapidly when used

Table 1.4 Resistance to antimalarial drugs [36].

Antimalarial drug	Introduction date	First reported resistance
Quinine	1632	1910
Chloroquine	1945	1957
Proguanil	1948	1949
Sulfadoxine + Pyrimethamine	1967	1967
Mefloquine	1977	1982
Halofantrine	1988	1993
Atovaquone	1996	1996
Artemisinin	1971	1980

alone, when combined with a second drug, such as proguanil (the combination used in Malarone™) or tetracycline, resistance develops more slowly [28]. Resistance is conferred by single point mutations in the cytochrome-b gene.

In one study, patients experiencing chloroquine treatment failure had recrudescent infections that tended to be less severe or even asymptomatic [29]. Schizont maturation may also be more efficient among resistant parasites [30, 31]. There is some evidence that certain combinations of drug-resistant parasites and vector species enhance transmission of drug resistance, while other combinations inhibit transmission of resistant parasites.

Many antimalarial drugs in current usage are closely related chemically, and development of resistance to one can facilitate development of resistance to others. Chloroquine and amodiaquine are both 4-aminoquinolines, and cross-resistance between these two drugs is well known [32, 33]. Development of resistance to mefloquine may also lead to resistance to halofantrine and quinine. Antifolate combination drugs have similar action, and widespread use of sulfadoxine/pyrimethamine (SP) for the treatment of malaria may lead to increased parasitological resistance to other antifolate combination drugs [34]. Development of high levels of SP resistance through continued accumulation of DHFR mutations may compromise the useful life span of newer antifolate combination drugs such as chlorproguanil/dapsone (LapDap) even before they are brought into use. This increased risk of resistance due to sulfadoxine–pyrimethamine (SP) use may even affect non-malarial pathogens; use of SP for treatment of malaria increased resistance to trimethoprim/sulfamethoxazole among respiratory pathogens [35] (Table 1.4).

1.4.1 Detection of Drug Resistance

In vivo test, *in vitro* test, animal models, molecular characterization, and additional methods such as case reports and case series are used for detection of drug resistance in malaria.

In an *in vivo* test, the symptomatic and parasitemia individuals are administered a known dose of drug and monitored over time to check for clinical response. In spite of *in vivo* tests offering reliable information on efficacy of antimalarial treatment, they do not necessarily reflect the actual level of antimalarial drug resistance. The *in vivo* test requires follow-up for a long period, but it has been modified to shorter period of 7–14 days as recurrence is more likely than reinfection. Hematological recovery can be checked as anemia that is a major effect of malaria [37].

The *in vitro* tests consist of collecting the parasite from a blood prick of an infected individual and exposing it to known quantities of drugs (microtiter) under suitable experimental conditions and checking for inhibition of maturation into schizonts. Several drugs can be assessed, but its correlation to actual clinical response in infected individuals was not found to be consistent. Prodrugs cannot be tested, and non-falciparum erythrocytic parasites cannot be generally evaluated by *in vitro* methods [38].

Animal model studies are a type of *in vivo* test but carried out on human models. This test allows testing of drugs not yet approved for human use, but only parasites adaptable to non-human primates can be tested.

Therefore, ACT, which is effective against chloroquine- and mefloquine-resistant strains, not only is active against the mature ring stage of *P. falciparum*, when the parasites are most metabolically active, but also targets the young ring stages of the parasites.

1.5 Newer Drugs Approved for Malaria Treatment

Besides the traditional drug discovery and development methods for the identification of new antimalarials that will be described below, there are a number of other ways in which a new antimalarial drug may be discovered. One way, as previously mentioned, is through the exploration of new combinations and formulations of current antimalarial drugs. This may help overcome issues with resistance to a particular component or may assist in the delivery of the drug allowing it to be more effective.

The new drug, Krintafel (tafenoquine), prevents relapse of malaria caused by *P. vivax*, one of several parasites that causes the disease.

Other Drugs Which are Under Clinical Trial

(1) **Tulane University researchers developed a new drug called AQ-13 and were able to clear the parasite responsible for disease within a week** [39]

It is a chloroquine (CQ) analogue with short side chain. It has a remarkable property of retrieving its activity against CQ resistant *P. falciparum*, and has a synonym Ro47-0543. CQ targets blood stage schizonts and interferes with heme detoxification within the food vacuole. CQ resistance is mediated by mutations in *P. falciparum* CQ resistance transporter gene (pfcrt) that leads to augmented efflux of CQ and restores hematin crystallization.

(2) **Methylene Blue** [40, 41]
Water-soluble dye, well absorbed from the GI tract. It was the first synthetic antimalarial to be used, which occurred in a German hospital some 120 years ago. Like 4-aminoquinolines, it also interacts with the polymerization of heme to hemozoin.

(3) **Fosmiomycin** [42]
A phosphoric acid derivative, which blocks a key enzyme 1-deoxy-D-xylulose 5-phosphate (DOXP) reductoisomerase, thus interferes in the DOXP pathway thereby inhibiting the growth of multi-drug-resistant strain.

(4) **Imtainib** [43]
Like all tyrosine-kinase inhibitors, it works by preventing a tyrosine kinase enzyme. It inhibits the phosphorylation of erythrocyte membrane band 3 by an erythrocyte tyrosine kinase. Since tyrosine phosphorylation of band 3 causes a destabilization of the erythrocyte membrane required for parasite to move out of erythrocytes, inhibition of the erythrocyte tyrosine kinase leads to parasite entrapment and termination of the malaria infection.

(5) **Sevuparin** [44]
A heparin analogue having low anticoagulant activity thus has anti-adhesive properties. It inhibits sequestration of late-stage infected erythrocyte to uninfected erythrocyte. Sevaparin is developed by Dilaforette AB, a Swedish pharmaceutical company founded by researchers of the Karolinska Institute. It is under Phase II clinical study, and probable further trials will show if this adds to therapy of severe malaria.

1.6 Current Approaches to Developing a Malaria Vaccine

Although there have been many efforts and substantial progress to control malaria, combination therapy is available to treat the resistance against the *P. falciparum*, but the disease is still a critical problem in endemic areas, affecting millions of children and adults. Vaccines aimed at different stages in the *Plasmodium* life cycle are in development, and in the future, successful candidates could be combined to achieve the greatest activity. One candidate, the RTS, -S vaccine that targets pre-erythrocytic stage parasites, has been implemented in three African countries.

1.6.1 Hope for Vaccine Lies in the Parasite Itself

The *Plasmodium* parasite leads a strange and complicated life, crisscrossing between two "host" species – humans and mosquitoes. Within the short span of just a few weeks, the organism cycles through a half dozen radically different sizes and shapes and alternatively makes its home in the human liver, a person's bloodstream, the insect stomach, and a mosquito's spit [45].

For years scientists knew that the most fruitful way to fight the parasite would be to target the form in which it exists in the bloodstream, since that is where the majority of clinical symptoms occur. Existing drugs, such as quinine and ART, both target the parasite in the blood.

About 15 years ago, scientists discovered a potential new source of drug targets in a tiny, factory-like enveloped organelle called an apicoplast that exists within the parasite. It was unlike anything found normally in the human body, which suggested that drugs designed to interfere with it might kill the parasite while essentially leaving people unharmed.

In the last decade, the evolutionary history of this strange organelle has unfolded. The apicoplast is the strange remnant of collisions between competing cells far back in evolutionary history. Scientists reason that through the course of evolution, the apicoplast arose from its origin as a stand-alone bacterium into its current form through a series of at least two endosymbiotic events, in which one cell engulfs and permanently acquires genetic material and cellular machinery of another for its own benefit.

The discovery of this strange organelle in modern *Plasmodium* immediately suggested that there might be ways to target it with new drugs. However, even after extensive research revealed the genes of this apicoplast, efforts to raise new drugs against it were mostly fruitless – largely because nobody knew what the organelle actually did while the parasite was inside the human bloodstream.

Now DeRisi and Yeh have shown that the sole essential function of the apicoplast while the parasite is in the blood to produce a single chemical known as isopentenyl pyrophosphate (IPP), a necessary building block the parasite uses to construct a variety of other molecules.

They discovered this by growing samples of *P. falciparum* within red blood cells in the test tube. If they treated the parasite with antibiotic drugs that kill the apicoplast, the parasites would all die. If they fed the parasites IPP at the same time, they lived – even though the parasites lost the organelle completely over time.

The work provides a new tool for probing the basic biology of the *Plasmodium* parasite, and it also suggests a new way of discovering promising new drugs to fight malaria. While many previous drug-screening efforts have identified multitudes of compounds that appear to inhibit growth of the parasites, most are without a known target within the parasites. Knowing the target of a drug greatly enables the necessary process of medicinal chemistry, in which the compound is optimized with respect to the target. Now, DeRisi and Yeh's discovery has provided a simple tool to determine whether any particular drug candidate targets the apicoplast [46].

The attenuated form of the parasite also provides an intriguing hypothetical vaccine candidate – and one that would be relatively cheap to produce, DeRisi said. However, he cautioned, the history of malaria control is filled with failed efforts, and several past vaccines have fallen short. Only time and clinical trials will tell if this is a viable solution to the problem. "This parasite has clearly evolved to be an immune system escape artist," DeRisi said. "It's no surprise that the simple approaches have not worked." (Table 1.5).

The idea of a pre-erythrocytic vaccine took shape with the landmark observation by Ruth Nussenzweig that vaccination of mice with irradiated sporozoites resulted in protection [47] and, further, that protection could be achieved by immunization

Table 1.5 Vaccine candidates that target each stage.

1. Pre-erythrocytic stages (Sporozoites)	**Anti-infection vaccines** Subunit vaccines: RTS, -S/AS01E, R21, full-length CSP Whole sporozite vaccines: PfSPZ vaccine, chemoprophylaxis vaccination, genetically attenuated sporozoites
2. Asexual blood stages (Merozoites)	**Blood stage vaccines** Merozoite antigens: AMA1, MSP1, MSP3, EBA-175, PfRh5, AMA1-RON2 complex Other antigens: PfSEA1, PfGARP, chemically attenuated parasites Placental malaria: VARCSA
3. Mosquito sexual stages (Gametocytes)	**Transmission blocking vaccines** Pfs25, Pfs230, Pfs48/45, Pvs230

with the CS protein (CSP) alone [48]. Development of human pre-erythrocytic vaccines began with the cloning of the *P. falciparum* CSP and the entry of SmithKline with the Walter Reed Army Institute of Research (WRAIR) into vaccine development in 1985. This research led to the development of the RTS, -S vaccine, which consists of hepatitis B surface antigen (HBsAg) particles with 25% of the HBsAg fused to the central repeat and thrombospondin domain of the CSP formulated in the adjuvant AS01 [48, 49].

1.7 Conclusion: The Path Forward

Vaccines for malaria are an important measure for prevention of the disease and minimize malaria transmission. Intense efforts by many groups in this field have happened over the last few decades. In spite of this, currently there is no malaria vaccine available. Many approaches have been worked upon to develop a malaria vaccine. The task of development of malaria vaccine is difficult due to the complexity of the malaria parasite.

About 275 000 children have received their first dose of the RTS, -S malaria vaccine through the pilot implementation program initiated in Ghana, Kenya, and Malawi in 2019. The malaria vaccine is the first vaccine that can significantly reduce malaria in children – the group at highest risk of dying from malaria.

1.7.1 RTS, -S Vaccine: A New Tool with Potential for Africa

Since 2000, the scale-up of proven interventions, such as insecticide-treated bed nets, has driven down malaria illness and death, but progress has slowed, particularly in Africa. Efforts are underway to increase the use of the tools we have, but even with scale-up of existing tools, there is a critical need for new tools to further drive down malaria illness and deaths – the RTS, -S malaria vaccine may be one of those tools. The malaria vaccine can reduce malaria in children, including cases of severe malaria, related hospital admissions, and the need for blood transfusions. The current pilot program will help guide and optimize the vaccine's future use.

References

1 WHO (2020). Malaria fact sheet. https://www.who.int/news-room/fact-sheets/detail/malaria (accessed 01 September 2020). CDC.

2 Gardner, M.J., Hall, N., Fung, E. et al. (2002). Genome sequence of the human malaria parasite *Plasmodium falciparum*. *Nature* 419 (6906): 498–511.

3 Achan, J., Talisuna, A.O., Erhart, A. et al. (2011). Quinine, an old anti-malarial drug in a modern world: role in the treatment of malaria. *Malaria Journal* 10: 144.

4 WHO (2015). Core vector control methods. https://apps.who.int/iris/bitstream/handle/10665/310862/9789241550499-eng.pdf (accessed 01 September 2020).

5 WHO (2011). 2011 world malaria report. https://www.mmv.org/newsroom/news/world-malaria-report-2011-highlights-fragile-progress (accessed 01 September 2020).

6 NIH (2016). Malaria parasite, mosquito, and human host. https://www.niaid.nih.gov/diseases-conditions/malaria-parasite (accessed 01 September 2020).

7 WHO (2019). World Malaria Report 2019. https://www.mmv.org/newsroom/publications/world-malaria-report-2019 (accessed 01 September 2020).

8 WHO (2015). Global technical strategy for malaria 2016–2030.

9 CDC (2020). https://www.cdc.gov/malaria/about/biology/ (accessed 01 September 2020).

10 (2011). https://www.ucsf.edu/news/2011/08/103884/progress-fighting-malaria-timeline (accessed 05 September 2020).

11 Willcox, M.L. and Bodeker, G. (2004). Traditional herbal medicines for malaria. *BMJ* 329 (7475): 1156–1159.

12 Tse, E.G., Korsik, M., and Todd, M.H. (2019). The past, present and future of anti-malarial medicines. *Malaria Journal* 18: 93.

13 Pussard, E. and Verdier, F. (1994). Antimalarial 4-aminoquinolines: mode of action and pharmacokinetics. *Fundamental and Clinical Pharmacology* 8 (1): 1–17.

14 White, N.J. (1996). The treatment of malaria. *The New England Journal of Medicine* 335: 800–806.

15 Foley, M. and Tilley, L. (1997). Quinoline antimalarials: mechanisms of action and resistance. *International Journal of Parasitology* 27 (2): 231–240.

16 Smith, C.C., Ihrig, J., and Menne, R. (1961). Antimalarial activity and metabolism of biguanides. *The American Journal of Tropical Medicine and Hygiene* 10 (5): 694–703.

17 Hitchings, G.H. Mechanism of action of trimethoprim-sulfamethoxazole. I. *Journal of Infectious Diseases* 128 (Suppl): 433–436.

18 Meshnick, S.R., Taylor, T.E., and Kamchonwongpaisan, S. (1996). Artemisinin and the antimalarial endoperoxides: from herbal remedy to targeted chemotherapy. *Micrological Reviews* 60 (2): 301–315.

19 Saifi, M.A., Beg, T., Harrath, A.H. et al. (2013). Antimalarial drugs: mode of action and status of resistance. *African Journal of Pharmacy and Pharmacology* 7 (5): 148–156.

20 Gemma, L.N., Moss, D.M., Shone, A.E. et al. (2013). Antimalarial pharmacology and therapeutics of atovaquone. *Journal of Antimicrobial Chemotherapy* 68 (5): 977–985.

21 Bruce-Chwatt, L.J., Black, R.H. et al. (1986). *Chemotherapy of Malaria*. Geneva: World Health Organization.

22 Lobel, H.O. and Campbell, C.C. (1986). Malaria prophylaxis and distribution of drug resistance. *Clinics in Tropical Medicine and Communicable Diseases* 1: 225–242.

23 Thaithong, S. (1983). Clones of different sensitivities in drug resistant isolates of *Plasmodium falciparum*. *Bulletin of the World Health Organization* 61: 709–712.

24 Krogstad, D.J., Gluzman, I.Y., Kyle, D.E. et al. (1987). Efflux of chloroquine from *Plasmodium falciparum*: mechanism of chloroquine resistance. *Science* 238: 1283–1285.

25 Martin, S.K., Oduola, A.M., and Milhous, W.K. (1987). Reversal of chloroquine resistance in *Plasmodium falciparum* by verapamil. *Science* 235: 899–901.

26 Plowe, C.V., Kublin, J.G., and Duombo, O.K. (1998). *P. falciparum* dihydrofolate reductase and dihydropteroate synthase mutations: epidemiology and role in clinical resistance to antifolates. *Drug Resistance Updates* 1: 389–396.

27 Ittarat, I., Asawamahasakda, W., and Meshnick, S.R. (1994). The effects of antimalarials on the *Plasmodium falciparum* dihydroorotate dehydrogenase. *Experimental Parasitology* 79: 50–56.

28 Looareesuwan, S., Viravan, C., Webster, H.K. et al. (1996). Clinical studies of atovaquone, alone or in combination with other antimalarial drugs for the treatment of acute uncomplicated malaria in Thailand. *American Journal of Tropical Medicine and Hygiene* 54: 62–66.

29 Handunnetti, S.M., Gunewardena, D.M., Ekanayake, K. et al. (1996). Features of recrudescent chloroquine-resistant *Plasmodium falciparum* infections confer a survival advantage on parasites and have implications for disease control. *Transactions of the Royal Society of Tropical Medicine & Hygiene* 90: 563–567.

30 Wernsdorfer, W.H., Walther, H., Landgraf, B. et al. (1995). Chloroquine resistance of *Plasmodium falciparum*: a biological advantage? *Transactions of the Royal Society of Tropical Medicine & Hygiene* 89: 90–91.

31 Warsame, M., Abdillahi, A., Nur Duale, O. et al. (1991). Susceptibility of *Plasmodium falciparum* in vitro to chloroquine, mefloquine, quinine and sulfadoxine/pyrimethamine in Somalia: relationships between the responses to the different drugs. *Transactions of the Royal Society of Tropical Medicine & Hygiene* 85: 565–569.

32 Basco, L.K. (1991). Inefficacy of amodiaquine against chloroquine-resistant malaria. *Lancet* 338: 1460–1460.

33 Hall, A.P., Segal, H.E., Pearlmanet, E.J. et al. (1975). Amodiaquine resistant falciparum malaria in Thailand. *American Journal of Tropical Medicine and Hygiene* 24: 575–580.

34 Watkins, W.M., Mberu, E.K., Winstanleyet, P.A. et al. (1997). The efficacy of antifolate antimalarial combinations in Africa: a predictive model based on pharmacodynamic and pharmacokinetic analyses. *Parasitology Today* 13: 459–464.

35 Feikin, D.R., Dowell, S.F., Nwanyanwu, O.C. et al. (2000). Increased carriage of trimethoprim/sulfamethoxazole-resistant *Streptococcus pneumoniae* in Malawian children after treatment for malaria with sulfadoxine/pyrimethamine. *Journal of Infectious Diseases* 181: 1501–1505.

36 Sinha, S., Medhi, B., and Sehgal, R. (2014). Challenges of drug-resistant malaria. *Parasite* 21: 61.

37 Bloland, P.B., Lackritz, E.M., Kazembe, P.N. et al. (1993). Beyond chloroquine: implications of drug resistance for evaluating malaria therapy efficacy and treatment policy in Africa. *Journal of Infectious Diseases* 167: 932–937.

38 Golenda, C.F., Li, J., and Rosenberg, R. (1997). Continuous in vitro propagation of the malaria parasite *Plasmodium vivax*. *Proceedings of the National Academy of Sciences of the United States of America* 94: 6786–6791.

39 Mengue, J.B., Held, J., and Kreidenweiss, A. (2019). AQ-13 – an investigational antimalarial drug. *Expert Opinion on Investigational Drugs* 28 (3): 217–222.

40 Schirmer, R.H., Coulibaly, B., Stitch, A. et al. (2003). Methylene blue as an antimalarial agent. *Redox Report* 8 (5): 272–275.

41 Lu, G., Nagbanshi, M., Goldau, N. et al. (2018). Efficacy and safety of methylene blue in the treatment of malaria: a systematic review. *BMC Medicine* 16: 59.

42 Michel, A.M., Steffen, B., Schindler, A. et al. (2003). Fosmidomycin for malaria. *Lancet* 360 (9349): 1941–1942.

43 Kesely, K.R., Pantaleo, A., Turrini, F.M. et al. (2016). Inhibition of an erythrocyte tyrosine kinase with imatinib prevents *Plasmodium falciparum* egress and terminates parasitemia. *PLoS One* 11 (10): e0164895.

44 Held, J., Kreidenweiss, A., and Mordmüller, B. (2013). Novel approaches in antimalarial drug discovery. *Expert Opinion on Drug Discovery* 8 (11): 1325–1337.

45 Bardi, J. (2011). Malaria discovery gives hope for new drugs and vaccine. https://www.ucsf.edu/news/2011/08/10524/malaria-discovery-gives-hope-new-drugs-and-vaccines (accessed 10 September 2020).

46 Yeh, E. and DeRisi, J.L. (2011). Chemical rescue of malaria parasites lacking an apicoplast defines organelle function in blood-stage *P. falciparum*. *PLoS Biology A* https://doi.org/10.1371/journal.pbio.1001138.

47 Hoffman, S.L. (2018). Ruth Nussenzweig (1928–2018) malaria vaccine and immunology pioneer. *The American Journal of Tropical Medicine and Hygiene* 99 (2): 253–254.

48 Tan, Z., Zhou, T., Zheng, H. et al. (2015). Malaria DNA vaccine gp96NTD-CSP elicits both CSP-specific antibody and CD8+ T cell response. *Parasitology Research* 114 (6): 2333–2339.

49 RTS,S Clinical Trials Partnership, Agnandji, S.T., Lell, B. et al. (2011). First results of phase 3 trial of RTS,S/AS01 malaria vaccine in African children. *The New England Journal of Medicine* 365 (20): 1863–1875.

Part II

Challenges and Opportunities in Malaria Therapy

2

Scientific Challenges and Treatment Opportunities in the Face of Shifting Malaria Epidemiology

Ketaki Ramani

RK University, School of Science, Department of Microbiology, Bhavnagar Highway, Kasturbadham, Rajkot, Gujarat 360 020, India

2.1 Introduction

Malaria is known to us for almost a century now, and yet we have not been able to develop an effective treatment for it. The major reason for this is the life cycle of the plasmodium parasite; from development in infected female *Anopheles* mosquito's gut to blood stage and liver stage infections in humans. Parasite virulence, number, and host immune status determine the infection range from being asymptomatic to fatal. Malaria transmission depends mainly on climatic factors such as temperature, humidity, and rainfall. These factors encourage the survival and multiplication of *Anopheles* mosquitoes, enabling the plasmodium parasites to complete their growth cycle in the mosquitoes. World Health Organization (WHO) reports in 2018, an estimated 228 million malaria cases worldwide with 405 000 deaths of which 272 000 (67%) were children aged under five years [1]. Pregnant women are at almost three times higher risk of contracting malaria and developing severe disease, than other populations. Patients with other conditions such as HIV/AIDS and travelers with no prior exposure to malaria are also more susceptible to infection.

The last two decades have witnessed substantial progress in the fight against malaria. However, the disease remains a major and growing threat to the public health and economic development of countries in the tropical and subtropical regions of the world. Some of the major contributing risk factors of malaria infection are resistance to antimalarial drugs and insecticides, the decay of public health infrastructure, season where high transmission follows rainy season, sociodemographic characteristics, and environmental changes [2]. The tragic number of malarial cases not only affects the health of an individual but also brings down the economy of a country and stalls the overall progress of a nation. Expenses to individuals and their families include cost of drugs for treating malaria at home; expenses for travel to, charges for treatment at, dispensaries and clinics; expenses for preventive measures. Costs to governments include maintenance, supply and staffing of health facilities; purchase of drugs and supplies; public

Drug Development for Malaria: Novel Approaches for Prevention and Treatment, First Edition.
Edited by Pravin Kendrekar.

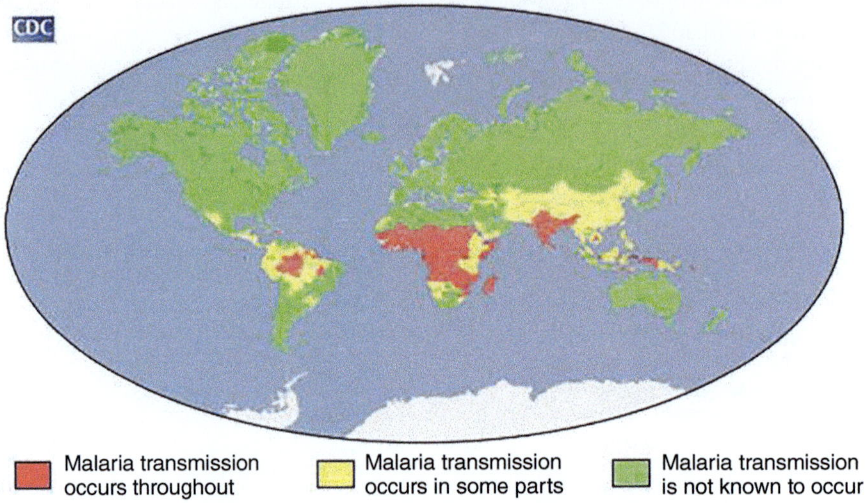

Figure 2.1 Global malaria transmissions reported by Centre for Disease Control and Prevention: https://www.cdc.gov/malaria/malaria_worldwide/impact.html.

health interventions against malaria, such as insecticide spraying or distribution of insecticide-treated bed nets. According to the economist Jeffery Sach, the economic growth of a malaria-ridden country decreases by 1.3% each year [3].

Epidemiological studies help to plan and evaluate schemes to prevent disease and provide patient management strategies in different groups of people. Epidemiological studies can confirm the resistance to a particular drug in the area and whether the treatment course of preventive measures can be continued or not. Malaria is predominant in tropical to temperate region accounting to 50% of the world's population at risk of malaria transmission (Figure 2.1). As per WHO data in 2018, the malaria cases in the African Region were 93%, 3.4% of the cases South-East Asia Region, and the Eastern Mediterranean Region with 2.1%. Sub-Saharan Africa and India carry almost 85% of the global malaria cases with major cases accounted in worldwide: Nigeria (25%), the Democratic Republic of the Congo (12%), Uganda (5%), and Côte d'Ivoire, Mozambique and Niger (4% each) [1].

2.2 The Scientific Challenges Against Malarial Drug

The world has been facing malaria for over centuries now but has also known to cure malaria since the 1600s. The first cure for malaria was discovered in the bark of the cinchona tree by Jesuit missionaries in Peru [4]. The bark of the cinchona tree contains quinine, which is still an effective treatment for malaria to this day. The transmission of malaria through the mosquito was discovered by British army surgeon Ronald Ross in 1897. And yet in 2020, there are about 228 million malaria cases and 0.5 million deaths from malaria. Malaria is still a threat to millions of lives due to the two unique characteristics of *Plasmodium falciparum* that make its elimination a challenge: (i) the parasite's unique pathogenesis where in it causes microvascular obstruction in vital organs, and (ii) ability to develop drug resistance. The plasmodium parasite spends half of its life cycle in cold-blooded invertebrate, while mosquito develops and reproduces in the warm-blooded vertebrate humans. The parasite has developed ways to not only survive in these environments but thrive in them by constantly evolving through various genetic mutations and developing resistance against the drugs. Each of the seven stages of parasite life cycle is totally different and has a completely different physiology. Hence the drugs that target one stage of a life cycle will be ineffective against the other.

2.3 Advances in Understanding and Managing Drug Resistance

Antimalarial drug discovery has substantially contributed to the gains achieved against malaria over the past two decades. Malaria treatment however is threatened by emerging drug resistance, and major gaps persist for most target compound profiles. Development and effectiveness of antimalarial drug rely on the vector–host–pathogen triad [5]. Artemisinin-based combination therapies, or ACTs, are currently the frontline treatments against *P. falciparum* malaria. As per the WHO reports [1], ACTs are effective in treating malaria in many countries, and yet there are growing concerns about developing resistance to ACTs. The number of available and effective antimalarial drugs is rapidly declining. This is mainly result of drug-resistance-associated mutations in malaria parasite genes, such as crt, mdr1, dhfr/dhps, and others, leading to resistance to all known classes of antimalarial compounds. Unfortunately, malaria parasites have started to exhibit some level of resistance in Southeast Asia even to the most recently introduced class of drugs, artemisinins. The Greater Mekong subregion (GMS) is a recurrent source of antimalarial drug resistance in *P. falciparum* malaria [6].

2.3.1 Vector and Its Control

The disease vector, *Anopheles* spp. is abundant and distributed all over the world. However, the efficacy of malaria transmission depends on the vector species and, therefore, varies considerably worldwide. There are hundreds of species of *Plasmodium* of this; six species are known to cause human malaria: *P. falciparum*, *P. vivax*, *P. ovalecurtisi*, *P. ovalewallikeri*, *P. malariae*, and *P. knowlesi* [7]. The majority of global deaths are caused by *P. falciparum*, which is the most prevalent species in sub-Saharan Africa. The other plasmodium species are not typically as life-threatening as *P. falciparum*. *P. vivax* is the second most significant species and is prevalent in Ethiopia and South America [5] and generally accounts for the majority of malaria cases in Central and South America [8]. *P. vivax* is the predominant parasite in the WHO Region of the Americas, representing 75% of malaria cases. *P. vivax* and *P. ovale* have the added complication of a dormant liver stage, which can be reactivated in the absence of a mosquito bite, leading to clinical symptoms. *P. ovale* and *P. malariae* represent only a small percentage of infections. *P. knowlesi* infects primates – has led to human malaria, but the exact mode of transmission remains unclear [6]. Coinfections between *P. falciparum* and *P. vivax* have been reported to cause malaria in up to 10–30% of patients living in areas where both parasites are prevalent [9]. Mixed infections can also include other species such as *P. ovale* and *P. malariae*, leading to the need in developing diagnostic methods to enable better assessment of the frequency and distribution of coinfection [10, 11].

Mosquito control can be achieved by insecticide-treated mosquito nets (ITNs) and indoor residual spraying (IRS). IRS involves spraying the inside walls of housing structures with insecticides, typically once or twice per year. Globally, the protection offered by IRS has declined from a peak of 5% in 2010 to 3% in 2017. This is due to development of resistance to dichlorodiphenyltrichloroethane (DDT) [12], an insecticide used for elimination of the vectors. From 2010 to 2018, some 81 countries reported data on insecticide resistance monitoring to WHO [1]. Several classes of insecticides such as organochlorine, carbamate, and pyrethroids are used in ITNs. The mosquitoes are however developing resistance to these insecticides. WHO 2018 reports [13] show that the resistance to organochlorines was detected for at least one malaria vector in almost two-thirds of the sites. Resistance to carbamates and organophosphates was less prevalent and was detected in 31% and 26% of the tested sites, respectively. Prevalence was highest for carbamates in the WHO South-East Asia Region and for organophosphates in the WHO South-East Asia Region and in the WHO Western Pacific Region. Currently pyrethroids are the only insecticide class used in ITNs. Resistance of malaria vectors to pyrethroids has been spreading throughout Africa over the last decade. An alternative option is to switch to a different class of insecticides with IRS, albeit at a higher cost, there are currently no alternatives to pyrethroids on ITNs. The piperonylbutoxide long-lasting insecticidal net and non-pyrethroid IRS interventions have decreased malaria transmission where pyrethroid resistance is prevalent [13]. Apart from IRS and ITNs, innovative vector control methods have been proposed in past such as antimosquito vaccines, genetic modification of mosquito vectors, and environmentally safe biological control agents [14].

2.3.2 Parasite and Its Control

Understanding the parasite life cycle can offer various treatment options. Each stage of the plasmodium life cycle is marked by expression of different proteins and/or location in the different sites in the host. This knowledge enables us to develop a target for the action of one or more antimalarial drugs. However, the emergence and spread of parasite resistance are not fully understood. Drug elimination half-life, parasite biomass, and malaria transmission intensity are some of the key contributing factors [15]. A high grade of parasitemia, along with low or inadequate drug levels, results in survival and propagation of resistant mutations. Epidemiological studies, advance diagnostic studies, and genomics of malaria parasites have contributed immensely to our understanding of parasite population dynamics, transmission, drug responses, and pathogenesis. The entire genome of *P. falciparum* was sequenced in 2002 [16]. The advance in genome sequencing techniques has resulted in the whole genome sequence of *P. falciparum* from dried blood spots [17] as well as dried erythrocyte spots [18]. This has changed the face and practice of malaria research opening up array of opportunities for the development of vaccines and drugs.

2.3.2.1 Malaria Vaccine

One of the most effective prophylactic tools for malaria prevention are vaccines. The landscape for malaria vaccines in 2020 is very different from that in the year 2000. http://ClinicalTrials.gov, a major venue to register clinical trials, maintains a repository of new malaria vaccine trails and has observed a steady rate of new malaria vaccine trial of ~10 trials each year [19]. Vaccines targeting various stages of malarial parasite such as pre-erythrocytic vaccine (PEV), whole sporozoite vaccine, blood stage vaccine, novel besifovir dipivoxil maleate (BSV) antigens, placental malaria vaccine, transmission blocking vaccine, vivax vaccines are being developed. The RTS, -S/AS01 vaccine and the PfSPZ vaccine products are two of the most promising malaria vaccine candidates to date [20].

The PEV product RTS, -S/AS01E (brand name Mosquirix™) has partial vaccine efficacy in pediatric phase [21] reducing clinical malaria in African children. The malaria vaccine RTS, -S/AS01E received a favorable opinion from the European Medicines Agency (EMA) in 2015. RTS, -S/AS01E contains a fusion protein including the central tandem repeat (NANP) and the C-terminal (C-term) regions of the *P. falciparum* circumsporozoite protein (CSP), and the hepatitis B virus surface antigen (HBsAg) [22].

2.3.2.2 Antimalarial Drugs

The use of antimalarial drugs has always been a central component of preventing malaria deaths. Quinine, derived from the bark of Cinchona trees, has been used as an antimalarial since as early as the seventeenth century [23]. Since then, different classes of compounds have been developed and deployed as therapeutic or preventive measures against malaria. These include the quinoline-type drugs (chloroquine [CQ], mefloquine, amodiaquine, and piperaquine), antifolates (sulfadoxine, proguanil, and pyrimethamine), naphthoquinones (atovaquone), and artemisinin-based compounds (dihydroartemisinin, artesunate, and artemether). Artemisinin and its derivatives have shown to rapidly eliminate parasite. The pairing of rapidly eliminated artemisinin derivatives and the slowly eliminated partner drugs shortens the course of treatment compared with artemisinin monotherapies [24]. Since 2006, WHO has recommended ACTs as the treatment of choice for uncomplicated *P. falciparum* malaria. Antimalarial chemotherapy and chemoprophylaxis have been key in reducing mortality and morbidity from malaria and therefore identifying and monitoring markers of adaptive mechanisms against antimalarials are of particular interest [25, 26].

2.4 Methods to Assess the Presence and Level of Drug Resistance

Early diagnosis and treatment of uncomplicated malaria with antimalarial drugs are the markers of disease control in endemic areas. Chloroquine (CQ) and sulfadoxine/pyrimethamine (SP) were the two inexpensive, first-line antimalarials for which *P. falciparum* has developed resistance [27, 28]. Resistance to several antimalarial drugs has originated from the GMS [29]. Epidemiological studies have revealed the declining efficacy of mefloquine-artesunate among Burmese migrants in western Thailand showing the spread of artemisinin resistance to the Thai–Burma border [30]. The list of other drugs that *P. falciparum* has developed resistance to includes quinine [31], amodiaquine, mefloquine, halofantrine, lumefantrine, atovaquone, cycloguanil/chlorcycloguanil, sulfonamides and sulfones [27], piperaquine [32], and recently, artemisinin and its derivatives [33, 34]. To counteract the spread of antimalarial drug resistance, surveillance systems capable to detect and track in real time, the emergence and spread need to be strengthened or in some places established. Currently, surveillance of antimalarial drug resistance is done by any of three approaches: (i) *in vivo* studies to assess the efficacy of drugs in patients; (ii) *in vitro/ex vivo* studies to evaluate parasite susceptibility to the drugs; and/or (iii) molecular assays to detect validated gene mutations and/or gene copy number changes that are associated with drug resistance [35]. It is important to understand the mechanism of the antimalarial drugs, as it is one of the key factors in the emergence and spread of drug resistance [36].

2.4.1 Therapeutic Efficacy of Antimalarial Drugs

The emergence of multidrug resistance, and ACTs, is a public health concern threatening the sustainability of the ongoing global effort to reduce the burden of malaria. Efficacy of antimalarial drug plays an important role in malaria control and elimination. Continuous efficacy monitoring is required to ensure early detection of, and response to, drug resistance for health officials and doctors to prescribe medicines to patients in malaria endemic countries. *In vivo* efficacy assessment consists of prescribing the required dose of antimalarial drugs (mono- or combination therapies) to patients infected with uncomplicated *Plasmodium* parasites. The WHO employs malaria surveillance in routine surveillance and is referred as therapeutic efficacy studies (TES) [37]. TES are conducted in a controlled environment where drug administration is supervised, the results of microscopic examinations of blood films are validated, and the origin and quality of the drugs are verified. TES are prospective evaluations of patients' clinical and parasitological responses to directly observed treatment for uncomplicated malaria. Studies at regular intervals at the same sites allow for the early detection of resistance. Findings also provide evidence for guiding national malaria treatment policy. Therapeutic outcomes are assessed on the final day of the study (day 28 or day 42 for drugs with longer elimination half-lives). In the current therapeutic efficacy protocol, systematic genotyping is recommended for clinical or parasitological failure, to distinguish recrudescence from re-infections, using three highly polymorphic genes: merozoite surface protein

1 (*msp1*), merozoite surface protein 2 (*msp2*), and glutamate-rich protein (*glurp*) [38]. Other methods have been developed to distinguish recrudescent and new infections, using microsatellite markers [39], DNA recoveries from rapid diagnostic tests (RDTs) [40]. While TES can help to predict the likelihood of antimalarial drug resistance, additional tools are needed to confirm its presence, such as *in vitro* tests, molecular analysis, and measurements of drug concentrations.

2.4.2 Molecular Markers Associated with *P. falciparum*

In an effort to combat the development and spread of drug resistance, various methods have been implemented to identify genetic markers that are associated with the parasite's sensitivity to antimalarial drugs. Molecular markers of malarial drugs resistance greatly facilitate surveillance of drug-resistant *P. falciparum* and improve the early detection and monitoring of drug resistance by *P. falciparum*. They are useful in monitoring epidemiological surveillance of drug resistance including their emergence and spread monitoring. Molecular markers for several antimalarial drugs have been identified and are constituted of either single nucleotide substitution or concatenated SNP in genes involved in parasite interaction with drugs. Next-generation sequencing (NGS) technologies provide new and effective ways of tracking drug-resistant malaria parasites. Global database on antimalarial drug efficacy includes data on the geographical distribution of molecular markers associated with *P. falciparum* drug resistance, including: *PfKelch13* (artemisinin resistance) [41], *Pfplasmepsin 2–3* copy number (piperaquine resistance) [42], *Pfmdr1* copy number (mefloquine and halofantrine resistance) [43] and *Pfcrt* (chloroquine, amodiaquine, quinine resistance) [44, 45], *Pfcytb* (atovaquone) [46], *Pfdhps* (sulfonamides, and sulfones, including sulfadoxine), *Pfdhfr* (pyrimethamine, cycloguanil and chlorcycloguanil) [47].

Deletions in the *pfhrp2* and *pfhrp3* (*pfhrp2/3*) genes of the parasite render parasites undetectable by RDTs based on histidine-rich protein 2 (HRP2). The prevalence of dual *pfhrp2* and *pfhrp3* among symptomatic patients reached as high as 80% in Eritrea and Peru. *PfKelch13* mutations have been identified as molecular markers of partial artemisinin resistance. *PfKelch13* mutations associated with artemisinin resistance are widespread in the GMS and have also been detected at a significant prevalence (over 5%) in Guyana, Papua New Guinea, and Rwanda [1]. More information about molecular markers of resistance and *in vitro* susceptibility antimalarials can be found in a website of WorldWide Antimalarial Resistance Network (WWARN) [48]. Frances Rocamora and Elizabeth A. Winzeler have enlisted a detailed review on linkage mapping, population-based drug resistance studies, and whole genome sequence analysis to drug resistance in malaria [23].

2.5 Antimalarial Drugs Currently in Use and in the Pipeline

Significant contributions to the antimalarial drug discovery pipeline are being made by companies, academic institutions, and nonprofit organizations located in malaria-endemic countries. Several drug molecules are used for prevention and cure of malaria. Uncomplicated malaria and severe malaria are treated differently. Antimalarial drugs are classified into three broad categories according to their chemical structure and mode of action (Table 2.1): (i) Aryl aminoalcohol compounds: quinine, quinidine, chloroquine, amodiaquine, mefloquine, halofantrine, lumefantrine, piperaquine, tafenoquine; (ii) Antifolate compounds ("antifols"): pyrimethamine, proguanil, chlorproguanil, trimethoprim; and (iii) Artemisinin compounds (artemisinin, dihydroartemisinin, artemether, artesunate). The mode of action involves the various stages of parasite development in vector and host. Malaria infection involves cyclic infection of humans and female *Anopheles* mosquitoes. In humans, the parasites grow and multiply first in the liver cells and then in the red cells of the blood. In the blood, successive broods of parasites grow inside the red cells and destroy them, releasing daughter parasites ("merozoites") that continue the cycle by invading other red cells. The blood stage parasites are those that cause the symptoms of malaria. When certain forms of blood stage parasites (gametocytes, which occur in male and female forms) are ingested during blood feeding by a female *Anopheles* mosquito, they mate in the gut of the mosquito and begin a cycle of growth and multiplication in the mosquito. After 10–18 days, a form of the parasite called a sporozoite migrates to the mosquito's salivary glands. When the *Anopheles* mosquito takes a blood meal on another human, anticoagulant saliva is injected together with the sporozoites, which migrate to the liver, thereby beginning a new cycle [49]. Antimalarials that target each of these stages are developed to prevent the parasite as shown in Table 2.1. A detailed review on the mechanism of antimalarial drug resistance has been published by Giancarlo A. Biagini and Stephen A. Ward [50].

WHO recommends ACTs for the treatment of uncomplicated malaria caused by the *P. falciparum* parasite. ACTs are the most effective antimalarial medicines available today as it combines two active molecules with different mechanisms of action. Five ACTs are recommended for use against *P. falciparum* malaria by WHO. The choice of ACT is based on the results of TESs against local strains of *P. falciparum* malaria. In recent years, access to ACTs has expanded substantially. Table 2.2 shows some of the ACTs available in market for malaria treatment. By the end of 2016, ACTs had been adopted as first-line treatment policy in 80 countries. An estimated 409 million treatment courses of ACT were procured by countries in 2016, an increase from 311 million in 2015. Over 69% of these procurements were reported to have been made for the public sector. The number of ACT treatments distributed through the public sector increased from 192 million in 2013 to 198 million in 2016. Most (99%) occurred in the WHO African Region.

Artemisinin resistance is the delayed parasite clearance, as the drug affects only ring-stage parasites and leads to partial clearance. Delayed parasite clearance after treatment with an ACT is of prime concern to WHO. In the GMS, high treatment failure rates following treatment with an ACT have almost always been observed in areas where there is concomitant resistance to artemisinin and the partner drug. Outside the GMS, treatment failure with ACTs (artemether–lumefantrine, artesunate–amodiaquine, and artesunate–sufadoxine–pyrimethamine) has occurred in the absence of artemisinin resistance

Table 2.1 List of currently used antimalarial drugs along with its mode of action, inhibitor coefficient (IC_{50}), and half-life.

Sr. No.	Drug	Mechanism of action	IC_{50}	Half life
1	*Artemisinin derivatives: artesunate, artemether, dihydroartemisinin*	Not fully understood. Active against blood-stage parasites, from the ring stages to early schizonts as well as young gametocytes, involving cation-mediated generation of reactive intermediates and reduction of the peroxide bridge		0.5–2.0 h (artesunate, dihydroartemisinin); 5–7 h (artemether)
2	*Quinine*	Active against large rings and trophozoites by inhibiting intraparasitic haem detoxification in the parasite's digestive vacuole. Active against gametocytes (except for *Plasmodium falciparum*)	IC_{50} > 500–800 nm	3–36 h
3	*Chloroquine*	Active by inhibiting intraparasitic haem detoxification in the parasite's digestive vacuole. Chloroquine may also act on the biosynthesis of nucleic acids	IC_{50} > 100 nm	5–12 d (chloroquine and monodesthylchloroquine)
4	*Amodiaquine*	Active by accumulation in the parasite's digestive vacuole and inhibition of the haem detoxification	Amodiaquine > 80 nm monodesethylamodiaquine IC_{50} > 60 nm	3–12 h (amodiaquine); 4–10 d (monodesethylamodiaquine)
5	*Mefloquine*	Active by inhibiting intraparasitic haem detoxification in the parasite's digestive vacuole and endocytosis of the cytosol by the parasite	IC_{50} > 30 nm	8–15 d
6	*Lumefantrine*	Active by inhibiting intraparasitic haem detoxification in the parasite's digestive vacuole and endocytosis of the cytosol by the parasite		2–11 d
7	*Sulfadoxine*	Active by inhibiting the enzyme dihydropteroate synthase (DHPS), a component of the folate biosynthetic pathway and the replication of the parasite DNA		4–11 d
8	*Pyrimethamine*	Active by inhibiting the bifunctional dihydrofolate reductase–thymidylate synthase activity, blocking the pyrimidine synthesis and the replication of the parasite DNA		2–19 d
9	*Proguanil*	Active through its active triazine metabolite (cycloguanil) by inhibiting the bifunctional dihydrofolate reductase–thymidylate synthase activity, blocking the pyrimidine synthesis and the replication of the parasite DNA	IC_{50} > 15 nm	Proguanil (8–18 h); cycloguanil (16–23 h)
10	*Atovaquone*	Active by inhibiting the transport of several parasite enzymes and by interfering with the cytochrome electron transport system, resulting in the collapse of the mitochondrial membrane potential	IC_{50} > 10 nm	1–6 d

Table 2.2 List of drugs combinations currently available for malaria treatment.

Drug combination/ formulations	Brand name	Company	Structure	
Artemether–lumefantrine	Coartem Dispersible	Novartis	Artemether 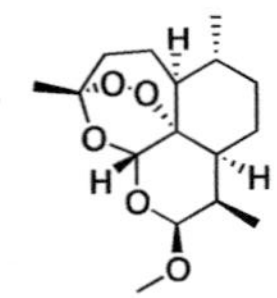	Lumefantrine 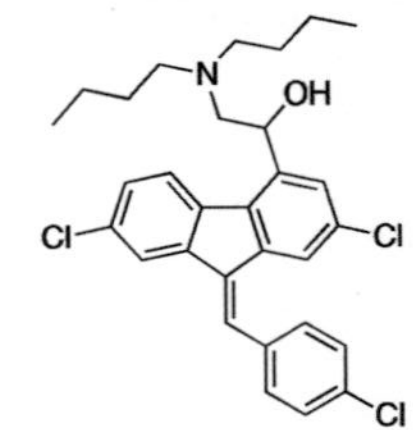
Artesunate	Artesun	Guilin Pharmaceuticals	Artesunate 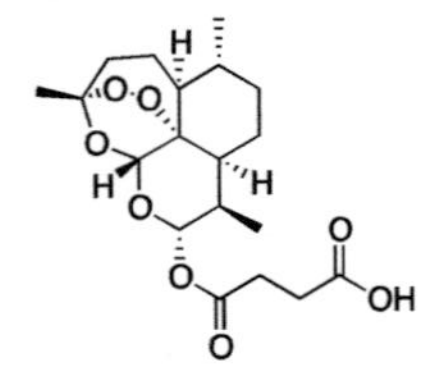	
Artesunate–amodiaquine	ASAQ Winthrop	Sanofi	Artesunate 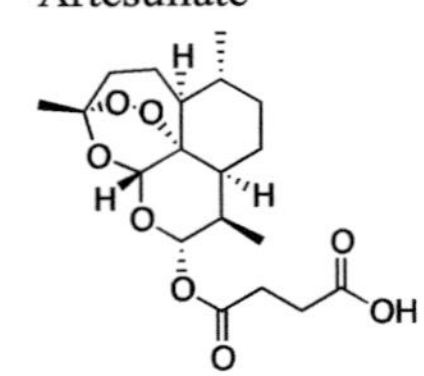	Amodiaquine 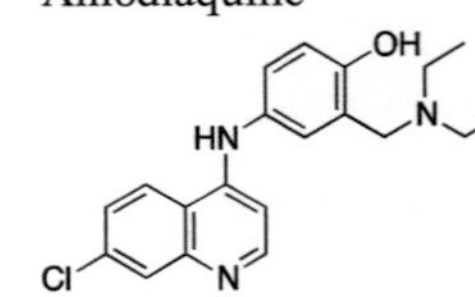
Pyronaridine–artesunate	Pyramax (granules)	Shin Poong	Pyronaridine 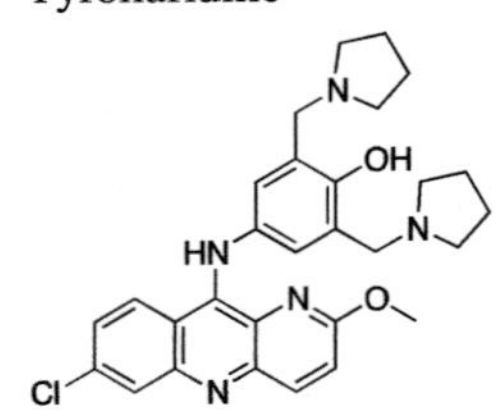	Artesunate 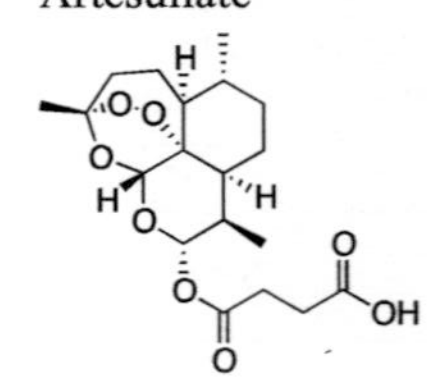

Artesunate–mefloquine	ASMQ	Cipla	Artesunate 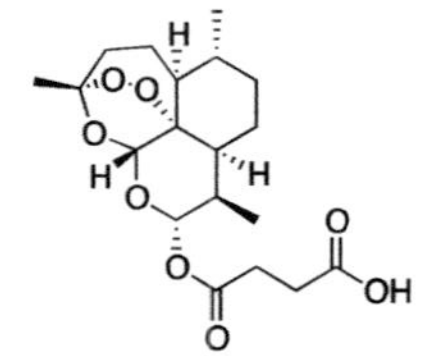	Mefloquine 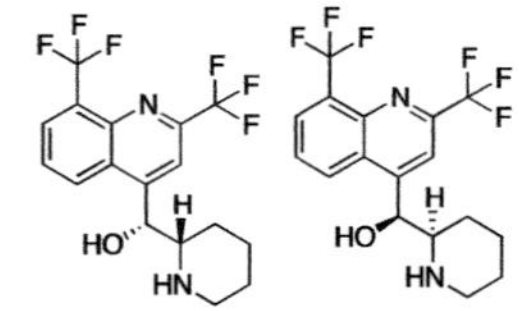
Tafenoquine	Krintafel	GlaxoSmithKline	Tafenoquine 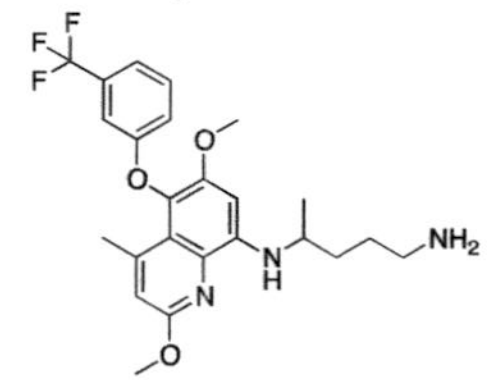	
Atovaquone–proguanil	Malarone	GlaxoSmithKline	Atovaquone 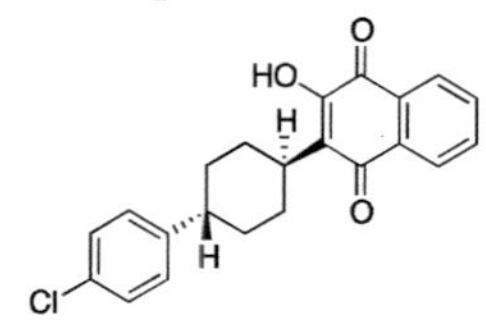	Proguanil 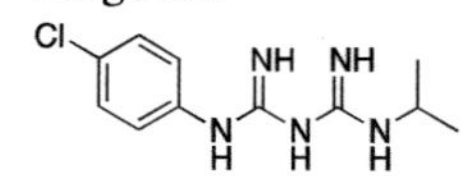
Pyrimethamine/ sulfadoxine	SPAQ-CO	Guilin Pharmaceuticals	Pyrimethamine 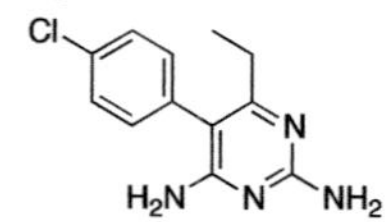	Sulfadoxine 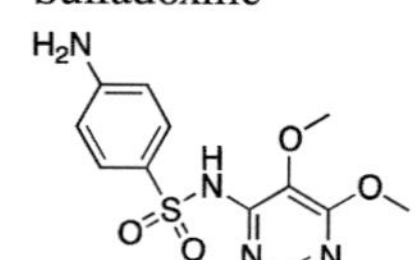
Dihyroartemisinin–piperaquine	Euratesim	Alfasigma/Pierre Fabre	Dihyroartemisisinin 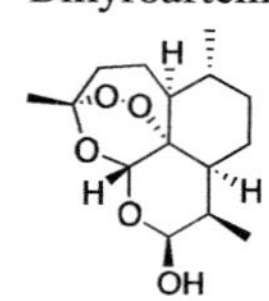	Piperaquine 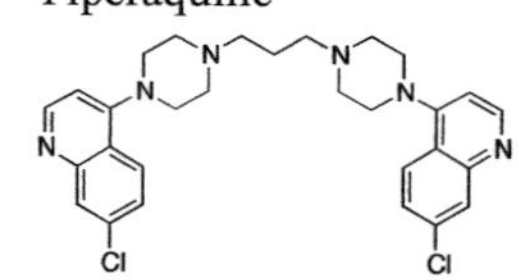

mainly due to partner drug resistance. Creative combination of existing drugs, including triple combination therapies, can be used until new effective antimalarial drugs or vaccines are available.

Several sources provide information in real time on the global antimalarial drug-resistance situation. The WHO maintains a network of sentinel sites in malaria-endemic countries performing TESs of first- and second-line antimalarial drugs using a standard protocol. The WHO website is regularly updated with the findings from national malaria control programs [51]. The WWARN provides updated maps on antimalarial drug resistance from clinical and laboratory studies, including molecular markers [52].

Past decade has seen development of new, less costly, and more sophisticated phenotypic screens leading to new drug candidates and antimalarial targets. Many of these molecules are now entering clinical development. Four new molecules with unprecedented modes of action are currently in Phase II trials for blood-stage treatments: KAE609 (also known as cipargamin), OZ439 (also known as artefenomel), KAF156 (also known as GNF156), and DSM265. These molecules have a potential to shorten the current 3-day regimen of artemisinin combination therapies. A new translational tool has been developed whereby antimalarial pharmacodynamics is studied in subclinically infected volunteers. The model is now routinely used for evaluating new drug candidates, resulting in significant time and cost savings for development [53]. Suporn et al. have developed TaqMan Array Card 87 assays. This enables detection of *P. falciparum* mutations associated with drugs such as chloroquine, atovaquone, pyrimethamine, sulfadoxine, and artemisinin resistance, and for neutral single nucleotide polymorphism (SNP) genotyping, all in a single reaction [54]. Medicines for Malaria Venture [55] is a product development partnership with academic and industries, has brought forward 11 new antimalarial medicines including Krintafel/Kozenis* (tafenoquine), a single-dose anti-relapse treatment developed with Glaxo Smith Kline (GSK) and for uncomplicated malaria, Pyramax® and Pyramax® Granules for children (pyronaridine–artesunate) with Shin Poong, Eurartesim® (dihydroartemisinin–piperaquine) with Sigma-Tau, as well as child-friendly formulation, Coartem® Dispersible (artemether–lumefantrine), with Novartis (Figure 2.2)

2.6 Future

The global battle against malaria has shown some positive signs. While the sub-Saharan Africa and India struggle with malaria, Algeria, Argentina, Paraguay, and Uzbekistan have been declared malaria-free by WHO. As a prophylactic measure, the PEV RTS, -S/AS01E has shown promising results. Upon completion of ongoing implementation programs in 2022 in three African countries, the results will be reviewed by international bodies including WHO and RTS, -S/AS01E will be considered by national policy decision-makers for broader use in Africa. WHO recommends exploring other tools that could help reach the public health goals of malaria control [56].

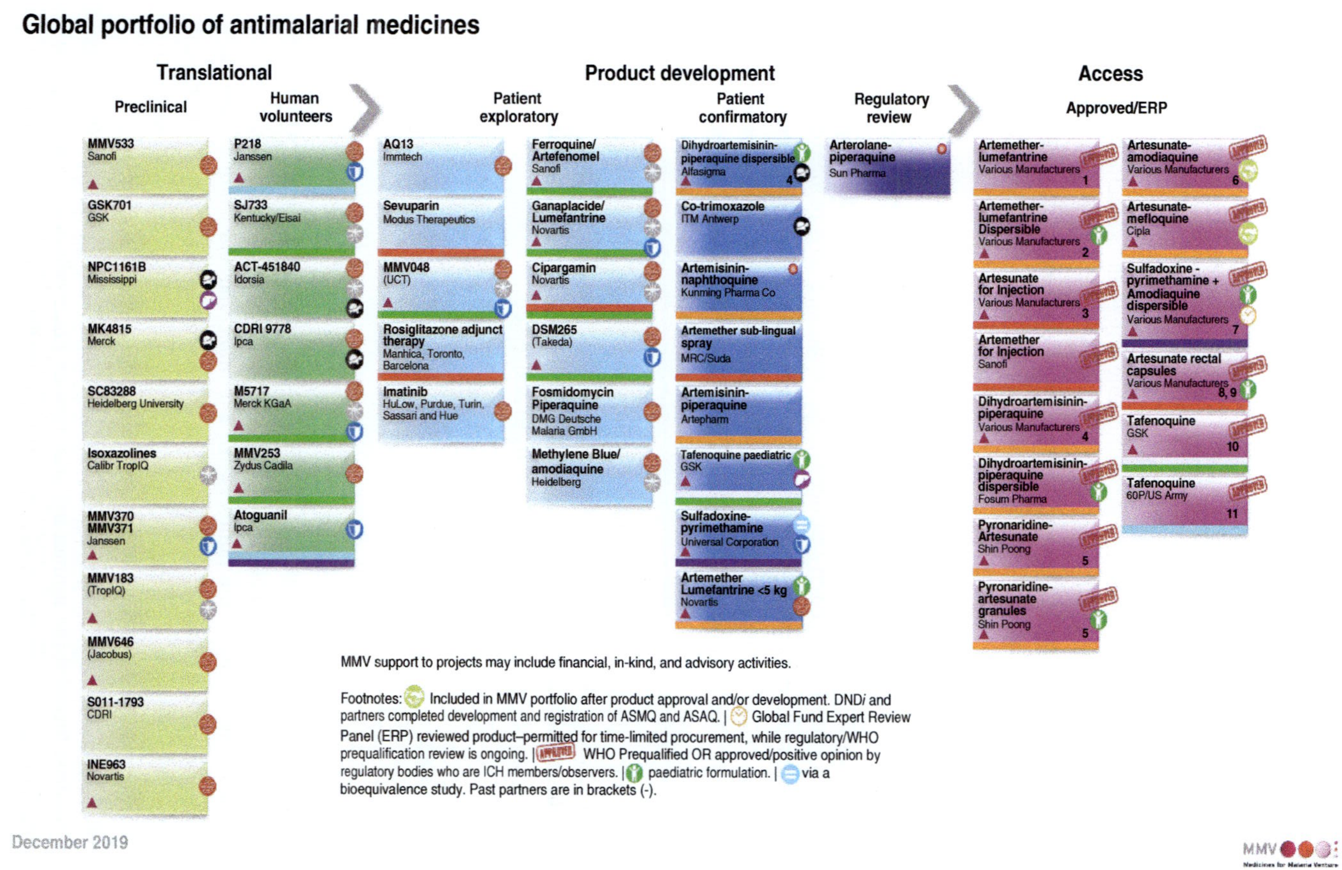

Figure 2.2 Shows the global antimalarial drugs under trails at various clinical phases at Medicines for Malaria Venture (MMV): https://www.mmv.org/research-development/mmv-supported-projects.

Parasite and host dynamics is an area that still needs to be investigated to better understand the pathogenesis and transmission dynamics. Symptomatic, asymptomatic, and subclinical disease reservoirs contribute to the transmission cycle, and laboratory, field, and modeling efforts have shown that the infectiousness of the host can be an important determinant of transmission [57, 58]. These are important considerations for vector-oriented research in the near future. If the parasite reservoir is going to be eliminated, medicines have to demonstrate a level of safety such that they can be given to people who are infected with extremely low levels of parasite and are asymptomatic. New molecules that can either prevent relapses from infection or that can provide chemoprotection for vulnerable populations, including expectant mothers, are also needed.

Malaria eradication will take many decades: the challenge is to consistently find innovative ways of targeting the parasite. The past decade has seen an immense progress in the research and development for malaria treatment with an increased collaboration between academia and industry with a focus on finding new drugs by screening directly against the parasite. We are awash with technology, advance imaging and omics approaches need to be conducted to deepen our knowledge on the complexity of *Plasmodium* biology, host–parasite interactions, population structures, mosquito infectivity, antigenic variation, and targets for treatment and immunization. The decrease in cost and increase in sensitivity of whole-genome sequencing technologies, real-time genomic surveillance of malaria-infected regions have now become more feasible. Computational approaches can be used to design better-informed, population-specific policies for combination therapy and recognize early indicators of resistance as well as new antimalarial drugs. This will advance our understanding of malaria pathogenesis, epidemiology, and evolution and will support work to develop new medicines and vaccines. Efforts to eliminate use of sub-standard and fake medicines need to be made and advancing access to life-saving severe malaria medicines needs to addressed.

References

1 WHO (2019). *World Malaria Report 2019*. Geneva: World Health Organization Licence: CC BY-NC-SA 3.0 IGO.

2 Greenwood, B. and Mutabingwa, T. (2002). Malaria in 2002. *Nature* 415: 670–672.

3 Breman, J.G., Egan, A., and Keusch, G.T. (2001). The intolerable burden of malaria: a new look at the numbers. In: *The Intolerable Burden of Malaria: A New Look at the Numbers: Supplement to Volume 64(1) of the American Journal of Tropical Medicine and Hygien* (ed. J.G. Breman, A. Egan and G.T. Keusch). Northbrook, IL: American Society of Tropical Medicine and Hygiene.

4 Sutherland, C.J., Tanomsing, N., Nolder, D. et al. (2010). Two nonrecombining sympatric forms of the human malaria parasite *Plasmodium ovale* occur globally. *The Journal of Infectious Disease* 201 (10): 1544–1550. https://doi.org/10.1086/652240.

5 Sinka, M.E., Bangs, M.J., Manguin, S. et al. (2011). The dominant *Anopheles* vectors of human malaria in the Asia-Pacific region: occurrence data, distribution

maps and bionomic précis. *Parasites & Vectors* 4: 89. https://doi.org/10.1186/1756-3305-4-89.

6 Imwong, M., Suwannasin, K., Kunasol, C. et al. (2017). The spread of artemisinin-resistant *Plasmodium falciparum* in the greater Mekong subregion: a molecular epidemiology observational study. *The Lancet Infectious Disease* 17: 491–497.

7 White, N.J. (2008). *Plasmodium knowlesi*: the fifth human malaria parasite. *Clinical Infectious Diseases* 46 (2): 172–173.

8 Sinka, M.E., Rubio-Palis, Y., Manguin, S. et al. (2010). The dominant *Anopheles* vectors of human malaria in the Americas: occurrence data, distribution maps and bionomic précis. *Parasites & Vectors* 3: 72. https://doi.org/10.1186/1756-3305-3-72.

9 Kotepui, M., Kotepui, K.U., De Jesus Milanez, G. et al. (2020). *Plasmodium* spp. mixed infection leading to severe malaria: a systematic review and meta-analysis. *Scientific Reports* 10: 11068. https://doi.org/10.1038/s41598-020-68082-3.

10 Yamamoto, T., Hashimoto, M., Nagatomi, K. et al. (2020). Development of a quantitative, portable, and automated fluorescent blue-ray device-based malaria diagnostic equipment with an on-disc SiO_2 nanofiber filter. *Scientific Reports* 10: 6585. https://doi.org/10.1038/s41598-020-63615-2.

11 Srisutham, S., Saralamba, N., Malleret, B. et al. (2017). Four human *Plasmodium* species quantification using droplet digital PCR. *PLoS One* 12: 0175771.

12 World Health Organization Report 2011

13 Protopopoff, N., Mosha, J.F., Lukole, E. et al. (2018). Effectiveness of a long-lasting piperonylbutoxide-treated insecticidal net and indoor residual spray interventions, separately and together, against malaria transmitted by pyrethroid resistant mosquitoes: a cluster, randomised controlled, two-by-two factorial design trial. *The Lancet* 391 (10130): 1577–1588. https://doi.org/10.1016/S0140-6736(18)30427-6.

14 Oaks, S.C. Jr.,, Mitchell, V.S., Pearson, G.W., and Charles, C.J. (1991). *Malaria. Obstacles and Opportunities*. Institute of Medicine (US) Committee for the Study on Malaria Prevention and Control; Carpenter. Washington, DC: National Academies Press (US).

15 Talisuna, A.O., Bloland, P., and D'Alessandro, U. (2004). History, dynamics, and public health importance of malaria parasite resistance. *Clinical Microbiology Reviews* 17: 235–254.

16 Gardner, M., Hall, N., Fung, E. et al. (2002). Genome sequence of the human malaria parasite *Plasmodium falciparum*. *Nature* 419: 498–511. https://doi.org/10.1038/nature01097.

17 Oyola, S.O., Ariani, C.V., Hamilton, W.L. et al. (2016). Whole genome sequencing of *Plasmodium falciparum* from dried blood spots using selective whole genome amplification. *Malaria Journal* 15: 597. https://doi.org/10.1186/s12936-016-1641-7.

18 Nag, S., Kofoed, P., Ursing, J. et al. (2018). Direct whole-genome sequencing of *Plasmodium falciparum* specimens from dried erythrocyte spots. *Malaria Journal* 17: 91. https://doi.org/10.1186/s12936-018-2232-6.

19 ClinicalTrials.gov https://clinicaltrials.gov.

20 Centers for Disease Control and Prevention: CDC https://www.cdc.gov/malaria/malaria_worldwide/reduction/vaccine.html.

21 Sánchez, L., Vidal, M., Jairoce, C. et al. (2020). Antibody responses to the RTS,S/AS01$_E$ vaccine and *Plasmodium falciparum* antigens after a booster dose within the phase 3 trial in Mozambique. *Nature Partners Journals: Vaccines* 5: 46. https://doi.org/10.1038/s41541-020-0192-7.

22 Cohen, J., Nussenzweig, V., Vekemans, J., and Leach, A. (2010). From the circumsporozoite protein to the RTS,S/AS candidate vaccine. *Human Vaccines* 6: 90–96.

23 Rocamora, F. and Winzeler, E.A. (2020). Genomic approaches to drug resistance in malaria. *Annual Review of Microbiology* 74 (1): 761–786. https://doi.org/10.1146/annurev-micro-012220-064343.

24 White, N.J., Hien, T.T., and Nosten, F.H. (2015). A brief history of qinghaosu. *Trends in Parasitology* https://doi.org/10.1016/j.pt.2015.10.010.

25 World Health Organization (2012). Seasonal malaria chemoprevention (SMC) for *Plasmodium falciparum* malaria control in highly seasonal transmission areas of the Sahel sub-region in Africa. Geneva.

26 World Health Organization (2015). Global Malaria Programme. The role of mass drug administration, mass screening and treatment, and focal screening and treatment for malaria: recommendations. Geneva.

27 White, N.J. (2004). Antimalarial drug resistance. *The Journal of Clinical Investigations* 113 (8): 1084–1092. https://doi.org/10.1172/JCI21682.

28 Hastings, I.M. (2003). Malaria control and the evolution of drug resistance: an intriguing link. *Trends in Parasitology* 19: 70–73. https://doi.org/10.1016/S1471-4922(02)00017-X.

29 Imwong, M., Dhorda, M., Tun, K.M. et al. (2020). Molecular epidemiology of resistance to antimalarial drugs in the Greater Mekong subregion: an observational study. *The Lancet, Infectious Disease* .

30 Nosten, F., Luxemburger, C., terKuile, F.O. et al. (1994). Treatment of multidrug-resistant *Plasmodium falciparum* malaria with 3-day artesunate-mefloquine combination. *The Journal of Infectious Diseases* 170 (4): 971–977. https://doi.org/10.1093/infdis/170.4.971.

31 Bunnag, D. and Harinasuta, T. (1987). The current status of drug resistance in malaria. *International Journal of Parasitology* 17 (1): 169–180. https://doi.org/10.1016/0020-7519(87)90038-5.

32 Eastman, R.T., Dharia, N.V., Winzeler, E.A., and Fidock, D.A. (2011). Piperaquine resistance is associated with a copy number variation on chromosome 5 in drug-pressured *Plasmodium falciparum* parasites. *Antimicrobial Agents and Chemotherapy* 55 (8): 3908–3916. https://doi.org/10.1128/AAC.01793-10.

33 Noedl, H., Se, Y., Schaecher, K. et al. (2008). Evidence of artemisinin-resistant malaria in western Cambodia. *The New England Journal of Medicine* 359 (24): 2619–2620. https://doi.org/10.1056/NEJMc0805011.

34 Cui, L., Mharakurwa, S., Ndiaye, D. et al. (2015). Antimalarial drug resistance: literature review and activities and findings of the ICEMR network. *The*

American Society of Tropical Medicine and Hygiene 93 (3 Suppl): 57–68. https://doi.org/10.4269/ajtmh.15-0007.

35 Nsanzabana, C., Djalle, D., Guérin, P.J. et al. (2018). Tools for surveillance of anti-malarial drug resistance: an assessment of the current landscape. *Malaria Journal* 17 (1): 75. https://doi.org/10.1186/s12936-018-2185-9.

36 Antony, H.A. and Parija, S.C. (2016). Antimalarial drug resistance: an overview. *Tropical Parasitology* 6 (1): 30–41. https://doi.org/10.4103/2229-5070.175081.

37 World Health Organization (2018). *Malaria Surveillance, Monitoring & Evaluation: A Reference Manual.* Licence: CC BY-NC-SA 3.0 IGO.

38 Mathema, V.B., Nakeesathit, S., Pagornrat, W. et al. (2020). Polymorphic markers for identification of parasite population in *Plasmodium malariae. Malaria Journal* 19: 48. https://doi.org/10.1186/s12936-020-3122-2.

39 Figan, C.E., Sá, J.M., Mu, J. et al. (2018). A set of microsatellite markers to differentiate *Plasmodium falciparum* progeny of four genetic crosses. *Malaria Journal* 17: 60. https://doi.org/10.1186/s12936-018-2210-z.

40 Nguyen, T.T., Nzigou Mombo, B., Lalremruata, A. et al. (2019). DNA recovery from archived RDTs for genetic characterization of *Plasmodium falciparum* in a routine setting in Lambaréné, Gabon. *Malaria Journal* 18: 336. https://doi.org/10.1186/s12936-019-2972-y.

41 Ariey, F., Witkowski, B., Amaratunga, C. et al. (2014). A molecular marker of artemisinin-resistant *Plasmodium falciparum* malaria. *Nature* 505 (7481): 50–55. https://doi.org/10.1038/nature12876.

42 Leroy, D., Macintyre, F., Adoke, Y. et al. (2019). African isolates show a high proportion of multiple copies of the *Plasmodium falciparum* plasmepsin-2 gene, a piperaquine resistance marker. *Malaria Journal* 18 (1): 126. https://doi.org/10.1186/s12936-019-2756-4.

43 Price, R.N., Uhlemann, A.C., Brockman, A. et al. (2004). Mefloquine resistance in *Plasmodium falciparum* and increased *pfmdr1* gene copy number. *Lancet* 364 (9432): 438–447. https://doi.org/10.1016/S0140-6736(04)16767-6.

44 Fidock, D.A., Nomura, T., Talley, A.K. et al. (2000). Mutations in the *P. falciparum* digestive vacuole transmembrane protein PfCRT and evidence for their role in chloroquine resistance. *Molecular Cell* 6 (4): 861–871. https://doi.org/10.1016/s1097-2765(05)00077-8.

45 Folarin, O.A., Bustamante, C., Gbotosho, G.O. et al. (2011). In vitro amodiaquine resistance and its association with mutations in pfcrt and pfmdr1 genes of *Plasmodium falciparum* isolates from Nigeria. *Acta Tropica* 120 (3): 224–230. https://doi.org/10.1016/j.actatropica.2011.08.013.

46 Siregar, J.E., Kurisu, G., Kobayashi, T. et al. (2015). Direct evidence for the atovaquone action on the *Plasmodium* cytochrome bc_1 complex. *Parasitology International* 64 (3): 295–300.

47 Kublin, J.G., Dzinjalamala, F.K., Kamwendo, D.D. et al. (2002). Molecular markers for failure of sulfadoxine-pyrimethamine and chlorproguanil-dapsone treatment of *Plasmodium falciparum* malaria. *The Journal of Infectious Diseases* 185 (3): 380–388. https://doi.org/10.1086/338566.

48 Worldwide Antimalarial Resistance Network (WWARN). http://www.wwarn.org/tracking-resistance.

49 Centers for Disease Control and Prevention: Malaria Biology. https://www.cdc.gov/malaria/about/biology/index.html.

50 Biagini, G.A. and Ward, S.A. (2017). Mechanisms of antimalarial drug resistance. In: *Antimicrobial Drug Resistance* (ed. D. Mayers, J. Sobel, M. Ouellette, et al.). Cham: Springer https://doi.org/10.1007/978-3-319-46718-4_41.

51 World Health Organization (WHO). http://www.who.int/topics/malaria/en.

52 WorldWide Antimalarial Resistance Network (WWARN). www.wwarn.org.

53 Wells, T., van Huijsduijnen, R., and Van Voorhis, W. (2015). Malaria medicines: a glass half full? *Nature Reviews Drug Discovery* 14: 424–442. https://doi.org/10.1038/nrd4573.

54 Pholwat, S., Liu, J., Stroup, S. et al. (2017). The malaria TaqMan array card includes 87 assays for *Plasmodium falciparum* drug resistance, identification of species, and genotyping in a single reaction. *Antimicrobial Agents and Chemotherapy* 61 (5): e00110–e00117. https://doi.org/10.1128/AAC.00110-17.

55 Medicines for Malaria Venture. https://www.mmv.org/research-development/mmv-supported-projects.

56 World Health Organization (2019). Malaria vaccine pilot launched in Malawi.

57 Gonçalves, B.P., Kapulu, M.C., Sawa, P. et al. (2017). Examining the human infectious reservoir for *Plasmodium falciparum* malaria in areas of differing transmission intensity. *Nature Communications* 8 (1): 1133. https://doi.org/10.1038/s41467-017-01270-4.

58 Vantaux, A., Samreth, R., Piv, E. et al. (2018). Contribution to malaria transmission of symptomatic and asymptomatic parasite carriers in Cambodia. *The Journal of Infectious Diseases* 217 (10): 1561–1568. https://doi.org/10.1093/infdis/jiy060.

3

Emerging Formulation Technologies Against Malaria Resurgence

Kinjal Parikh[1], Rakhee Kapadia[2], Rohan Pai[3], Mahendra Prajapati[4], and Ganesh Shevalkar[5]

[1] *The Maharaja Sayajirao University of Baroda, Faculty of Pharmacy, Kalabhavan, Vadodara, Gujarat 390020, India*
[2] *SAGE University, SIRT-Pharmacy, Sahara Bypass Road, Katara Hills, Extension, Bhopal, Madhya Pradesh 462022, India*
[3] *Shobhaben Pratapbhai Patel School of Pharmacy & Technology Management, SVKM's NMIMS, V.L. Mehta Road, Vile Parle (W), Mumbai 400056, India*
[4] *School of Pharmacy & Technology Management, SVKM's NMIMS, Babulde, Shirpur, Maharashtra 425405, India*
[5] *R. C. Patel Institute of Pharmaceutical Education and Research, Department of Pharmaceutics, Shirpur, Maharashtra 425405, India*

List of Abbreviations

ACT	artemisinin-based combination therapy
AgNP	silver nanoparticles
ART-NE	arteether nanoemulsion
AS	artesunate
AuNP	gold nanoparticles
CNT	carbon nanotubes
CS	chitosan
DNA	deoxyribonucleic acid
ds RNA	double-stranded ribonucleic acid
EMA	European Medical Agency
FDA	Food and Drug Administration
GDL	glyceryl dilaurate
GNO	groundnut oil
GQD	graphene quantum dots
HDAC	histone deacetylase
HPH	high-pressure homogenization
HRP2	histidine-rich protein 2
IP	intellectual property
IV	intravenous
LbL	layer by layer

Drug Development for Malaria: Novel Approaches for Prevention and Treatment, First Edition.
Edited by Pravin Kendrekar.

NLC	nanostructured lipid carriers
NP	nanoparticle
PCL	polycaprolactone
PEG	polyethylene glycol
PLA	poly(D,L-lactide)
PLGA	poly(lactic-*co*-glycolic acid)
pNIPAm	poly(*N*-isopropyl acrylamide)
PVA	polyvinyl alcohol
QD	quantum dots
RBC	red blood cells
RNA	ribonucleic acid
SEDDS	self-emulsifying drug delivery system
SLN	solid lipid nanoparticle
SMEDDS	self-microemulsifying drug delivery system
SNEDDS	self-nanoemulsifying drug delivery system
TGA	Therapeutic Goods Administration
WHO	World Health Organization
ZBS	zinc basic salt
Zn-DFO	zinc desferrioxamine
ZnO-NP	zinc oxide nanoparticles

3.1 Introduction

Malaria is a life-threatening disease caused by *Plasmodium* parasites that entered in a person's blood through the bites of infected female *Anopheles* mosquitoes. After they come into the blood, the parasite travels along with blood and reaches the liver, where they mature and reproduce [1].

Mainly five species of *Plasmodium*, namely, *P. falciparum*, *P. vivax*, *P. ovale*, *P. malariae*, and *P. knowlesi*, spread malaria humans [2]. Among these, most deaths are caused by *P. falciparum*, while the other four cause the milder form of malaria. In 2018, worldwide 228 million cases and 405 000 deaths were reported because of malaria. Children below five years are the most susceptible to malaria; in 2018, around 6.7%, i.e. 272 000 deaths of children, were reported because of malaria. The African region carries a high number of malarial cases compared with the rest of the world. In 2018, 93% of malaria cases and 94% of deaths were reported in this region [3].

3.1.1 Major Pathological Hallmarks of Malaria

Malaria is commonly characterized by an acute febrile illness, which generally shows symptoms within 10–15 days when the nonimmune individual bite by an infective mosquito. Initially, it shows symptoms such as fever, headache, and chills. Sometimes these symptoms are mild and hence become difficult to diagnose as malaria. If not treated within 24 hours, *P. falciparum* malaria produces severe illness, which may lead to death also. At the same time, improper treatment causes recurrences of the disease [4].

3.1.2 Current Treatment Strategies

Vector control: It is an essential attribute that helps to prevent malarial transmission. It can be done by various means such as the use of body repellents, insecticides, nets, and mosquito coils. Maintenance of cleanliness around the houses and personal hygiene also helps to prevent transmission of malaria [5].

Monotherapies: Malaria can primarily be treated with the monotherapy of drugs such as quinine, chloroquine (CQ), and amodiaquine. However, the use of monotherapy rapidly develops resistance to malarial parasites. Thus it restricts its use in the treatment of malaria [6].

Combination therapies: As the malaria parasite's resistance develops to monotherapies, a combination of drugs having different mechanisms of action is suggested to provide a satisfactory cure rate and delayed resistance. At present, artemisinin-based combination therapy (ACT) is used to treat malaria as it offers high efficacy, fast action, and the reduced possibility of developing resistance. In this combination therapy, the fast-acting artemisinin-analogs such as dihydroartemisinin, artesunate (AS), and artemether are combined with other antimalarial drugs such as lumefantrine, amodiaquine, mefloquine, and piperaquine [7].

3.2 Pitfalls of the Current Treatment Regimen

Despite the high usefulness of ACTs, the drawbacks, such as low aqueous solubility and poor bioavailability, high doses, and high cost, limit its usage. In addition, conventional antimalarial therapy has limitations such as stability and the occurrence of resistance in parasites. Hence all together, antimalarial treatment faces several shortcomings that include drug resistance, a bulky dose, long-term treatment, and recurrence of disease [5].

3.2.1 Drug Resistance

Drug resistance develops when parasite strain no longer responds to a drug that previously treated them effectively. Malarial parasites have shown resistance against all classes of the antimalarial agent, which eventually affected public health and also increased the economic burden. The occurrence of resistance in parasites depends on many factors, including (i) the rate of mutation in the parasite, (ii) the overall parasite load, (iii) selected drug strength, and (iv) the treatment compliance.

Higher mutation rates in parasites result in the development of rapid mutation that helps the parasites to adapt to the changing environment quickly [8, 9]. Strong drug selection pressure decreases the prevalence of competing sensitive wild-type parasites; this accelerates the emergence of resistance. The primary reason for the development of drug resistance is the exposure of the parasite to sub-therapeutic drug concentration. Drug resistance can also occur due to improper dosing, poor pharmacokinetic properties, fake drugs, or infection acquired during treatment results in inadequate drug exposure to the parasites [10].

3.2.2 High Drug Dose

Low oral bioavailability, short half-life, drug resistance, and sub-therapeutic drug concentration demand larger doses of antimalarial. The high drug concentrations kill partially resistant or drug-tolerant parasites that occur after adequate treatment doses. However, suboptimal doses and the drug concentration during the terminal elimination phase are not sufficient to kill the parasites [11]. Thus, sub-therapeutic drug levels increase the risk of treatment failure and provide selection pressure for resistant parasites, whereas the highest concentration is more likely to produce toxicity [12]. Reports have also shown that a high dose of primaquine, which is used to treat multidrug-resistant *P. falciparum* malaria and to prevent relapse of *P. vivax* malaria, causes hemolysis in healthy individuals [13, 14].

Most of the antimalarial drugs have low aqueous solubility and high lipophilicity, which affect the oral bioavailability of the antimalarial drug. This is the key cause for large interindividual variability in blood concentration that increases the risk of sub-therapeutic levels of drugs [7]. In combination-drug therapy, high doses of drugs and excipients are mixed to form a single unit dosage form, which increases the bulkiness of the dosage form, and such dosage form becomes challenging to administer.

3.2.3 Long-Term Treatment

For a complete cure, the antimalarial medicines need to be taken for at least four asexual cycles (seven days). Hence, for an effective treatment, the therapeutic level of the drug should exist for at least four cycles [15, 16]. Artemisinin and its derivatives have a shorter half-life that results in their rapid absorption and elimination. Quinine is also absorbed and eliminated within one parasite life cycle (11 hours half-life). Hence with such types of drugs, long-term treatment is necessary.

3.2.4 Recurrence and Reversion of Diseases

Recurrence of malaria existed in the past, but it is most prevalent in recent times, irrespective of the geographical or human host range [17]. The recurrence of malaria mainly depends on the half-life of the drug. For the drugs that have extended half-life, such as mefloquine, recurrence of malaria occurs after 63 days or even longer [18].

Hence there is a need to develop new treatment strategies that will overcome the limitations of conventional antimalarial therapy. This chapter aims to discuss the applications and advantages of various nano-platforms, such as liposomes, polymeric nanoparticles (NPs), self-nano emulsifying drug delivery systems (SNEDDS), solid lipid nanoparticles (SLNs), and so forth in the treatment of malaria.

This chapter deals with the emerging formulation strategies for the treatment of malaria and to prevent a malarial resurgence and other limitations associated with conventional treatment therapy. The section also includes selected case studies to explain the advantage of nano-platform in drug delivery.

3.3 Nanotechnology-Based Strategies for Targeting in Antimalarial Therapy

Nanomedicine is the medical application of the knowledge and tools of nanotechnology for designing nanomaterials, nanoparticles, or even nanodevices for diagnosis or delivery of therapeutics [19]. One of the significant advantages of the nanotechnology-based drug delivery systems is their ability to enhance the stability and bioavailability of drug substances, thereby improving or prolonging their pharmacokinetic profiles [20]. This is particularly beneficial in antimalarial therapy wherein the duration, as well as the dose of the drugs prescribed during the illness, is significantly higher. The other important aspect of nanotechnology-based delivery systems that could be beneficial in antimalarial therapy is their interaction with red blood cells (RBCs), their cell-adhesion properties, and interaction with the parasite membrane [5].

3.3.1 Passive Targeting

Passive targeting relies heavily on the disease pathophysiology and pharmacology to accumulate the drugs at the target site. In context to malaria, wherein the target site, i.e. the infected host RBCs, which are not phagocytic or endocytic, cannot be passively targeted conventionally. Thus, passive targeting for infected RBC in malaria, although less exploited, mainly involves modifying the surface of the nanocarriers with hydrophilic polymers, e.g. polyethylene glycol (PEG), polyvinyl alcohol (PVA), poloxamers, polyacrylamide, and polyvinyl pyrrolidone. The surface modification of nanocarriers with such polymers enhances circulation time, prolonging drug half-life, and prevents their uptake by opsonization, thus improving drug pharmacokinetics. Such long-circulating nanocarriers increase the contact with the infected RBC for the drugs to take effect. On the other hand, conventional unmodified nanocarriers could be used for passively targeting the dormant forms of the parasite *P. vivax* located in the hepatocytes alongside the Kupffer cells [21].

3.3.2 Active Targeting

Active targeting is achieved by modifying conventional nanocarrier with the ligand, i.e. carbohydrates, proteins or peptides, and even antibodies. The ligands are cell-specific or target specifically toward a diseased cell. However, this approach can be successful only if the receptors at the surface of the infected cells are expressed uniquely or overexpressed compared with the healthy cells. The one major drawback of such an approach is that the ligand may induce an immunological response due to its proteinaceous nature. Nevertheless, active targeting using target-specific ligands has been widely explored for actively targeting the two primary targets, i.e. the erythrocytes in the bloodstream and the hepatocytes in the liver. Further, in recent times this strategy has also been utilized for the management and treatment of cerebral malaria by targeting the brain [22].

3.3.2.1 Hepatocyte Targeting

After entering the bloodstream, the malarial parasites are taken up by the hepatocytes in the liver, wherein the sporozoite stage of the *Plasmodium* begins within a few hours. Thus, interfering with the schizonts within the hepatocyte before their rupture into the bloodstream can help to alleviate the severity of the symptoms. The organ specificity of the sporozoites is attributed to two surface proteins on their surface, i.e. the circumsporozoite protein (CSP) and thrombospondin-related anonymous protein. The amino acid sequences, namely KLKQP in the peptide "region I plus," are believed to be associated with binding of the *Plasmodium* to the hepatocytes [23].

3.3.2.2 Erythrocyte Targeting

All major pathologies and the clinical symptoms of malaria arise during the intra-erythrocytic stage of the parasite. Hence, the RBC is of prime importance for targeting of the therapeutics to attenuate the malarial symptoms. Several targeting moieties are utilized for delivering therapeutics to the infected RBCs using active targeting methods. Antibodies have been effectively used to differentiate between normal and infected RBC. Carbohydrates such as glycosamine, a negatively charged polysaccharide, have also been used to target the infected RBC. Proteins such as heparin sulfate and heparin-like molecules target the infected RBC by forming small rosette-like clusters around them. However, the use of heparin is mostly limited due to the tendency of intracranial bleeding owing to its intracranial activity. Lipids such as glyceryl dilaurate (GDL) have also been used to target the *Plasmodium*-infected RBC [24].

3.3.2.3 Brain Targeting

A rare instance of an extreme clinical symptom of malaria is the entry of the parasite in the meninges of the brain. Thus, for the timely treatment of cerebral malaria, the drug is required to reach the brain in sufficient quantities. Conventionally, cerebral malaria is addressed with parenteral administration of either artemisinin or quinine. However, the short half-life of artemisinin and toxicity of quinine limit their use. Moreover, most of the drug molecules are unable to cross the blood–brain barrier due to the presence of the tight junctions of epithelial cells. Thus, nanoplatforms can be made to actively target the brain using receptor functionalization, like in the case of transferrin receptors, which are expressed on the luminal membrane of endothelial cells of the brain. These receptors are involved in mediating endocytosis of transferrin into the cells, thereby assisting in receptor-mediated endocytosis of the transferrin decorated nanocarrier from the blood to the brain [24].

3.3.3 Rapid Diagnosis and Vector Control

One of the major reasons for the deaths in cases with malaria is generally delaying in its diagnosis. The use of nanotechnology has also led to the emergence of rapid and accurate diagnosis techniques for timely detection and treatment of malaria. An ideal diagnostic method for malaria is expected to be simple, safe, accurate, cost-effective, relatively fast, sensitive, and specific. Nanotechnology-based platforms can satisfy these requirements and provide a rapid and sensitive method for diagnosis owing to their uniqueness in surface functionalities. In recent times, microfluidic technologies, in conjunction with lab-on-chip devices, have emerged as a new and promising tool for not only diagnosis but also monitoring of the malarial pathogen during the treatment [25].

3.4 Nano Formulations for Malarial Treatment

Nanomaterials provide a larger surface area and can be used to adsorb multiple drugs. The smaller size helps to reach inaccessible areas that conventional drug delivery systems cannot. With the reduction in the dose of active pharmaceutical ingredient, it lessens the side effects and increases therapeutic effectiveness. Various therapeutic nanoplatforms that are being used for antimalarial delivery are shown in Figure 3.1. Although these nano-formulations are in the research phase, they have the potential to revolutionize the antimalarial delivery strategy (Figure 3.2).

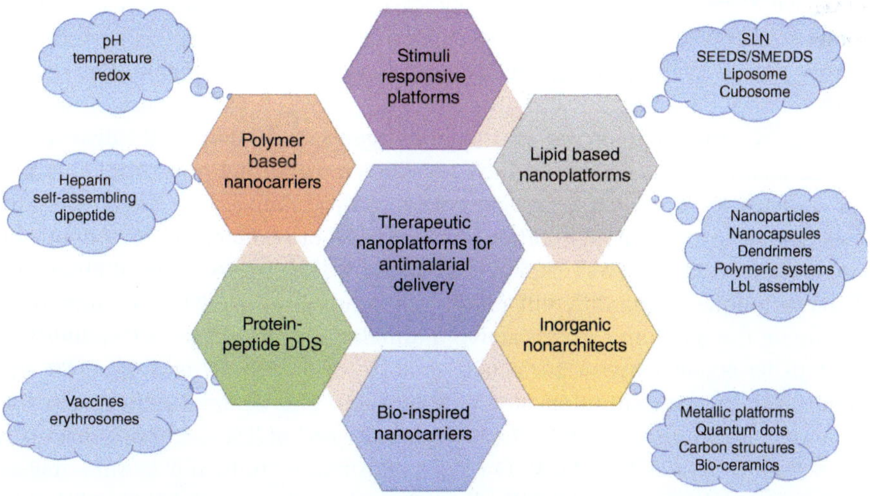

Figure 3.1 Therapeutic nanoplatforms for antimalarial delivery.

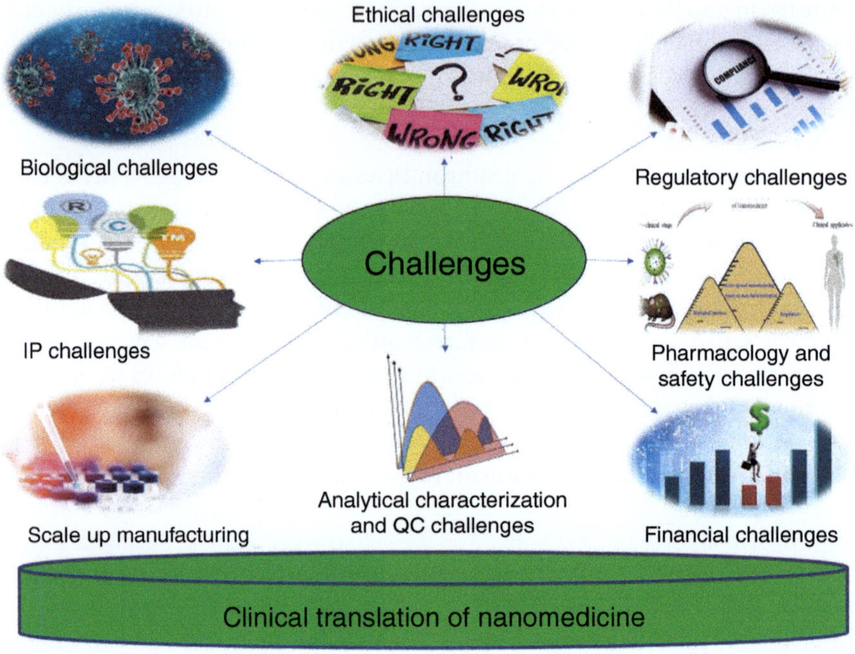

Figure 3.2 Challenges in clinical translation of nanomedicine.

3.4.1 Lipid-Based Nanoplatforms

3.4.1.1 Nanoemulsion

Nanoemulsion is an isotropic delivery system that is thermodynamically stable. They have a size range of approximately 50–1000 nm in diameter concerning the droplet size. In the past few decades, nanoemulsion has emerged as a promising delivery system for improving the dissolution rate and bioavailability of several poorly water-soluble antimalarial agents [26].

The most prominent of the antimalarial agents and structurally diverse are the artemisinin class of drugs, which are known to be highly hydrophobic and thus difficult to formulate using conventional drug delivery systems. This also raises the issue of their dissolution and variable bioavailability. Nanoemulsion of Arteether (ART-NE) was explored by using a high-pressure homogenization (HPH) technique, using different ratios of groundnut oil (GNO) and surfactants to improve the solubility of the active antimalarial agent [27]. The system was found to be stable when a surfactant mixture of Tween 80 and Span 80 was employed in the concentration of 0.5% w/w each. This optimal ratio resulted in maximum drug loading of $93 \pm 7.4\%$, a globule size of 156 ± 10.2 nm, having a zeta potential of -23.3 ± 3.4 mV. On the performance front, the *in vitro* release profile of the developed ART-NE showed a phenomenal improvement in the dissolution of arteether, with around 62% of the drug released within 12 hours. The biopharmaceutical studies of the developed ART-NE in Sprague–Dawley rats showed enhanced oral bioavailability in comparison to ART dissolved in GNO, demonstrating superior *in vivo* pharmacokinetics, evident from the area under curve (AUC) of ART-NE was found to be more than threefold higher than ART in GNO. The improved pharmacokinetic profile was also seen to impact the C_{max} of arteether nanoemulsion (1506 ± 161.22 ng/ml) system, which was also significantly higher than that of ART in GNO (175.2 ± 16.54 ng/ml) and even when ART was given intramuscularly (278.05 ± 38.59 ng/ml). The significant improvements in the biopharmaceutical parameters directly translated to a higher antimalarial efficacy and survival rate of mice administered with the developed ART-NE, exhibiting cure rate of nearly 80% at a dose of 12.5 mg/kg for five days as compared with merely 30% cure rate at the same daily dose for ART in GNO. Moreover, as compared with the intramuscularly administered ART at the same dose and frequency, a 100% cure rate was achieved at a 12.5 mg/kg dose of ART-NE given for five days.

On similar lines, in one study, oil-in-water nanoemulsion loaded with another efficient antimalarial drug of the quinine class, primaquine was evaluated for their efficacy against *Plasmodium berghei*, which was infected Swiss albino mice model. The developed nanoemulsion exhibited a significant 25% reduction in the therapeutic dose of primaquine when compared with the oral dose. Further, the *in vivo* studies indicated a substantial decrease in the parasite progression and an overall increase in the survival period, even at that reduced dose. The outcome of the developed nanoemulsion was compared with plain drug solution, and it was observed that the pharmacokinetic and biodistribution studies showed an improvement in not only the oral bioavailability but also in the accumulation of significant concentration of primaquine in the liver [28]. In addition to this, the nanoemulsion also enhanced the stability of the entrapped primaquine and was reported to be more stable in serum, exhibiting a controlled release from the carrier [29].

3.4.1.2 Self-Emulsifying Drug Delivery System (SEDDS)

Like nanoemulsions, self-emulsifying drug delivery system (SEDDS) are also isotropic and mixtures of oils and surfactants, sometimes including cosolvents, which self-emulsify under gentle means of agitation. Such a condition would be similar to the environment that would be encountered in the gastrointestinal tract. One of the important advantages of SEDDS is that the highly hydrophobic drugs can often be easily encapsulated as unit dosage forms for per-oral administration by dissolving them in SEDDS [30].

SNEDDS of arteether has been widely reported as it efficiently enhances the oral bioavailability of the artemisinin class of the drugs [31]. This has been demonstrated by a study wherein the antimalarial efficacy and safety of the SNEDDS were tested in an animal model infected with the *Plasmodium yoelii*. The relative bioavailability (% RB) of arteether was found to drastically increase by 257% when administered in the form of SNEDDS as against its aqueous suspension and the GNO solution. Moreover, the arteether-loaded SNEDDS showed a higher antimalarial activity as compared with that of GNO solution, at even the lower dose of 12.5 mg/kg administered for five days.

In another such study, a self-microemulsifying drug delivery system (SMEDDS) formulation was developed of the antimalarial drug artemether, and the antimalarial activity of the developed SMEDDS was compared with the marketed formulation (Larither) having the globule size of around 100 nm. The *in vivo* antimalarial activity of the developed SMEDDS was significantly higher than the marketed formulation as evidenced from the promising survival and suppression of parasitemia progression [32].

3.4.1.3 Solid Lipid Nanoparticles (SLNs) and Nanostructured Lipid Carriers (NLCs)

SLNs are a type of a lipid-based nanocarrier system having a submicron size range between 50 and 1000 nm. One of the major advantages of the SLNs is that they are composed of lipid components, which are not only physiologically compatible but also in a solid state at room temperature. The example of such lipids includes the triglycerides, glyceride mixtures, and waxes, all of which are highly purified for pharmaceutical use [33, 34]. The advancements in SLNs or their next generation are referred to as nanostructured lipid carriers (NLCs), which are also composed of solid lipid, but with a fraction of the oil blended in with it, making them more dynamic and flexible as compared with the SLN [34]. NLCs are fabricated to overcome the few major drawbacks of SLNs mainly related to the expulsion of the active ingredient owing to the polymorphic changes that occur in the highly crystalline nature of the lipids usually used in their preparation [35].

SLNs of arteether containing glyceryl monostearate as the solid lipid matrix and Pluronic F68, and soya lecithin as the surfactant, and cosurfactant, respectively, were prepared using the HPH technique [36]. The optimized SLNs achieved an average particle size of 100 ± 11.2 nm, zeta potential value of -23.3 ± 3.2 mV, and entrapment efficiency of $69 \pm 4.2\%$. In one of the *in vivo* studies, arteether-SLNs were compared against arteether in GNO and arteether in aqueous suspension with respect to the percent relative bioavailability. It was observed that arteether-SLN was found to attain a percent relative bioavailability of 7461%, which was drastically higher as compared with the other two groups.

Similarly, for the NLCs, several antimalarial drugs were evaluated by encapsulating them in a glyceryl-dilaurate (GDL-NLCs) to target the actives to the *Plasmodium*-infected RBCs using the NLC, wherein GDL was used as the targeting moiety [37]. GDL-NLCs were found to be localized within the mitochondrion of the concerned parasite, further leading to Ca^{2+} ion accumulations and the polarization of the mitochondrial membrane. The localization was also seen to release the reactive oxidative species, resulting in the selective lysis of the stage-specific infected RBCs alone. Thus, complete parasite clearance was reported at a significantly lower dose of a combination of antimalarial drugs, namely the artemether–clindamycin and artemether–lumefantrine combinations.

3.4.1.4 Liposome

Liposomes are one of the most widely accepted and extensively studied nanocarrier systems and fundamentally are vesicles using phospholipids surrounding an inner aqueous core by one or several bilayers. The aqueous cavity can conveniently incorporate the hydrophilic drugs, whereas the lipophilic drugs are imbibed into the phospholipid bilayer [38]. Thus, liposomes have been rightly explored for improving the efficacy of the hydrophobic antimalarial agents.

The potential of liposomes as a delivery system for antimalarials was explored for the intravenous (IV) delivery of curcuminoids in a mouse model. The liposomes of soy phosphatidylcholine (soy PC) loaded with curcuminoids alone and in combination with α/β arteether were formulated and evaluated intravenously in *P. berghei* infected mice for their antimalarial efficacy. The outcome of the study showed a high survival rate along with a very low parasitemia in animals treated with curcuminoid-loaded liposomes as compared with that of the control groups (saline and free curcuminoids treated). Moreover, such a combination therapy of the antimalarial drug with α/β arteether along with the curcuminoids-loaded liposomes was successfully able to cure and prevent recrudescence in the tested mice model [39].

More recently, liposomes loaded with chloroquine and primaquine, further conjugated with thiolated polyclonal antibodies against MAH-RP121-40 peptide, were formulated and evaluated for their ability to actively target the infected RBCs. The conjugated immune-liposomes liposomes containing the neutral saturated phospholipids were developed using the widely employed thin-film hydration method. Chloroquine and primaquine, which are chemically weakly basic drugs, were loaded in the liposomes using a pH gradient loading method. The developed liposomes were evaluated for their entrapment efficiency, which exceeded more than 96%. The developed immune-liposomes were capable of targeting the *Plasmodium*-infected RBCs at even a low concentration of only 0.5 μM. Moreover, concerning the targeting potential, it was seen that around 95% of the delivered liposomes were successfully retained on the surface of the RBCs. In brief, the prepared immune-liposomes containing chloroquine possessed 40 times more antimalarial activity than free chloroquine as evidenced by their ability to arrest the growth of the parasite in their early stage [40].

3.4.2 Polymer-Based Nanoplatforms for Malaria

The employment of polymeric nanoparticulate carrier systems is among the emerging trends in the management and recovery of malaria [41]. Nanoparticulate carrier systems include various carriers such as nanoparticles (NPs), nanogels, nanocapsules, dendrimers, layer by layer assembly systems, etc. For antimalarial nanoparticulate drug delivery, various natural polymers such as polysaccharides – chitosan (CS) and proteins such as gelatin, albumin, or the synthetic polymers such as Eudragit (L100-55 and S100), poly(lactic-*co*-glycolic acid) (PLGA), poly(D,L-lactide) (PLA), polycaprolactone (PCL), etc. are used, wherein the drug can either be encapsulated or conjugated to surface by functional group.

3.4.2.1 Nanoparticles

3.4.2.1.1 Chitosan

Among the various natural polymers, CS is the most widely used polymer for different nanoformulation preparations of antimalarial drugs/biologicals such as ds-RNA,

DNA, and protein. It is a linear polysaccharide composed of D-glucosamine and *N*-acetyl-D-glucosamine [42].

Chitosan Nanoparticles for Drugs To minimize the dose-related blood toxicities and improved liver targeting, CS nanoparticles of primaquine phosphate (Size 287–686 nm) were prepared by Rajera et al. [43]. The drug-loaded NPs have significantly lower toxicity as compared with pure drug solution as revealed from *in vivo* acute toxicological study in mice [43]. In yet another study, a dose and duration-dependent antimalarial study of prepared chloroquine-conjugated CS NP (nanochloroquine) against *P. berghei* infection in Swiss mice was performed. The results showed that the novel formulation has a maximum effect at 250 mg/kg bodyweight concentration in 15 days treatment and can also act as an antioxidant agent [44]. The same research group has also reported that chloroquine-conjugated CS NP is more effective in combating the parasite infection, oxidative stress, and DNA damage in lymphocytes as compared with the free drug [45]. This group also studied the efficacy of chloroquine-conjugated CS NP on reactive oxygen species (ROS) mediated caspase activation and apoptosis in the liver during *P. berghei* NK65 infection. Results showed that the malarial damage due to apoptosis was significantly reduced by conjugating the drug to CS NP [46].

In yet another study, curcumin-bound CS NPs were developed for improving its chemical instability and bioavailability after oral administration in *P. yoelii* infected mice. Data of *in vitro* study suggest that curcumin bound CS NPs can inhibit hemozoin synthesis in the parasite. After its administration, the mice survived for five more days as compared with untreated mice [47].

Chitosan Nanoparticles for Double-Stranded Ribonucleic Acid (ds RNA) Delivery In the development of novel antimalarials, DNA/RNA has played an important role, and their incorporation into CS NPs can further increase the efficacy of these nucleic acids as antimalarials. In a study, for the inhibition of malaria parasite growth and development, long PfHDAC-1 double-stranded (ds) RNA was used against parasite histone deacetylase (HDAC) enzyme, which plays an essential role in maintaining histone protein concentrations, which are the new target for the development stage antimalarial drugs. Histones play crucial roles in transcriptional regulation, cell cycle progression, and development events in eukaryotes after posttranslational acetylation and deacetylation modifications. Two families of enzymes, histone acetyltransferase and HDAC, control the acetylation state of histones. In this study, chloroquine and pyrimethamine (PMA)-resistant *P. falciparum*, K1 strain was exposed to ds-RNA loaded nanoparticles, and it inhibits 47% growth in a culture, which secures its place for a safe antimalarial agent [48]. Based on the same strategy, CS NPs complexed long ds RNA targeting the coding region of *P. falciparum* DNA topoisomerase II enzyme (required for DNA replication) was studied to inhibit the growth and development of the parasite in culture. Results of the study showed CS NPs complexed with ds-RNA inhibits 71% growth of the parasite in culture, suggesting the potential of CS NPs to deliver ds-RNA [49]. In a recent study, CS/ds RNA NPs have been developed as a pest control strategy for the *Aedes aegypti* mosquito. The ability to repress the expression of *vg* gene responsible for wing development of *Ae. aegypti* mosquito was studied for CS/ds-RNA NPs. Results showed that NPs caused significant mortality, delayed growth development, and caused adult wing malformation of mosquito, suggesting the use of these carriers as a novel platform for pest control [50].

3.4.2.1.2 Human Serum Albumin Nanoparticles

The use of albumin-based carriers provides a unique advantage for antimalarials delivery, as it targets the infected erythrocytes and is selectively taken up and degraded by parasitized RBCs [51, 52]. For chloroquine-resistant malaria, Ibrahim et al. have developed albumin-bound indolone-*N*-oxides NPs. In *P. berghei* infected mice and *P. falciparum*-infected "humanized" mice, the novel formulation achieved complete cure with 99.1% and 97.5% of parasitemia inhibition [51]. The same researchers have developed albumin-bound artemisinin NPs for intravenous administration. The antimalarial efficiency was studied in *P. falciparum*-infected "humanized" mice, and results showed 96% parasitemia inhibition at 10 mg/kg/day dose, suggesting its utility as an intravenous formulation [52]. In a recent study, artemether intravenous formulation was developed by employing albumin-bound (nab) technology. NPs are prepared by the emulsification and desolvation approach to obtain a particle size of less than 50 nm. NPs displayed significantly enhanced dissolution properties over raw artemether [53].

3.4.2.1.3 Other Polymers

Cryptolepine hydrochloride-loaded gelatin nanoparticles have been developed, and the antimalaria activity was evaluated in Wistar mice after intravenous administration. Improved pharmacokinetics and *in vivo* antiplasmodial activity with NPs compared with free Cryptolepine hydrochloride indicated its effectiveness [54].

A carboxylic ionophore, monesin, was encapsulated in PLGA nanoparticles, and *in vitro* antimalarial activity was evaluated by inhibition of growth of *P. falciparum*. Results showed that monesin-loaded PLGA nanoparticles were 10 times more effective in inhibiting the growth of *P. falciparum in vitro* as compared with monesin alone [55].

Recently, for increasing the curcumin efficacy for malarial infection, it was loaded in eudragit nutriosomes prepared using eudragit, phospholipid vesicles, and Nutriose® FM06. The curcumin-loaded eudragit nutriosomes showed excellent results in Caco-2 cell lines (*in vitro*) and *in vivo* studies in malaria-infected mice, which was attributable to the increased ability of curcumin to counteract the oxidative stress [56].

Chloroquine-conjugated polyamidoamine nanoparticles were prepared for oral administration, and their efficacy was tested for parasite growth inhibition, hemolysis, and unspecific cytotoxicity assays. Results showed nanoparticles reached the blood circulation of *P. yoelii* infected mice and helped in building up immunity against malarial infection. These carriers also target the mosquito stages of *Plasmodium* and thus can be effective carriers for antimalarial drugs [57].

Poly(diethylmethylidene malonate) nanoparticles loaded with primaquine diphosphate were prepared, and the toxicity of the free drug, empty, and primaquine phosphate-loaded nanoparticles was studied in Naval Medical Research Institute (NMRI) mice. Results showed primaquine phosphate-loaded nanoparticles showed an increased life span index for mice [58].

3.4.2.2 Nanocapsules

3.4.2.2.1 Polycaprolactone Nanocapsules

Polysorbate-80-coated PCL nanocapsules were developed for the co-encapsulation of curcumin and quinine as monotherapy for drug-resistant malaria. The developed nanoformulation was evaluated for their *in vitro* schizonticidal activity and safety on *P. falciparum* and *Caenorhabditis elegans*, respectively. These nanocapsules showed a significant reduction in *P. falciparum* parasitemia. Compared with free drug, safety evaluation of nanocapsules in worms showed higher survival and longevity and no decrease in their reproductive capacity indicating the minimum toxic effect of nanocapsules in *C. elegans* worm [6].

3.4.2.2.2 Poly(D,L-Lactide) Nanocapsules

PEG-grafted PLA nanocapsules of halofantrine were prepared for parenteral administration. The efficacy and pharmacokinetics were studied in *P. berghei* infected mice. Results showed that PEG coating and encapsulation of halofantrine in PLA nanocapsules reduce the IV dose and toxicity of the drug, thus suggesting the use of formulation in severe malaria [59].

3.4.2.3 Dendrimers

Dendrimers are nano-sized globular structures resembling the architecture of trees. It has an initiator core and terminal groups at the end of repetitive layers that start radially from the core [60]. Drugs/biological molecules (DNA, RNA, and proteins), other polymers (carbohydrates, PEG), or targeting structures (folic acid, carbohydrates) can either be attached covalently to their peripheral portion by covalent linkage or by ionic interaction into their internal space. For reducing the reported hemolytic toxicity of chloroquine phosphate, two dendrimer formulations are reported.

In the first study, uncoated and chondroitin sulfate-A coated PEGylated Poly-L-lysine-based dendrimers of chloroquine phosphate were prepared. Results showed that coated dendrimers have significantly reduced hemolytic toxicity and cytotoxicity of chloroquine phosphate as compared with uncoated dendrimers [61].

In another study, D-galactose-coated chloroquine phosphate encapsulated poly-L-lysine dendrimers were prepared, which also shows reduced hemolytic toxicity along with the controlled release of chloroquine phosphate [62].

PEGylated peptide-based dendritic nanoparticulate systems of artemether were prepared for sustained and controlled delivery of the drug. They were found active against *P. falciparum* infection in rats [63]. In yet another study, primaquine phosphate polypropyleneimine dendrimers coated with galactose were prepared, which showed improved hemolytic toxicity, blood level, and hematological profile of primaquine phosphate after coating [64].

3.4.2.4 Micelles

PMA-loaded poloxamer-407 nano micelles were developed for evaluating their effect against *P. berghei* National Institute for Communicable Disease (NICD) strain for human malaria. Prepared nano micelles possessed a potent antimalarial activity and can be an effective candidate for the antimalarial drug [65]. Artemisinin micelles of PCL–PEG–PCL triblock polymers were prepared for the improved bioavailability, water solubility, and antiplasmodial property of artemisinin. The antiplasmodial activity of artemisinin-loaded micelles was measured against *P. berghei* infected Swiss albino mice, *in vivo*. Results indicated that micelles could prolong the circulation time and therapeutic efficacy of artemisinin [66].

3.4.2.5 Polymeric Hydrogel Nanoparticles

Hydrogel nanoparticles of curcumin were prepared using hydroxyl propyl methyl cellulose and polyvinyl pyrrolidone for enhanced absorption and prolonging the rapid clearance of curcumin by the reticuloendothelial system. *In vivo* antimalarial, acute, subacute toxicity, and genocytic studies performed to evaluate the novel formulation showed that it was safe as an adjunct antimalarial therapy [67].

3.4.2.6 Nanosuspension

In an attempt to combat malaria, nanosuspension of proguanil hydrochloride and atovaquone was prepared and studied in a murine model. Results show that the combination significantly reduced the drug dose and cost of therapy. This combination can be promising as it can act at multiple stages of the malaria lifecycle. Also, a twofold increase in bioavailability was observed due to the atovaquone suspension formulation [68].

3.4.3 Organized Layer-by-Layer Assembly

Layer-by-Layer (LbL) self-assembled thin films fabricated from CS and heparin sodium salt were loaded with 1,3,5-trisubstituted-2-pyrazolines. LbL film was fabricated with biocompatible and biodegradable polyelectrolytes. CS is a cationic polysaccharide owing to $-NH_2$ groups, whereas heparin is an anionic mucopolysaccharide, having high positive charge density due to sulfonyl hydroxide (SO_3H) and carboxyl (COOH) groups. Thin-film formation takes place via electrostatic interactions between the oppositely charged polyelectrolyte molecules. The *in vitro* release indicated sustained release of the drug molecule. Prophylactic drug delivery of the drug in a controlled release manner can effectively address the drug resistance against malarial parasites [69].

3.4.4 Inorganic Nano-architectonics

The architecture of nano-sized materials, also known as nano-architectonics, represents specifically engineered nanomaterials. The use of inorganic nanomaterials, such as metals and nonmetals, has been evolved in the detection and smart release and targeting of malarial parasites.

3.4.4.1 Metallic Platforms

Metallic nanocarriers such as gold, silver, iron, zinc, ruthenium, copper, cadmium, and bimetallic nanoparticles and drug–metal complex have been widely used for targeted drug delivery. These biocompatible, biodegradable, and nontoxic scaffolds are used to break the life cycle of the malarial parasite.

Green synthesis of silver nanoparticles (AgNPs) using soil fungus *Aspergillus niger* 2587 (20–70 nm size), when tested against larvae and pupae of *Culex quinquefasciatus*, showed 100% mortality within one hour [70]. In a similar synthesis of AgNP from *Artemisia nilagirica* plant having <30 nm size indicated larvicidal and pupicidal action against developmental stages of *Anopheles stephensi* and *Ae. aegypti* [71]. Some bacteria such as *Calothrix pulvinata, Anabaena flosaquae, Vibrio alginolyticus, Aeromonas* spp. SH10, *Plectonema boryanum* UTEX 485, and *Lactobacillus* spp. also have the potential to generate intracellular and extracellular AgNP [42, 72–76].

To boost *Plasmodium* immunity, DNA vaccine encoding *P. yoelii* merozoite surface protein $MSP1_{19}$ was delivered via magnetofection using supramagnetic nanoparticles coated with polyethyleneimine polymer. The study reported that *in vitro* transfection efficiency for DNA vaccine into eukaryotic cells was increased by magnetic nanoparticles under the external magnetic field [77]. Surface-modified iron oxide nanoparticles fortified with artesunate when tested against *P. falciparum* and experimental mouse model indicated effectiveness against multidrug-resistant malaria. The nanoparticles showed sustained pH-dependent release of Fe^{2+} within parasitic food vacuole for enhanced ROS generation. The study indicated that 1/8th concentration of fortified nanoparticles was as effective as the artesunate. *In vivo* study also suggested that a significant reduction in parasitemia can be obtained with an 8–10-fold reduced dose of artesunate when fortified with iron oxide nanoparticles [78].

Green synthesis of zinc oxide nanoparticles (ZnO-NPs) from *Plectranthus amboinicus* leaf extract, having an average size of around 20–50 nm, showed 100% mortality against mosquito larvae of *An. stephensi* and *C. quinquefasciatus* at the concentration of 8 and 10 μg/ml. Histopathological analysis for *An. stephensi* and *C. quinquefasciatus* larvae showed that the midgut, hindgut, muscles, and nerve ganglia were highly affected tissues in larvae [79]. Similarly, green synthesis of ZnO-NP from seaweed having face-centered cubic geometry reduced the fitness and reproduction of the malaria vector *An. stephensi* [80]. The complex of zinc metal with desferrioxamine (Zn–DFO complex) was also found to be superior to metal-free DFO. Zn–DFO complex was found to be more permeative into parasitized erythrocytes and exchanges its zinc for ferric ions, hence, rendering the iron unavailable for parasite functioning [81]. Similarly, zinc–quinine complex showed better therapeutic activity against malaria compared with chloroquine diphosphate [82, 83]. Synthesis of ZnO-NP by coprecipitation method from exopolysaccharide of probiotic *Bacillus licheniformis* indicated nearly 100% mortality against *Ae. Aegypti* and *An. stephensi* larvae [84].

Ruthenium–chloroquine complex was found to be two to fivefold more active than chloroquine alone. It was suggested that the complex rapidly hydrolyzed to its active species in an aqueous solution, which binds to hematin and inhibits its aggregation at pH ~ 5 [85]. Copper(II) nanohybrid solids were reported to exhibit *in vitro* antimalarial activity against *P. falciparum* [86]. Copper NP synthesized by polyol process also showed mosquito larvicidal activity [87]. Palladium NP, synthesized by biological reduction process using palladium acetate and aqueous extract of *Eclipta prostrata*, indicated dose-dependent suppression of parasitemia in Swiss albino mice [88].

Similar to previously described metal–drug complexes, the gold–chloroquine complex was also found to be more effective against two chloroquine-resistant strains of *P. falciparum* and *P. berghei*. *In vivo* activity of the synthesized complex against *P. berghei* infected female BALB/c mice indicated 84% more parasitemia suppressing ability compared with chloroquine [89].

Nano-vaccine is an emerging nanomedicine technology for the efficient delivery of immunogenic material. A nano-vaccine prepared by attaching *P. falciparum* antigen Pfs25 to gold nanoparticle (AgNP) blocked malaria transmission by blocking the sexual stages of the parasite. The study reported that AgNPs as an adjuvant might have enhanced uptake of antigen to antigen-presenting cells and elicit more immune response. Owing to tunable particle size, easy surface modification, and biocompatibility, AgNP serves as an efficient and cost-effective approach for vaccine delivery [90].

A comparative study of the effectiveness of bimetallic nanoparticles of Cu–Zn and Ag–Cu prepared using aqueous extract of *Ocimum sanctum* against mosquito larva indicated superior performance of Ag–Cu bimetallic nanoparticles [91].

3.4.4.2 Quantum Dots

Semiconductor-based nanoplatform, also known as quantum dots (QDs), is very useful for antimalarial drug delivery owing to its ultra-small size ranging from 1 to 10 nm and high surface area. These semiconductor nanocrystals exhibit exceptional characteristics such as size-tunable optical properties, anti-photo bleach properties, and excitation of various fluorescence colors. There are different types of QD, such as core type, core–shell type, and alloyed type (bimetallic). Core-type QD contains a single inorganic metal core or chalcogenides metal core, whereas core–shell type QD contains inorganic elemental central core and inorganic shell, e.g. CdTe/CdSe, CdSe/CdS. Alloyed QD is synthesized by allowing two semiconductors with different bandgap energies [92]. Highly sensitive and photo-bleaching resistant CdTe/Cds and CdSe/CdS QD were employed to stain *Plasmodium ookinete* to study its *in vivo* interaction in the midgut of mosquito. The study showed that QD staining of ookinetes remained permanent and indicated massive binding potency of concanavalin-A coated QD to the midgut wall of the mosquito vector. This result indicated that QDs were biocompatible and suitable luminescent marker to study *Plasmodium* penetration to the midgut of mosquito strain *P. berghei*. Hence, QD can be used to study the life cycle mechanism and invasion mechanism of the *Plasmodium* parasite into the mosquito vector [93]. A study reports that QD barcode microbeads exhibited enhanced stability and sensitivity for the multiplexed bio-sensing study. The metal nanoshell-coated single and mixed polymer microbeads, when used for multiplexed bio-detection for differentiation of *P. falciparum* from other non-lethal species, indicated its specificity, especially for detection of *P. falciparum* parasite even at low parasitemia.

Moreover, it concluded that the bead assay is an ultrasensitive high-throughput bio-sensing assay as compared with currently used clinical diagnosis [94]. Another study suggests that the *in vitro* antiplasmodial potential of graphene quantum dots (GQDs) is higher than chloroquine (CQ) itself. IC_{50} for GQD was found to be 82.43 μg/ml, whereas, for CQ, it was 90 μg/ml. *In vivo* studies carried out in male albino rats after oral administration of GQD indicated dose-dependent suppression of parasitemia [95].

3.4.4.3 Carbon Nanostructures

Carbon nanostructures can be divided into three groups depending on their dimensions: zero dimensional (0D), one dimensional (1D), and two dimensional (2D). Fullerene, nanodiamonds are 0D, whereas carbon nanotubes (CNTs) are 1D. Widely explored graphene is a 2D material. These materials are widely used for drug delivery due to their excellent mechanical, electrical, and thermal properties. Moreover, ease of functionalization over the high surface area and elasticity are favorable parameters for targeted drug delivery [96]. Currently, only CNTs are explored antimalarial drug delivery. Other carbon nanostructures for antimalarial are not yet reported till date.

CNTs are the hexagonal arrangement of carbon atoms in a cylindrical manner, i.e. graphene arranged in a roll. It can be either single-walled carbon nanotubes (SWCNTs) or multiwalled carbon nanotubes (MWCNTs). Generally, CNTs are capped by fullerenes, i.e. hemispherical arrangements of carbon networks [97]. Drugs are loaded in the cavity of the CNTs either during the synthesis of CNTs or by the equilibrium dialysis method after the synthesis of CNTs [98]. Owing to its nanostructure and larger surface area, targeting to subcellular structures by attaching functional groups is also possible.

A theoretical nanotechnological approach indicated SWCNTs conjugated with antimalarial drug artemisinin, and its derivatives could serve as a suitable inhibitor of *P. falciparum* [2]. A study reported that mannosylated MWCNTs loaded with artesunate effective targeting to the brain to treat cerebral malaria. The conventional therapy for cerebral malaria needs higher dose requirements and subsequent intolerable toxicity. D-Mannose conjugation of MWCNTs targets the brain cells having the mannose receptor, and thereby by the endocytosis-mediated delivery will effectively treat the disease. *In vivo* biodistribution study in albino Wistar rats indicated that IV administered formulations of artesunate loaded in Mannose conjugated MWCNTs were highly accumulated in the brain as compared with IV solution of pure drug. This observation shows that the use of mannosylated MWCNTs can deliver drug at the desired site with improved therapeutic margin [99].

3.4.4.4 Bio-ceramics

Ceramics are inorganic materials having ionic and covalent bonding. These nano-sized porous structures are widely explored for drug delivery. It includes calcium phosphatase-based drug delivery systems made from hydroxyapatite, tricalcium phosphates, and calcium phosphate cement. Similarly, from silica-based ceramics, bioactive glass and mesoporous silica are explored. Other bio-ceramics include alumina, zirconia, and non-oxide ceramics, such as silicon nitride and silicon carbide [100]. Among available ceramics, major research work is reported only on mesoporous silica nanoparticles for antimalarial delivery.

Well-ordered drug carriers MCM-41 and 3-phenyl propyl silane organo functionalized MCM-41 (pMCM-41) types of mesoporous silica were loaded with antimalarial drugs artesunate and quinine. *In vitro* drug release indicated the controlled release of drug from the carrier. *In vivo* studies showed high intracellular uptake of mesoporous silica nanocarriers (MSNs), thereby even at a 240-fold lesser dose of quinine in mesoporous silica was more effective than non-encapsulated quinine. Similarly, for artesunate, 20 times lesser dose was needed to inhibit parasite growth compared with the parent drug [101]. In a similar study, the SBA-15 type of mesoporous silica was used as a nanocarrier for artesunate and mefloquine drugs. Confinement of drugs in the mesoporous structures led to amorphization of the crystalline active pharmaceutical ingredient (API) and increased dissolution of the drugs. The study reported that co-formulation of both the drugs in SBA-15 carrier prepared by spray drying led to spatial confinements of the drugs in the pore structure of SBA-15.

Moreover, the hydrophilicity of the SBA-15 contributed to enhanced dissolution [102]. In another research, artemisinin was loaded in the SBA-15 mesoporous silica using a co-spray drying technique. Contact angle measurement as a means of wettability indicated that pure drug artemisinin had a contact angle of $70.1 \pm 3.0°$, whereas artemisinin loaded in SBA-15 showed only $21.2 \pm 2.8°$. The results indicated significant improvement in the wettability of solid dispersion due to hydrophilicity and capillary effect of carrier and amorphization of SBA-15. Moreover, *in vitro* cytotoxicity study in the Caco-2 cell line indicated nontoxic and biocompatible behavior of pure SBA-15 and artemisinin loaded SBA-15, as survival rate was found to be more than 90% [103].

3.4.5 Bio-inspired Nanocarriers

Although synthetic drug carriers are widely under development and in use, it is essential to consider natural particulates. The natural particulates will provide targeted drug delivery to achieve the maximal therapeutic effect [104]. Bio-engineered strategies based on pathogens (bacteria, virus), eukaryotic cells (erythrocytes, macrophages, lymphocytes, stem cells) are explored by researchers for drug delivery.

3.4.5.1 Vaccines Based on Bio-inspired Nanocarriers

Virus-like particles (VLPs) are self-assembled particles of capsid proteins that are structurally similar to viruses. Hence, these structures mimicking VLPs generate a robust humoral response [105]. RTS,S/AS01 Mosquirix™ developed with collaborative efforts between GlaxoSmithKline and Walter Reed Army Institute of Research, is the only extensively tested vaccine for preventive measures against malaria caused by *P. falciparum*. Phase 3 trials indicated its efficacy and safety among children aged 5–17 months and infants aged 6–12 weeks [106].

3.4.5.2 Bio-engineered Strategy Based on Erythrocytes

Erythrocytes, as drug carriers, offer advantages over other drug carriers concerning biocompatibility [107]. Nano-erythrosomes, a derivative of erythrocyte ghost, is explored to deliver the antimalarial drug, PMA [108–110]. As senescent cells are removed from circulation by phagocytosis action of Kupffer cells of the liver, the nano-erythrosomes would be readily taken up in the liver – where actual targeting of the antimalarial drug is required. Glutaraldehyde cross-linked PMA on the nanoerythrosomes displayed controlled drug release and more than 40% target in the liver tissue as compared with the free drug [108]. Artesunate-loaded nanoerythrosomes showed zero-order drug release up to eight hours [109]. Similarly, encapsulated drug primaquine also showed increased hepatic localization.

3.4.6 Protein–Peptide-Based Drug Delivery System

Self-assembling dipeptide (phenylalanine–dehydrophenylalanine) NPs loaded with curcumin were found to be effective for the treatment of malaria. Curcumin-loaded dipeptide NPs were found to be non-cytotoxic and non-hemolytic. *In vitro* cytotoxicity study carried out in mouse fibroblast L929 cell line by lactate dehydrogenase (LDH) release assay indicated dipeptide NPs were safe. *In vivo* antimalarial activity of curcumin-loaded dipeptide NP in *P. berghei* infected BALB/c mice showed a significant decrease in parasitemia and increased life span [111].

Artesunate–heparin conjugates were prepared, which were self-assembled as nanocapsules at low critical micelle concentration of 20 μg/ml concentration owing to the hydrophobic and hydrophilic structures of artesunate and heparin, respectively. These self-assembled nanocapsules showed a higher release rate of artesunate in a simulated acidic microenvironment, which mimics the acidic parasitic food vacuole of *P. falciparum*. Results of *in vivo* pharmacokinetics showed the extended half-life of nanocapsules in blood and thus can act as a promising carrier for antimalarial therapy [112].

Lumefantrine encapsulated in zein protein NPs achieved 20–30 times higher supersaturation levels in dissolution studies. The zein protein NPs were prepared by spray drying using casein as an electrostatic stabilizer. *In vitro* drug release indicated faster dissolution kinetics in simulated fasted or fed conditions compared with pure drug. This significant observation eliminated the bioavailability variation of the pure lumefantrine [113].

3.4.7 Stimuli-Responsive Platforms for Malaria

This is a novel drug delivery approach, wherein materials sensitive to external stimuli such as temperature, pH, light, redox, etc. are employed. In response to external stimuli, change occurs in either their structure or properties, which was exploited for treatment and diagnosis of malaria [114].

3.4.7.1 pH-Responsive Formulations

Recently a group has developed a zinc basic salt (ZBS) of artesunate (AS) to overcome the major physicochemical problems of the drug, such as poor solubility and decomposition in the acidic pH of the stomach. The ZBS-AS was developed by encapsulating the artesunate in the interlayer space of ZBS by a coprecipitation method. These were further coated with Eudragit L-100 polymer to form a ZBS-AS-L100 drug-polymer hybrid, which increased aqueous solubility and 5.5-time higher oral bioavailability than the pure drug. Due to pH selectivity and higher bioavailability, the developed system has a potential for antimalarial formulation [115].

In another study, the pH-sensitive hydrogel of an antimalarial drug methylene blue was prepared by the co-polymerization of two monomers methacrylamide and methacrylic acid. The prepared hydrogel was investigated for oral delivery and the drug release in gastric and intestinal fluid. Results showed 75% drug release at basic pH, which was attributable to the electrostatic repulsion between the similarly charged groups at this pH, resulting in bigger pores and high drug release. In comparison, only 29% of the drug was released at acidic pH due to the unionized group at this pH resulting in compact pores and slower drug release [116].

3.4.7.2 Thermo-Responsive Formulations

The use of thermo-responsive platforms in the treatment of malaria can be beneficial in certain conditions. Some researchers have developed thermosensitive gels of quinine for rectal administration, particularly for small children. They have used a thermosensitive polymer-poloxamer 407 and a bio-adhesive polymer hydroxy propyl methyl cellulose (HPMC) along with propanediol-1,2, which avoids the phase separation of two polymers and helps to form stable formulation [117].

3.4.7.3 Redox State Responsive Substances

For combating malaria parasites, the utilization of redox mechanisms is an emerging trend in malaria treatment strategies. Redox cyclers, are redox-active substances that can act as catalysts and inhibitors of multiple targets of the parasite *P. falciparum*. Some examples of redox recyclers are methylene blue and plasmodione. Recently, new potent antimalarial agents have been identified by researchers, such as derivatives of 3-benzylmenadiones class [118] and 1,4-naphthoquinones class compounds [119], which act as redox cycler. Both classes of compounds act by forming a less digestive form of hemoglobin by employing a redox mechanism, which accumulates in the parasite and ultimately results in its death.

3.4.7.4 Stimuli-Responsive Liquid Crystalline Materials

Recently, researchers have developed lyotropic liquid crystalline preconcentrates of drugs arteether and lumefantrine as a combination therapy for *falciparum* malaria. The distinguishing features of these preconcentrates are that they are less viscous and easily injectable, unlike the liquid crystalline phase, which is highly viscous and has lower diffusion coefficients. In the presence of water *in situ*, these lyotropic liquid crystalline preconcentrates convert themselves into the liquid crystalline phase of the drug [120].

3.5 Diagnostics

Identification and detection of biological markers of malaria, such as the antigens, from the body fluids such as plasma and urine at an early stage can be very helpful in combating malaria. Attempts have been made in the last few years to incorporate stimuli-sensitive technology to develop efficient and sensitive diagnostic agents.

3.5.1 Stimuli-Responsive Iron Oxide and Gold Nanoparticle Reagent System

Recently, a group has developed AuNPs coated with a thermally responsive diblock containing a poly(*N*-isopropyl acrylamide) (pNIPAm) segment and a gold-binding block composed of NIPAm-*co*-*N*,*N*-dimethyl aminoethyl acrylamide, to finally obtain AuNP coated with a diblock polymer, which was then attached with streptavidin containing antibodies, which will detect the antigens present in the plasma. These AuNP systems were then co-aggregated and separated on the application of a magnetic field in the presence of iron oxide nanoparticles. These large-sized "half sandwiches" are then applied on lateral flow strips to obtain a sensitive detection kit [121].

In another study, a porous membrane grafted with the stimuli-responsive polymer–antibody conjugate has been developed, which can efficiently purify and detect the malaria antigen *P. falciparum* histidine-rich protein 2 (PfHRP2) from spiked human plasma at clinically relevant concentrations [122].

3.5.2 Immunological Adjuvants

"Adjuvants" is the term given to pharmacological or immunological that can be added to vaccines as an adjuvant to boost the immune responses. Examples of adjuvants are alum, paraffin oil, etc. In the direction of malaria research, Verma et al. have developed a highly specific murine monoclonal antibody (mAb) against recombinant truncated HRP2 of *P. falciparum* by using a smart polymer pNIPAm and Complete Freund's Adjuvant, which was very sensitive and useful for the diagnosis of malaria [123].

3.5.3 Nanofibers

An ultrasensitive method was developed in which the antigen HRP2 released by *P. falciparum* parasite in the bloodstream can be detected in atto-gram/ml. The nano biosensor consisted of mercapto propyl phosphonic acid functionalized copper doped zinc oxide nanofibers and worked on the principle of the immunoassay technique. These nanofibers are promising candidates for developing commercial diagnostic kits of malaria as they can quantify the lowest detection limit of the malarial parasite [124].

3.6 Challenges in Clinical Translation of Nanomedicine

Nanomedicines are a very complex system in comparison to conventional medicine. Clinical translation of nanomedicine is challenging, expensive, and time-consuming [125]. The major challenges in clinical translation include biological challenges, biocompatibility and safety issue, challenges in manufacturing and scale-up, regulatory challenge, intellectual property (IP) issues, and high cost. The above problems severely limit the translation of nanomedicine into the market [126, 127].

3.6.1 Biological Challenges

Potential reasons behind the failure of nanomedicines in clinical translation include physiological barriers in the body, formulation issues, target accessibility, receptor expression level, and ligand concentration on the nanocarrier surface [128]. Understanding the relationship between disease pathophysiology and nanomedicine technology is an essential prerequisite for the successful translation of nanomedicines [129]. Preclinical studies of nanomedicine should be designed appropriately and evaluated in multiple animal models for effective clinical translation.

3.6.2 Biocompatibility and Safety

The toxicological evaluation of nanomedicine is essential for clinical translation. Regulatory bodies also recommend carrying out the toxicological assessment of nanomedicines to assure their safety [130]. The antimalarial drugs for which little or no information available, a meticulous clinical evaluation will be required for determining its efficacy and safety. Appropriate design of clinical trials and mobile clinical trial networks are required (for example, measurement of gametocyte prevalence and infectivity in malaria-exposed populations) to evaluate drug efficacy for blocking transmission and preventing relapse [131]. The increased complexity of nanomedicine significantly affects the biocompatibility and safety of nanomedicines [132]. Extensive *in vitro* and *ex vivo* assays are required to assess the potential risk of cytotoxicity, immunotoxicity, and genotoxicity of nanoformulations [133]. Although currently available assays are limited for nanotoxicology evaluations, many experimental malaria techniques are more specific for nanomedicines to evaluate drugs and vaccines. Standard regulatory protocols need to be followed to determine any toxicity caused by the therapeutic compounds entrapped within nanomedicine [134].

3.6.3 Challenges in Manufacturing Scale-Up and Reproducibility

The nanoformulation requires a complex and laborious method of preparation, which has limited clinical translation potential. Potential issues with nanomedicine manufacturing at large scale are (i) poor quality control (QC); (ii) formulation complexities; (iii) incomplete and challenging purification; (iv) high costs; (v) low yield; (vi) poor reproducibility, and final product stability during storage (e.g. uniformity in particle size distribution, surface charge, porosity, and mass). Thus, there is a need of techniques that can produce a large number of nanomaterials having desirable quality and reproducibility [135, 136].

Several industrially scalable methods have been successfully developed for the preparation of nanotechnology-based drug delivery systems without the need of multiple manufacturing steps. The challenges become more prominent with increased complexity. For example, surface modification with ligands, the insertion of multiple targeting moieties, or adding two or more drugs. The incorporation of many components into a single nanocarrier involves multiple steps, which unavoidably create problems in manufacturing, scale-up, and make more difficult quality assurance (QA) and quality control (QC) evaluation [126, 137]. The formulation characteristics of developed nanomedicines should be well defined and reproducible to allow their clinical translation.

3.6.4 Analytical Characterization and Quality Control Challenges of Nano-Formulations

Because of the complex structure, it is difficult to characterization nanomedicines. Batch-to-batch variability of nanomedicine leads to significant changes in physicochemical, pharmacokinetic, and/or pharmacodynamics properties. Nanoformulation should possess sufficiently high stability during manufacturing, storage, and in clinical settings. Therefore, an appropriate analytical method is required to characterize physicochemical and biological properties [138]. These challenges are from the development and regulatory perspective. It is of prime importance to extensively evaluate the nanomedicines using *in vitro* and *in vivo* models under clinically relevant conditions [136].

3.6.5 Regulatory Challenges

From the last two decades, nanomedicines are marketed, still regulations not in place to ensure their quality, safety, and efficacy for clinical use. In the past, regulatory bodies (FDA and EMA) have approved several nanomedicines. However, addressing the vast scientific and regulatory gap is challenging for nanomedicine. Nanomedicine is currently regulated in each country by its regulatory authority (e.g. FDA, TGA, and EMA). The regional and national differences in regulatory requirement among countries have affected the successful nanomedicine development and clinical translation [139]. Nanomedicines, which are intended to be marketed worldwide, should be governed by the same regulatory standards [140]. Extensive evaluation of nanomedicine with proper documentation, quality control, and handling environmental issues as per industrial standards are needed. There is an urgent requirement for refined, integrated, and standardized regulatory approaches from regulatory bodies to approve safe, effective, and quality nanomedicine products.

3.6.6 Other Challenges

Researchers from academic institutions, small and medium industry faced difficulty in managing the required finances for clinical translations. Academic scientists apply for grants to different government bodies and pursue basic science research with received funding. However, its clinical translation requires huge funds that they cannot manage. The licensing of technology may be used to solve this purpose.

Another issue that arises with nanomedicine is IP rights. There is clarity required for intellectual property in nanotechnology as they have a very complex structure. The increased complexity of nanomedicine makes the IP situation more confusing. Like, the invention is related to the existing drugs in combination with newer nanotechnologies or innovation involving nanomedicine of existing drugs with existing nanotechnology, but intended for a new medical application. Other issues such as the inclusion of multiple patents with one single technology, cross-licensing, time involved in the negotiation, collaboration, and licensing agreements cause a delay in the translation of nanomedicine from innovation to commercialization. Therefore, improvement in IP strategies is needed to make an easy path for reducing the processing time and expenditure.

Other than financial and IP issues, ethical issue is also hampering the clinical translation of nanomedicines. In early clinical trials, assessment of risks and benefits, understanding, and knowledge of nanomedicine are most critical. The regulatory bodies and ethical committees need to be careful as patient safety is their responsibility. However, the fine balance between risk and benefit needs to be swing [141]. Patients have a vital role to play in translational research. It is challenging to explain to patients about trial design and risks/benefits. Significant challenges were to provide information without destroying their hope [142].

3.7 Summary and Future Perspective

It is challenging to predict the future of nanotechnology in addressing malaria and other infectious diseases. Nanotechnology has a primary focus on the delivery of drugs in the form of multifunctional nanocarrier to target the cluttered sites in the parasite and thereby to control the drug resistance and subsequent toxicity. Problems associated with malaria can be prevented by developing advanced portable integrated nanodevices that will perform functions such as identification and separation between normal cells and parasitized cells, calculation of parasitemia percentage, and identification of drug-resistant parasites. The development of cost-effective, simple, and acceptable nanotechnology devices or delivery systems is expected in the future from scientists to control the spread of disease.

3.8 Conclusion

The advent of drug resistance in malaria parasites has endangered the lives of millions of people. The primary cause of the resistance is exposure to a suboptimal concentration of drugs due to various underlying reasons of conventional therapy. The development of a new chemical entity is not economical as it needs a lot of time and resources. Here, a novel drug delivery system, i.e. therapeutic nanoplatforms, provides smart and targeted delivery of an antimalarial drug. Prophylactic vaccines, bio-inspired nanocarriers, surface-modified nanoplatforms, stimuli-responsive platforms, inorganic nano-architects, lipid/polymer/protein–peptide-based nanocarriers can be potentially used to treat malaria either by active or passive targeting mechanism. The successful transformation of nanomedicines from the research lab to the clinic requires the development of simple, safe, reproducible, eco-friendly, and cost-effective methods for their synthesis and in-depth understanding of the safety control mechanisms, as well as the bio-distribution and pharmacokinetics of nanoplatforms in clinical applications.

Acknowledgments

Authors are thankful to the R. C. Patel Institute of Pharmaceutical Education and Research (RCPIPER), Shirpur, Maharashtra, The Maharaja Sayajirao University of Baroda, Kalabhavan, Vadodara, Gujarat, India, Shobhaben Pratapbhai Patel School of Pharmacy & Technology Management, SVKM's NMIMS, V.L. Mehta Road, Vile Parle (W), Mumbai, India. and Oriental College of Pharmacy, Oriental Education Society, Sanpada, Navi Mumbai, Maharashtra, India, for providing the facilities for writing this chapter.

References

1 *CDC – Malaria – About Malaria – Biology* [Internet]. [cited 3 December 2021]. Available from: https://www.cdc.gov/malaria/about/biology/index.html.

2 Singh, S.P. and Konwar, B.K. (2013). Carbon nanotube assisted drug delivery of the anti-malarial drug artemesinin and its derivatives—a theoretical nanotechnology approach. *Journal of Bionanoscience* 7 (6): 630–636. https://doi.org/10.1166/jbns.2013.1168.

3 WHO (2014). *World Health Organization: World Malaria Report 2014*. Google Scholar, 2014. World Health Organization.

4 Wassmer, S.C., Taylor, T.E., Rathod, P.K. et al. (2015). Investigating the pathogenesis of severe malaria: a multidisciplinary and cross-geographical approach. *The American Journal of Tropical Medicine and Hygiene*. American Society of Tropical Medicine and Hygiene 93 (3_Suppl): 42–56. https://doi.org/10.4269/ajtmh.14-0841.

5 Garg, A., Bhalala, K., Tomar, D.S., and Wahajuddin, M. (2017). *Nanomedicine: Emerging Trends in Treatment of Malaria, Antimicrobial Nanoarchitectonics: From Synthesis to Applications*. Elsevier Inc. https://doi.org/10.1016/B978-0-323-52733-0.00017-3.

6 Velasques, K., Maciel, T.R., de Castro Dal Forno, A.H. et al. (2018). Co-nanoencapsulation of antimalarial drugs increases their in vitro efficacy against *Plasmodium falciparum* and decreases their toxicity to *Caenorhabditis elegans*. *European Journal of Pharmaceutical Sciences* 118: 1–12. https://doi.org/10.1016/j.ejps.2018.03.014.

7 White, N. (1999). Antimalarial drug resistance and combination chemotherapy. *Philosophical Transactions of the Royal Society of London. Series B: Biological Sciences*. Edited by R.M. Anderson. Royal Society 354 (1384): 739–749. https://doi.org/10.1098/rstb.1999.0426.

8 Paget-McNicol, S. and Saul, A. (2001). Mutation rates in the dihydrofolate reductase gene of *Plasmodium falciparum*. *Parasitology* 122 (5): 497–505. https://doi.org/10.1017/S0031182001007739.

9 Sniegowski, P.D., Gerrish, P.J., Johnson, T. et al. (2000). The evolution of mutation rates: separating causes from consequences. *BioEssays* 22 (12): 1057–1066. https://doi.org/10.1002/1521-1878(200012)22:12<1057::AID-BIES3>3.0.CO;2-W.

10 Barnes, K.I., Watkins, W.M., and White, N.J. (2008). Antimalarial dosing regimens and drug resistance. *Trends in Parasitology* 24 (3): 127–134. https://doi.org/10.1016/j.pt.2007.11.008.

11 Hastings, I. and Watkins, W. (2006). Tolerance is the key to understanding antimalarial drug resistance. *Trends in Parasitology* 22 (2): 71–77.

12 Watkins, W.M. and Mosobo, M. (1993). Treatment of *Plasmodium falciparum* malaria with pyrimethamine-sulfadoxine: selective pressure for resistance is a function of long elimination half-life. *Transactions of the Royal Society of Tropical Medicine and Hygiene*. Oxford Academic 87 (1): 75–78. https://doi.org/10.1016/0035-9203(93)90431-O.

13 Duparc, S. and Beutler, E. (2007). Glucose-6-phosphate dehydrogenase deficiency and antimalarial drug development. *The American Journal of Tropical Medicine and Hygiene* 77 (4): 779–789. https://doi.org/10.4269/ajtmh.2007.77.779.

14 Phophak, N., Brittenham, G.M., Looareesuwan, S. et al. (2008). High-dose primaquine regimens against relapse of *Plasmodium vivax* malaria. *The American Journal of Tropical Medicine and Hygiene* 78 (5): 736–740. https://doi.org/10.4269/ajtmh.2008.78.736.

15 White, N.J. (1997). Assessment of the pharmacodynamic properties of antimalarial drugs in vivo. *Antimicrobial Agents and Chemotherapy* 41 (7): 1413–1422.

16 White, N.J. (1998). Why is it that antimalarial drug treatments do not always work? *Annals of Tropical Medicine and Parasitology*. Informa UK Limited 92 (4): 449–458. https://doi.org/10.1080/00034983.1998.11813303.

17 Morens, D.M., Folkers, G.K., and Fauci, A.S. (2004). The challenge of emerging and re-emerging infectious diseases. *Nature* 430 (6996): 242–249. https://doi.org/10.1038/nature02759.

18 Smithuis, F.M., van Woensel, J.B., Nordlander, E. et al. (1993). Comparison of two mefloquine regimens for treatment of *Plasmodium falciparum* malaria on the northeastern Thai-Cambodian border. *Antimicrobial Agents and Chemotherapy* 37 (9): 1977–1981. https://doi.org/10.1128/AAC.37.9.1977.

19 Soares, S., Sousa, J., Pais, A., and Vitorino, C. (2018). Nanomedicine: principles, properties, and regulatory issues. *Frontiers in Chemistry* 6 (Aug): 1–15. https://doi.org/10.3389/fchem.2018.00360.

20 Patra, J.K., Das, G., Fraceto, L.F. et al. (2018). Nano based drug delivery systems: recent developments and future prospects. *Journal of Nanobiotechnology*. BioMed Central Ltd. 16 (1): 71. https://doi.org/10.1186/s12951-018-0392-8.

21 Sinnis, P. and Kim Lee Sim, B. (1997). Cell invasion by the vertebrate stages of *Plasmodium*. *Trends in Microbiology*. Elsevier Ltd 5 (2): 52–58. https://doi.org/10.1016/S0966-842X(97)84657-4.

22 Santos-Magalhães, N.S. and Mosqueira, V.C.F. (2010). Nanotechnology applied to the treatment of malaria. *Advanced Drug Delivery Reviews*. Elsevier B.V. 62 (4, 5): 560–575. https://doi.org/10.1016/j.addr.2009.11.024.

23 Ancsin, J.B. and Kisilevsky, R. (2004). A binding site for highly sulfated heparan sulfate is identified in the N terminus of the circumsporozoite protein. *Journal of Biological Chemistry* 279 (21): 21824–21832. https://doi.org/10.1074/jbc.M401979200.

24 Juillerat-Jeanneret, L. (2008). The targeted delivery of cancer drugs across the blood–brain barrier: chemical modifications of drugs or drug-nanoparticles? *Drug Discovery Today* 13 (23, 24): 1099–1106. https://doi.org/10.1016/j.drudis.2008.09.005.

25 Tangpukdee, N., Duangdee, C., Wilairatana, P., and Krudsood, S. (2009). Malaria diagnosis: a brief review. *The Korean Journal of Parasitology* 47 (2): 93. https://doi.org/10.3347/kjp.2009.47.2.93.

26 Jaiswal, M., Dudhe, R., and Sharma, P.K. (2015). Nanoemulsion: an advanced mode of drug delivery system. *3 Biotech* 5 (2): 123–127. https://doi.org/10.1007/s13205-014-0214-0.

27 Dwivedi, P., Khatik, R., Chaturvedi, P. et al. (2015). Arteether nanoemulsion for enhanced efficacy against *Plasmodium yoelii* nigeriensis malaria: an approach by enhanced bioavailability. *Colloids and Surfaces B: Biointerfaces* 126: 467–475. https://doi.org/10.1016/j.colsurfb.2014.12.052.

28 Singh, K.K. and Vingkar, S.K. (2008). Formulation, antimalarial activity and biodistribution of oral lipid nanoemulsion of primaquine. *International Journal of Pharmaceutics* 347 (1, 2): 136–143. https://doi.org/10.1016/j.ijpharm.2007.06.035.

29 Dierling, A.M. and Cui, Z. (2005). Targeting primaquine into liver using chylomicron emulsions for potential vivax malaria therapy. *International Journal of Pharmaceutics* 303 (1, 2): 143–152. https://doi.org/10.1016/j.ijpharm.2005.07.015.

30 Pouton, C.W. (1997). Formulation of self-emulsifying drug delivery systems. *Advanced Drug Delivery Reviews* 25 (1): 47–58. https://doi.org/10.1016/S0169-409X(96)00490-5.

31 Dwivedi, P., Khatik, R., Khandelwal, K. et al. (2014). Self-nanoemulsifying drug delivery systems (SNEDDS) for oral delivery of arteether: pharmacokinetics, toxicity and antimalarial activity in mice. *RSC Advances* 4 (110): 64905–64918. https://doi.org/10.1039/C4RA09267H.

32 Mandawgade, S.D., Sharma, S., Pathak, S., and Patravale, V.B. (2008). Development of SMEDDS using natural lipophile: application to β-artemether delivery. *International Journal of Pharmaceutics* 362 (1, 2): 179–183. https://doi.org/10.1016/j.ijpharm.2008.06.021.

33 Manjunath, K., Reddy, J.S., and Venkateswarlu, V. (2005). Solid lipid nanoparticles as drug delivery systems. *Methods and Findings in Experimental and Clinical Pharmacology* 27 (2): 127. https://doi.org/10.1358/mf.2005.27.2.876286.

34 Mehnert, W. (2001). Solid lipid nanoparticles production, characterization and applications. *Advanced Drug Delivery Reviews* 47 (2, 3): 165–196. https://doi.org/10.1016/S0169-409X(01)00105-3.

35 Shevalkar, G. and Vavia, P. (2019). Solidified nanostructured lipid carrier (S-NLC) for enhancing the oral bioavailability of ezetimibe. *Journal of Drug Delivery Science and Technology*. Elsevier 53 (April): 101211. https://doi.org/10.1016/j.jddst.2019.101211.

36 Dwivedi, P., Khatik, R., Khandelwal, K. et al. (2014). Pharmacokinetics study of arteether loaded solid lipid nanoparticles: an improved oral bioavailability in rats. *International Journal of Pharmaceutics*. Elsevier 466 (1, 2): 321–327. https://doi.org/10.1016/j.ijpharm.2014.03.036.

37 Jain, S.A., Basu, H., Prabhu, P.S. et al. (2014). Parasite impairment by targeting *Plasmodium*-infected RBCs using glyceryl-dilaurate nanostructured lipid carriers. *Biomaterials* 35 (24): 6636–6645. https://doi.org/10.1016/j.biomaterials.2014.04.058.

38 Immordino, M.L., Dosio, F., and Cattel, L. (2006). Stealth liposomes: review of the basic science, rationale, and clinical applications, existing and potential. *International Journal of Nanomedicine* 1 (3): 297–315. https://doi.org/10.2217/17435889.1.3.297.

39 Aditya, N.P., Chimote, G., Gunalan, K. et al. (2012). Curcuminoids-loaded liposomes in combination with arteether protects against *Plasmodium berghei* infection in mice. *Experimental Parasitology* 131 (3): 292–299. https://doi.org/10.1016/j.exppara.2012.04.010.

40 Moles, E., Urbán, P., Jiménez-Díaz, M.B. et al. (2015). Immunoliposome-mediated drug delivery to *Plasmodium*-infected and non-infected red blood cells as a dual therapeutic/prophylactic antimalarial strategy. *Journal of Controlled Release*. Elsevier 210: 217–229. https://doi.org/10.1016/j.jconrel.2015.05.284.

41 Mhlwatika, Z. and Aderibigbe, B. (2018). Polymeric nanocarriers for the delivery of antimalarials. *Molecules* 23 (10): 2527. https://doi.org/10.3390/molecules23102527.

42 Rahman, K., Khan, S.U., Fahad, S. et al. (2019). Nano-biotechnology: a new approach to treat and prevent malaria. *International Journal of Nanomedicine* 14: 1401–1410. https://doi.org/10.2147/IJN.S190692.

43 Rajera, R., Nagpal, K., Singh, S.K., and Mishra, D.N. (2013). Toxicological study of the primaquine phosphate loaded chitosan nanoparticles in mice. *International Journal of Biological Macromolecules* https://doi.org/10.1016/j.ijbiomac.2013.08.019.

44 Tripathy, S., Das, S., Chakraborty, S.P. et al. (2012). Synthesis, characterization of chitosan–tripolyphosphate conjugated chloroquine nanoparticle and its in vivo anti-malarial efficacy against rodent parasite: a dose and duration dependent approach. *International Journal of Pharmaceutics* 434 (1, 2): 292–305. https://doi.org/10.1016/j.ijpharm.2012.05.064.

45 Tripathy, S., Mahapatra, S.K., Chattopadhyay, S. et al. (2013). A novel chitosan based antimalarial drug delivery against *Plasmodium berghei* infection. *Acta Tropica*. Elsevier 128 (3): 494–503. https://doi.org/10.1016/j.actatropica.2013.07.011.

46 Tripathy, S., Chattopadhyay, S., Dash, S.K. et al. (2015). Chitosan conjugated chloroquine: proficient to protect the induction of liver apoptosis during malaria. *International Journal of Biological Macromolecules* 74: 585–600. https://doi.org/10.1016/j.ijbiomac.2014.12.016.

47 Akhtar, F., Rizvi, M.M.A., and Kar, S.K. (2012). Oral delivery of curcumin bound to chitosan nanoparticles cured *Plasmodium yoelii* infected mice. *Biotechnology Advances* https://doi.org/10.1016/j.biotechadv.2011.05.009.

48 Sriwilaijaroen, N., Boonma, S., Attasart, P. et al. (2009). Inhibition of *Plasmodium falciparum* proliferation in vitro by double-stranded RNA directed against malaria histone deacetylase. *Biochemical and Biophysical Research Communications* 381 (2): 144–147. https://doi.org/10.1016/j.bbrc.2009.01.165.

49 Noonpakdee, W., Pothikasikorn, J., Nimitsantiwong, W., and Wilairat, P. (2003). Inhibition of *Plasmodium falciparum* proliferation in vitro by antisense oligodeoxynucleotides against malarial topoisomerase II. *Biochemical and Biophysical Research Communications* 302 (4): 659–664. https://doi.org/10.1016/S0006-291X(03)00246-8.

50 Ramesh Kumar, D., Saravana Kumar, P., Gandhi, M.R. et al. (2016). Delivery of chitosan/dsRNA nanoparticles for silencing of wing development vestigial (vg) gene in *Aedes aegypti* mosquitoes. *International Journal of Biological Macromolecules*. Elsevier B.V. 86: 89–95. https://doi.org/10.1016/j.ijbiomac.2016.01.030.

51 Ibrahim, N., Ibrahim, H., Dormoi, J. et al. (2014). Albumin-bound nanoparticles of practically water-insoluble antimalarial lead greatly enhance its efficacy. *International Journal of Pharmaceutics*. Elsevier 464 (1, 2): 214–224. https://doi.org/10.1016/j.ijpharm.2014.01.001.

52 Ibrahim, N., Ibrahim, H., Sabater, A.M. et al. (2015). Artemisinin nanoformulation suitable for intravenous injection: preparation, characterization and antimalarial activities. *International Journal of Pharmaceutics*. Elsevier 495 (2): 671–679. https://doi.org/10.1016/j.ijpharm.2015.09.020.

53 Boateng-Marfo, Y., Dong, Y., Loh, Z.H. et al. (2018). Intravenous human serum albumin (HSA)-bound artemether nanoparticles for treatment of severe malaria. *Colloids and Surfaces A: Physicochemical and Engineering Aspects*. Elsevier B.V. 536: 20–29. https://doi.org/10.1016/j.colsurfa.2017.08.016.

54 Kuntworbe, N., Ofori, M., Addo, P. et al. (2013). Pharmacokinetics and in vivo chemosuppressive activity studies on cryptolepine hydrochloride and cryptolepine hydrochloride-loaded gelatine nanoformulation designed for parenteral administration for the treatment of malaria. *Acta Tropica* 127 (3): 165–173. https://doi.org/10.1016/j.actatropica.2013.04.010.

55 Surolia, R., Pachauri, M., and Ghosh, P.C. (2012). Preparation and characterization of monensin loaded PLGA nanoparticles: *in vitro* anti-malarial activity against *Plasmodium falciparum*. *Journal of Biomedical Nanotechnology* 8 (1): 172–181. https://doi.org/10.1166/jbn.2012.1366.

56 Manconi, M., Manca, M.L., Escribano-Ferrer, E. et al. (2019). Nanoformulation of curcumin-loaded eudragit-nutriosomes to counteract malaria infection by a dual strategy: improving antioxidant intestinal activity and systemic efficacy. *International Journal of Pharmaceutics*. Elsevier B.V. 556: 82–88. https://doi.org/10.1016/j.ijpharm.2018.11.073.

57 Martí Coma-Cros, E., Biosca, A., Marques, J. et al. (2018). Polyamidoamine nanoparticles for the oral administration of antimalarial drugs. *Pharmaceutics* 10 (4): 225. https://doi.org/10.3390/pharmaceutics10040225.

58 Mbela, T.K.M., Poupaert, J.H., and Dumont, P. (1992). Poly(diethylmethylidene malonate) nanoparticles as primaquine delivery system to liver. *International Journal of Pharmaceutics* 79 (1–3): 29–38. https://doi.org/10.1016/0378-5173(92)90090-O.

59 Mosqueira, V.C.F., Loiseau, P.M., Bories, C. et al. (2004). Efficacy and pharmacokinetics of intravenous nanocapsule formulations of halofantrine in *Plasmodium berghei*-infected mice. *Antimicrobial Agents and Chemotherapy* 48 (4): 1222–1228. https://doi.org/10.1128/AAC.48.4.1222-1228.2004.

60 Dias, A.P., da Silva Santos, S., da Silva, J.V. et al. (2020). Dendrimers in the context of nanomedicine. *International Journal of Pharmaceutics*. Elsevier B.V. 573: 118814. https://doi.org/10.1016/j.ijpharm.2019.118814.

61 Bhadra, D., Bhadra, S., and Jain, N.K. (2006). PEGylated peptide dendrimeric carriers for the delivery of antimalarial drug chloroquine phosphate. *Pharmaceutical Research* 23 (3): 623–633. https://doi.org/10.1007/s11095-005-9396-9.

62 Agrawal, P., Gupta, U., and Jain, N.K. (2007). Glycoconjugated peptide dendrimers-based nanoparticulate system for the delivery of chloroquine phosphate. *Biomaterials*. Elsevier 28 (22): 3349–3359. https://doi.org/10.1016/j.biomaterials.2007.04.004.

63 Bhadra, D., Bhadra, S., and Jain, N.K. (2005). PEGylated peptide-based dendritic nanoparticulate systems for delivery of artemether. *Journal of Drug Delivery Science and Technology* 15 (1): 65–73. https://doi.org/10.1016/S1773-2247(05)50008-X.

64 Bhadra, D., Bhadra, S., and Jain, N.K. (2005). Glycodendrimeric nanoparticulate carriers of primaquine phosphate for liver targeting. *International Journal of Pharmaceutics* 295 (1, 2): 221–233. https://doi.org/10.1016/j.ijpharm.2005.01.026.

65 Pestehchian, N., Vafaei, M.R., Nematolahy, P. et al. (2020). A new effective antiplasmodial compound: nanoformulated pyrimethamine. *Journal of Global Antimicrobial Resistance* 20: 309–315. https://doi.org/10.1016/j.jgar.2019.08.002.

66 Ramazani, A., Keramati, M., Malvandi, H. et al. (2018). Preparation and in vivo evaluation of anti-plasmodial properties of artemisinin-loaded PCL–PEG–PCL nanoparticles. *Pharmaceutical Development and Technology* 23 (9): 911–920. https://doi.org/10.1080/10837450.2017.1372781.

67 Dandekar, P.P., Jain, R., Patil, S. et al. (2010). Curcumin-loaded hydrogel nanoparticles: application in anti-malarial therapy and toxicological evaluation. *Journal of Pharmaceutical Sciences*. John Wiley and Sons Inc. 99 (12): 4992–5010. https://doi.org/10.1002/jps.22191.

68 Kathpalia, H., Juvekar, S., Mohanraj, K. et al. (2020). Investigation of pre-clinical pharmacokinetic parameters of atovaquone nanosuspension prepared using a pH-based precipitation method and its pharmacodynamic properties in a novel artemisinin combination. *Journal of Global Antimicrobial Resistance* 22: 248–256. https://doi.org/10.1016/j.jgar.2020.02.018.

69 Bhalerao, U.M., Valiveti, A.K., Acharya, J. et al. (2015). Controlled release studies of antimalarial 1,3,5-trisubstituted-2-pyrazolines from biocompatible chitosan–heparin layer-by-layer (LbL) self assembled thin films. *Colloids and Surfaces B: Biointerfaces* 125: 151–159. https://doi.org/10.1016/j.colsurfb.2014.11.016.

70 Soni, N. and Prakash, S. (2013). Possible mosquito control by silver nanoparticles synthesized by soil fungus (*Aspergillus niger* 2587). *Advances in Nanoparticles* 02 (2): 125–132. https://doi.org/10.4236/anp.2013.22021.

71 Nalini, M., Lena, M., Sumathi, P., and Sundaravadivelan, C. (2017). Effect of phyto-synthesized silver nanoparticles on developmental stages of malaria vector, *Anopheles stephensi* and dengue vector, *Aedes aegypti*. *Egyptian Journal of Basic and Applied Sciences* 4 (3): 212–218. https://doi.org/10.1016/j.ejbas.2017.04.005.

72 Brayner, R., Barberousse, H., Hemadi, M. et al. (2007). Cyanobacteria as bioreactors for the synthesis of Au, Ag, Pd, and Pt nanoparticles via an enzyme-mediated route. *Journal of Nanoscience and Nanotechnology* 7 (8): 2696–2708. https://doi.org/10.1166/jnn.2007.600.

73 Fu, M., Li, Q., Sun, D. et al. (2006). Rapid preparation process of silver nanoparticles by bioreduction and their characterizations. *Chinese Journal of Chemical Engineering* 14 (1): 114–117. https://doi.org/10.1016/S1004-9541(06)60046-3.

74 Lengke, M.F., Fleet, M.E., and Southam, G. (2007). Biosynthesis of silver nanoparticles by filamentous cyanobacteria from a silver(I) nitrate complex. *Langmuir* 23 (5): 2694–2699. https://doi.org/10.1021/la0613124.

75 Nair, B. and Pradeep, T. (2002). Coalescence of nanoclusters and formation of submicron crystallites assisted by *Lactobacillus* strains. *Crystal Growth & Design* 2 (4): 293–298. https://doi.org/10.1021/cg0255164.

76 Singh, H., Du, J., Singh, P., and Yi, T.H. (2018). Extracellular synthesis of silver nanoparticles by *Pseudomonas* sp. THG-LS1.4 and their antimicrobial application. *Journal of Pharmaceutical Analysis* 8 (4): 258–264. https://doi.org/10.1016/j.jpha.2018.04.004.

77 Al-Deen, F.N., Ho, J., Selomulya, C. et al. (2011). Superparamagnetic nanoparticles for effective delivery of malaria DNA vaccine. *Langmuir* 27 (7): 3703–3712. https://doi.org/10.1021/la104479c.

78 Kannan, D., Yadav, N., Ahmad, S. et al. (2019). Pre-clinical study of iron oxide nanoparticles fortified artesunate for efficient targeting of malarial parasite. *eBioMedicine* 45: 261–277. https://doi.org/10.1016/j.ebiom.2019.06.026.

79 Vijayakumar, S., Vinoj, G., Malaikozhundan, B. et al. (2015). *Plectranthus amboinicus* leaf extract mediated synthesis of zinc oxide nanoparticles and its control of methicillin resistant *Staphylococcus aureus* biofilm and blood sucking mosquito larvae. *Spectrochimica Acta Part A: Molecular and Biomolecular Spectroscopy* 137: 886–891. https://doi.org/10.1016/j.saa.2014.08.064.

80 Murugan, K., Roni, M., Panneerselvam, C. et al. (2018). *Sargassum wightii*-synthesized ZnO nanoparticles reduce the fitness and reproduction of the malaria vector *Anopheles stephensi* and cotton bollworm *Helicoverpa armigera*. *Physiological and Molecular Plant Pathology* 101: 202–213. https://doi.org/10.1016/j.pmpp.2017.02.004.

81 Chevion, M., Chuang, L., and Golenser, J. (1995). Effects of zinc-desferrioxamine on *Plasmodium falciparum* in culture. *Antimicrobial Agents and Chemotherapy* 39 (8): 1902–1905. https://doi.org/10.1128/AAC.39.8.1902.

82 Ogunlana, O.O. (2012). Antiplasmodial activity of quinine-zinc complex and chloroquine: a comparative in vitro assessment. *African Journal of Pharmacy and Pharmacology* 6 (8): https://doi.org/10.5897/AJPP11.482.

83 Ogunlana, O.O., Ogunlana, O.E., and Ademowo, O.G. (2009). Comparative in vitro assessment of the antiplasmodial activity of quinine-zinc complex and quinine sulphate. *Scientific Research and Essay*. Academic Journals 4 (3): 180–184.

84 Abinaya, M., Vaseeharan, B., Divya, M. et al. (2018). Bacterial exopolysaccharide (EPS)-coated ZnO nanoparticles showed high antibiofilm activity and larvicidal toxicity against malaria and Zika virus vectors. *Journal of Trace Elements in Medicine and Biology*. Elsevier GmbH 45: 93–103. https://doi.org/10.1016/j.jtemb.2017.10.002.

85 Martínez, A., CSK, R., Naoulou, B. et al. (2008). The mechanism of antimalarial action of the ruthenium(II)–chloroquine complex $[RuCl_2(CQ)]_2$. *JBIC, Journal of Biological Inorganic Chemistry* 13 (5): 703–712. https://doi.org/10.1007/s00775-008-0356-9.

86 Mohapatra, S.C., Tiwari, H.K., Singla, M. et al. (2010). Antimalarial evaluation of copper(II) nanohybrid solids: inhibition of plasmepsin II, a hemoglobin-degrading malarial aspartic protease from *Plasmodium falciparum*.

JBIC, Journal of Biological Inorganic Chemistry. Springer 15 (3): 373–385. https://doi.org/10.1007/s00775-009-0610-9.

87 Ramyadevi, J., Jeyasubramanian, K., Marikani, A. et al. (2011). Copper nanoparticles synthesized by polyol process used to control hematophagous parasites. *Parasitology Research* 109 (5): 1403–1415. https://doi.org/10.1007/s00436-011-2387-3.

88 Rajakumar, G., Rahuman, A.A., Chung, I.-M. et al. (2015). Antiplasmodial activity of eco-friendly synthesized palladium nanoparticles using *Eclipta prostrata* extract against *Plasmodium berghei* in Swiss albino mice. *Parasitology Research* 114 (4): 1397–1406. https://doi.org/10.1007/s00436-015-4318-1.

89 Navarro, M., Pérez, H., and Sánchez-Delgado, R.A. (1997). Toward a novel metal-based chemotherapy against tropical diseases. 3. Synthesis and antimalarial activity in vitro and in vivo of the new gold–chloroquine complex $[Au(PPh_3)(CQ)]PF_6$. *Journal of Medicinal Chemistry*. American Chemical Society 40 (12): 1937–1939. https://doi.org/10.1021/jm9607358.

90 Kumar, R., Ray, P.C., Datta, D. et al. (2015). Nanovaccines for malaria using *Plasmodium falciparum* antigen Pfs25 attached gold nanoparticles. *Vaccine* 33 (39): 5064–5071. https://doi.org/10.1016/j.vaccine.2015.08.025.

91 Minal, S.P. and Prakash, S. (2016). Cu–Zn and Ag–Cu bimetallic nanoparticles as larvicide to control malaria parasite vector: a comparative analysis. In: *2016 IEEE Region 10 Humanitarian Technology Conference (R10-HTC)*, 1–6. IEEE https://doi.org/10.1109/R10-HTC.2016.7906817.

92 Bilan, R., Nabiev, I., and Sukhanova, A. (2016). Quantum dot-based nanotools for bioimaging, diagnostics, and drug delivery. *ChemBioChem* 17 (22): 2103–2114. https://doi.org/10.1002/cbic.201600357.

93 Basseri, H.R., Javazm, M.S., Farivar, L., and Abai, M.R. (2016). Lectin-carbohydrate recognition mechanism of *Plasmodium berghei* in the midgut of malaria vector *Anopheles stephensi* using quantum dot as a new approach. *Acta Tropica* 156: 37–42. https://doi.org/10.1016/j.actatropica.2016.01.003.

94 Chen, K., LYT, C., Song, F., and WCW, C. (2013). Fabrication of metal nanoshell quantum-dot barcodes for biomolecular detection. *Nano Today* 8 (3): 228–234. https://doi.org/10.1016/j.nantod.2013.04.009.

95 Murugan, K., Nataraj, D., Jaganathan, A. et al. (2017). Nanofabrication of graphene quantum dots with high toxicity against malaria mosquitoes, *Plasmodium falciparum* and MCF-7 cancer cells: impact on predation of non-target tadpoles, odonate nymphs and mosquito fishes. *Journal of Cluster Science* 28 (1): 393–411. https://doi.org/10.1007/s10876-016-1107-7.

96 Erol, O., Uyan, I., Hatip, M. et al. (2018). Recent advances in bioactive 1D and 2D carbon nanomaterials for biomedical applications. *Nanomedicine: Nanotechnology, Biology and Medicine* 14 (7): 2433–2454. https://doi.org/10.1016/j.nano.2017.03.021.

97 Herlem, G., Picaud, F., Girardet, C., and Micheau, O. (2019). Carbon nanotubes. *Nanocarriers for Drug Delivery*. Elsevier 469–529. https://doi.org/10.1016/B978-0-12-814033-8.00016-3.

98 Aderibigbe, B.A. and Mukaya, H.E. (2016). Nanobiomaterials architectured for improved delivery of antimalaria drugs. *Nanoarchitectonics for Smart Delivery and Drug Targeting*. Elsevier 169–200. https://doi.org/10.1016/B978-0-323-47347-7.00007-0.

99 Gulbake, A.S., Jain, A., Shilpi, S. et al. (2019). Mannosylated multiwalled carbon nanotubes assisted artesunate delivery for cerebral malaria. *International Journal of Applied Pharmaceutics* https://doi.org/10.22159/ijap.2019v11si2.32887.

100 Manzano, M. (2014). Ceramics for drug delivery. In: *Bio-ceramics with Clinical Applications* (ed. M. Vallet-Regí), 343–382. Chichester, UK: Wiley https://doi .org/10.1002/9781118406748.ch12.

101 Amolegbe, S.A., Hirano, Y., Adebayo, J.O. et al. (2018). Mesoporous silica nanocarriers encapsulated antimalarials with high therapeutic performance. *Scientific Reports* 8 (1): 3078. https://doi.org/10.1038/s41598-018-21351-8.

102 Letchmanan, K., Shen, S.C., Ng, W.K., and RBH, T. (2017). Dissolution and physicochemical stability enhancement of artemisinin and mefloquine co-formulation via nano-confinement with mesoporous SBA-15. *Colloids and Surfaces, B: Biointerfaces* https://doi.org/10.1016/j.colsurfb.2017.05.003.

103 Letchmanan, K., Shen, S.-C., Ng, W.K., and RBH, T. (2015). Enhanced dissolution and stability of artemisinin by nano-confinement in ordered mesoporous SBA-15 particles. *Journal of Microencapsulation* 32 (4): 390–400. https://doi.org/ 10.3109/02652048.2015.1035684.

104 Yoo, J.-W., Irvine, D.J., Discher, D.E., and Mitragotri, S. (2011). Bio-inspired, bioengineered and biomimetic drug delivery carriers. *Nature Reviews Drug Discovery* 10 (7): 521–535. https://doi.org/10.1038/nrd3499.

105 Roy, P. and Noad, R. (2009). Virus-like particles as a vaccine delivery system: myths and facts. *Advances in Experimental Medicine and Biology* 145–158. https://doi.org/10.1007/978-1-4419-1132-2_11.

106 RTS,S Clinical Trials Partnership (2015). Efficacy and safety of RTS,S/AS01 malaria vaccine with or without a booster dose in infants and children in Africa: final results of a phase 3, individually randomised, controlled trial. *The Lancet*. Lancet Publishing Group 386 (9988): 31–45. https://doi.org/10.1016/ S0140-6736(15)60721-8.

107 Talwar, N. and Jain, N.K. (1992). Erythrocytes as carriers of primaquine-preparation: characterization and evaluation. *Journal of Controlled Release* 20 (2): 133–141. https://doi.org/10.1016/0168-3659(92)90159-O.

108 Agnihotri, J. and Jain, N.K. (2013). Biodegradable long circulating cellular carrier for antimalarial drug pyrimethamine. *Artificial Cells, Nanomedicine and Biotechnology* https://doi.org/10.3109/21691401.2012.743901.

109 Agnihotri, J., Saraf, S., Singh, S., and Bigoniya, P. (2015). Development and evaluation of anti-malarial bio-conjugates: artesunate-loaded nanoerythrosomes. *Drug Delivery and Translational Research* 5 (5): 489–497. https://doi.org/10 .1007/s13346-015-0246-y.

110 Jain, N., Agnihotri, J., and Gajbhiye, V. (2010). Engineered cellular carrier nanoerythrosomes as potential targeting vectors for anti-malarial drug. *Asian Journal of Pharmaceutics* 4 (2): 116. https://doi.org/10.4103/0973-8398.68462.

111 Alam, S., Panda, J.J., Mukherjee, T.K., and Chauhan, V.S. (2016). Short peptide based nanotubes capable of effective curcumin delivery for treating drug resistant malaria. *Journal of Nanobiotechnology* 14 (1): 26. https://doi.org/10.1186/s12951-016-0179-8.

112 Ismail, M., Du, Y., Ling, L., and Li, X. (2019). Artesunate-heparin conjugate based nanocapsules with improved pharmacokinetics to combat malaria. *International Journal of Pharmaceutics* 562: 162–171. https://doi.org/10.1016/j.ijpharm.2019.03.031.

113 Feng, J., Zhang, Y., SA, M.M. et al. (2019). Amorphous nanoparticles by self-assembly: processing for controlled release of hydrophobic molecules. *Soft Matter* 15 (11): 2400–2410. https://doi.org/10.1039/C8SM02418A.

114 Debije, M.G. and Schenning, A.P.H.J. (2016). Stimuli-responsive liquid crystalline materials. *Reference Module in Materials Science and Materials Engineering*. Elsevier. https://doi.org/10.1016/B978-0-12-803581-8.04039-X.

115 Kim, J.-Y., Yang, J.-H., Lee, J.-H. et al. (2015). 2D inorganic-antimalarial drug-polymer hybrid with pH-responsive solubility. *Chemistry – An Asian Journal*. John Wiley and Sons Ltd 10 (10): 2264–2271. https://doi.org/10.1002/asia.201500347.

116 Bajpai, S.K. and Saggu, S.P.S. (2007). Controlled release of an anti-malarial drug from a pH-sensitive poly(methacrylamide-*co*-methacrylic acid) hydrogel system. *Designed Monomers and Polymers*. Taylor & Francis Group 10 (6): 543–554. https://doi.org/10.1163/156855507782401196.

117 Koffi, A.A., Agnely, F., Ponchel, G., and Grossiord, J.L. (2006). Modulation of the rheological and mucoadhesive properties of thermosensitive poloxamer-based hydrogels intended for the rectal administration of quinine. *European Journal of Pharmaceutical Sciences* 27 (4): 328–335. https://doi.org/10.1016/j.ejps.2005.11.001.

118 Sidorov, P., Desta, I., Chessé, M. et al. (2016). Redox polypharmacology as an emerging strategy to combat malarial parasites. *ChemMedChem* 11 (12): 1339–1351. https://doi.org/10.1002/cmdc.201600009.

119 Müller, T., Johann, L., Jannack, B. et al. (2011). Glutathione reductase-catalyzed cascade of redox reactions to bioactivate potent antimalarial 1,4-naphthoquinones – a new strategy to combat malarial parasites. *Journal of the American Chemical Society* 133 (30): 11557–11571. https://doi.org/10.1021/ja201729z.

120 Dawre, S., Pathak, S., Sharma, S., and Devarajan, P.V. (2018). Enhanced antimalalarial activity of a prolonged release in situ gel of arteether–lumefantrine in a murine model. *European Journal of Pharmaceutics and Biopharmaceutics* 123: 95–107. https://doi.org/10.1016/j.ejpb.2017.11.002.

121 Nash, M.A., Waitumbi, J.N., Hoffman, A.S. et al. (2012). Multiplexed enrichment and detection of malarial biomarkers using a stimuli-responsive iron oxide and gold nanoparticle reagent system. *ACS Nano*. ACS Nano 6 (8): 6776–6785. https://doi.org/10.1021/nn3015008.

122 Golden, A.L., Battrell, C.F., Pennell, S. et al. (2010). Simple fluidic system for purifying and concentrating diagnostic biomarkers using stimuli-responsive antibody conjugates and membranes. *Bioconjugate Chemistry* 21 (10): 1820–1826. https://doi.org/10.1021/bc100169y.

123 Verma, R., Ravichandran, R., Jayaprakash, N.S. et al. (2015). Adjuvant poly(*N*-isopropylacrylamide) generates more efficient monoclonal antibodies against truncated recombinant histidine-rich protein2 of *Plasmodium falciparum* for malaria diagnosis. *Biotechnology Journal* 10 (5): 772–782. https://doi.org/10.1002/biot.201400386.

124 Brince Paul, K., Kumar, S., Tripathy, S. et al. (2016). A highly sensitive self assembled monolayer modified copper doped zinc oxide nanofiber interface for detection of *Plasmodium falciparum* histidine-rich protein-2: targeted towards rapid, early diagnosis of malaria. *Biosensors and Bioelectronics* 80: 39–46. https://doi.org/10.1016/j.bios.2016.01.036.

125 Narang, A., Chang, R., and Hussain, M.A. (2013). Pharmaceutical development and regulatory considerations for nanoparticles and nanoparticulate drug delivery systems. *Journal of Pharmaceutical Sciences* 102 (11): 3867–3882. https://doi.org/10.1002/jps.23691.

126 Bawa, R., Bawa, S.R., and Mehra, R.N. (2016). The translational challenge in medicine at the nanoscale. In: *Handbook of Clinical Nanomedicine*, 1345–1400. Jenny Stanford Publishing.

127 Eleraky, N.E., Allam, A., Hassan, S.B., and Omar, M.M. (2020). Nanomedicine fight against antibacterial resistance: an overview of the recent pharmaceutical innovations. *Pharmaceutics* 12 (2): 142. https://doi.org/10.3390/pharmaceutics12020142.

128 Iqbal, J., Abbasi, B.A., Ahmad, R. et al. (2018). Nanomedicines for developing cancer nanotherapeutics : from benchtop to bedside and beyond. *Applied Microbiology and Biotechnology* .

129 Agrahari, V. and Agrahari, V. (2018). Facilitating the translation of nanomedicines to a clinical product: challenges and opportunities. *Drug Discovery Today*. Elsevier Ltd 23 (5): 974–991. https://doi.org/10.1016/j.drudis.2018.01.047.

130 Siegrist, S., Cörek, E., Detampel, P. et al. (2019). Preclinical hazard evaluation strategy for nanomedicines. *Nanotoxicology*. Taylor & Francis 13 (1): 73–99. https://doi.org/10.1080/17435390.2018.1505000.

131 The malERA Consultative Group on Drugs (2011). A research agenda for malaria eradication: drugs. *PLoS Medicine* 8 (1): e1000402. https://doi.org/10.1371/journal.pmed.1000402.

132 Li, X., Wang, L., Fan, Y. et al. (2012). Biocompatibility and toxicity of nanoparticles and nanotubes. *Journal of Nanomaterials* 2012: 1–19. https://doi.org/10.1155/2012/548389.

133 Dobrovolskaia, M.A. and McNeil, S.E. (2013). Understanding the correlation between in vitro and in vivo immunotoxicity tests for nanomedicines. *Journal of Controlled Release*. Elsevier B.V. 172 (2): 456–466. https://doi.org/10.1016/j.jconrel.2013.05.025.

134 Bahadar, H., Maqbool, F., Niaz, K. et al. (2016). Toxicity of nanoparticles and an overview of current experimental models. *Iranian Biomedical Journal* 20 (1): 1–11. https://doi.org/10.7508/ibj.2016.01.001.

135 Hua, S., de Matos, M.B.C., Metselaar, J.M., and Storm, G. (2018). Current trends and challenges in the clinical translation of nanoparticulate nanomedicines: pathways for translational development and commercialization. *Frontiers in Pharmacology* 9 (July): 1–14. https://doi.org/10.3389/fphar.2018.00790.

136 Ventola, C.L. (2017). Progress in nanomedicine: approved and investigational nanodrugs. *P & T: A Peer-Reviewed Journal for Formulary Management* 42 (12): 742–755.

137 Svenson, S. (2012). Clinical translation of nanomedicines. *Current Opinion in Solid State and Materials Science* 16 (6): 287–294. https://doi.org/10.1016/j.cossms.2012.10.001.

138 Mourdikoudis, S., Pallares, R.M., and Thanh, N.T.K. (2018). Characterization techniques for nanoparticles: comparison and complementarity upon studying nanoparticle properties. *Nanoscale*. Royal Society of Chemistry 10 (27): 12871–12934. https://doi.org/10.1039/C8NR02278J.

139 Foulkes, R., Man, E., Thind, J. et al. (2020). The regulation of nanomaterials and nanomedicines for clinical application: current and future perspectives. *Biomaterials Science*. Royal Society of Chemistry 8 (17): 4653–4664. https://doi.org/10.1039/D0BM00558D.

140 Halamoda-Kenzaoui, B., Holzwarth, U., Roebben, G. et al. (2019). Mapping of the available standards against the regulatory needs for nanomedicines. *Wiley Interdisciplinary Reviews: Nanomedicine and Nanobiotechnology* 11 (1): e1531. https://doi.org/10.1002/wnan.1531.

141 Resnik, D.B. and Tinkle, S.S. (2007). Ethics in nanomedicine. *Nanomedicine* 2 (3): 345–350. https://doi.org/10.2217/17435889.2.3.345.

142 Resnik, D.B. (2009). The clinical investigator–subject relationship: a contextual approach. *Philosophy, Ethics, and Humanities in Medicine* 4 (1): 16. https://doi.org/10.1186/1747-5341-4-16.

4

Targeted Drug Delivery for Antimalarial Therapy

Suha Zwayen[1,2], Tamara Zwain[1,3], and Kamalinder K. Singh[1,3,4]

[1]*University of Central Lancashire, School of Pharmacy and Biomedical Sciences, Faculty of Clinical and Biomedical Sciences, Fylde Rd, Preston PR1 2HE, UK*
[2]*Precision Nanosystems Inc., W Kent Ave N, Vancouver, BC V6P 6T7, Canada*
[3]*University of Central Lancashire, UCLan Research Centre for Smart Materials, Fylde Rd, Preston, Preston PR1 2HE, UK*
[4]*University of Central Lancashire, UCLan Research Centre for Translational Biosciences and Behaviour, Fylde Rd, Preston, Preston PR1 2HE, UK*

4.1 Introduction

Malaria is a widespread parasitic disease caused by protozoa of the *Plasmodium* genus. With a very widespread, effectual, and difficult to control vector, the mosquito, nearly half of the world's population is at risk of malaria. Hence malaria is considered as a one of the major global health priorities and listed in WHO's sustainable development goals, with WHO endeavouring to end the epidemics of AIDS, tuberculosis, malaria by 2030.

As per the WHO malaria report 2021, out of the total 241 million malaria cases and 627 000 related deaths in 2020 [1], 228 000 malaria cases were in Africa alone showing the widespread of the disease in this continent. Malaria, the disease of the tropics, is caused when any of the five species, *Plasmodium falciparum*, *Plasmodium vivax*, *Plasmodium malariae*, *Plasmodium ovale,* and recently identified *Plasmodium knowlesi*, are transmitted to human host by the bite of female vector mosquito species '*Anopheles gambiae*' [2]. The current disease distribution of human-pathogenic *Plasmodium* species shows the dominance of *P. falciparum* in tropical Africa and is responsible for most malaria deaths, while *P. vivax* is more prevalent in South America. Both *P. falciparum* and *P. vivax* are widespread in south-eastern Asia and the western Pacific [3, 4]. Generally, *P. vivax* has a wider geographical distribution than *P. falciparum*. *P. vivax* can progress in the *Anopheles* mosquito vector at lower temperatures (<20 °C) and can survive at higher altitudes [5]. It also has a dormant liver stage (hypnozoite) that can activate months after initial infection, causing a relapse of the symptoms. The latent stage enables *P. vivax* to survive in the human host for long periods when Anopheline mosquitoes are absent [6]. In Africa, the risk of *P. vivax* is very low owing to the absence of Duffy gene in most of the African populations, which serves as a chemokinase and

Drug Development for Malaria: Novel Approaches for Prevention and Treatment, First Edition.
Edited by Pravin Kendrekar.

receptor for *P. vivax* malaria parasite and enables it to invade red blood cells (RBCs) [7, 8]. Although *P. malariae* may occur in all malaria-endemic areas, its prevalence is generally low. In tropical Africa, *P. falciparum* and *P. malariae* co-infections are sometimes encountered [9]. *P. ovale* is widespread principally in tropical Africa [10].

Despite efforts for vector control and development of newer drugs to treat malaria, the disease is not declining in most malaria-prevalent areas of the world. Several new potential therapeutic drug candidates are being discovered or developed to treat malaria. However, their discovery is time-consuming and expensive. One of the major approaches to overcome this problem of inadequate funding and long research duration for new drug candidates, is the development of novel approaches of drug delivery to enhance the therapeutic potency of existing drugs by improving their absorption, distribution, metabolism, and excretion (ADME), reducing their toxicity, providing targeted drug delivery to the intracellular parasite and curtailing the frequency of administration to combat recrudesce and drug resistance.

The *P. falciparum* life cycle in humans includes the pre-erythrocytic stage, which initiates the infection; the asexual erythrocytic stage, which causes the disease; and the gametocyte stage, which infects mosquitoes that transmit the parasite. The malaria life cycle begins when the female *Anopheles* releases worm-like sporozoite into the human blood from its salivary gland. After invading the liver, each sporozoite multiplies over several days into tens of thousands of tiny merozoites packed into a single hepatocyte. No clinical signs or symptom occurs during the pre-erythrocytic stages. After completion of the pre-erythrocytic stage, hepatocyte is ruptured releasing merozoites into the circulation and initiates the 'blood stage' of malaria infection. This stage is responsible for the disease. Merozoites quickly invade RBCs or erythrocytes, where asexual multiplication takes place. Merozoites divide and grow within the RBCs and then finally burst the RBCs.

In malaria, infected red blood cells (iRBCs) are the main target for blood schizonticidal drugs and hepatocytes in the liver are the target for tissue schizonticidal drugs. The identification of new *Plasmodium* or infected cell targets can provide powerful strategies to modify existing drug delivery systems by employing nanotechnology to deliver antimalarial drug molecules more efficiently to the newly targeted sites of action.

4.2 Remodelling of Parasite-Infected Red Blood Cell (pRBC)

The parasite extensively modifies the host RBC, as required for its survival. Upon invasion, parasite alters the permeability and adhesive property of the erythrocyte. Several unusual structures appear over in the parasite infected red blood cell (pRBC), which are usually absent in non-infected RBC. Understanding the remodelling of host RBCs by the parasite for its survival and proliferation can provide powerful strategies for drug delivery and drug targeting to the pRBCs.

Mature erythrocytes do not show endocytosis while pRBCs are capable of endocytosis [11]. During the intraerythrocytic stage, the parasite is separated from

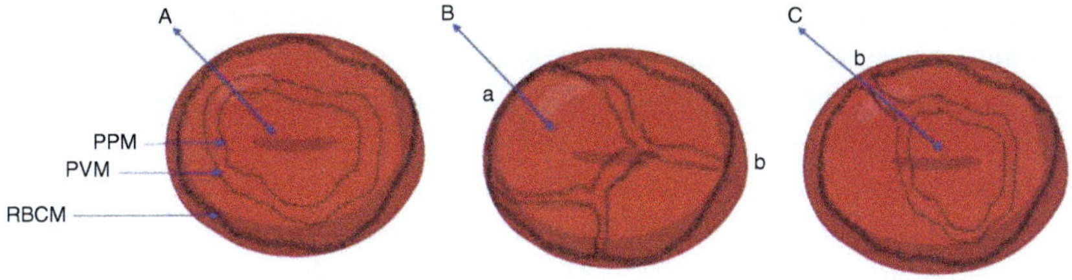

Figure 4.1 Remodelling in the red blood cell infected by *Plasmodium*. (A) An outlook of red blood cell membrane (RBCM), the parasitophorous vacuole membrane (PVM), and the parasite plasma membrane (PPM). (B, C) Parallel pathways allow solutes without passing through the erythrocyte cytosol to pass to the parasite, where (a) refers to a range of channels and transporters, and (b) tubulovesicular network structures (TVNs).

the extracellular medium by the red blood cell membrane (RBCM), the parasitophorous vacuole membrane (PVM), and the parasite plasma membrane (PPM) (Figure 4.1).

4.2.1 The Red Blood Cell Membrane (RBCM)

Upon invasion of the RBC by the merozoite, the parasite is captured within the parasitophorous vacuole. The pRBC then undergoes rapid morphological changes. At the same time, the pRBC metabolic activity and permeability increase due to the presence and formation of transporters and channels to aid the parasite survival and proliferation [12]. *Plasmodium* induces New Permeability Pathways (NPPs) to transport essential nutrient for parasite development and proliferation [13, 14]. This parasite-induced permeability shows to be blocked by a range of pharmacological agents, especially ion transport inhibitors (e.g. furosemide, niflumate) [13] and other various compounds such as biotin derivative [15]. The increase in the flux of low-molecular-weight solutes across the parasite-infected RBCM is thought to be via NPPs, which are non-saturable ion-selective channels. It has been reported that NPPs facilitate the entry and exit of both metabolic biosynthetic substrate and the catabolites, respectively [13]. An increase in the rate of solutes transported through the NPPs includes monosaccharide sugar alcohols, amino acids, peptides, nucleosides, monocarboxylate, small quaternary ammonium compounds, and monovalent inorganic cations and ions [16]. At least four types of ion channels have been identified after a patch-clamp of single-channel pRBC: (i) very low conductance inwardly rectifying CIC-2 anion channels, (ii) inwardly rectifying anion channels (IR), (iii) outwardly rectifying anion channels (OR), and finally (iv) non-selective cation channels. OR was permeable for organic osmolytes and activated by human serum albumin as OR activity was reduced when cells were washed with free-serum albumin culture media [17].

4.2.2 The Parasitophorous Vacuole Membrane (PVM)

The PVM transport properties have been reported after conducting patch-clamp studies. The PVM channel presented in a very high density, and it is highly permeable to a range of unrelated solutes, anions, and cations with a minimum ability to distinguish between them (e.g. Tris, glutamate, lysine, Mg^{2+}, and Ca^{2+}). Electrophysiological studies suggested that PVM acts as a molecular sieve allowing free passage to all of the low-molecular-weight solutes [16]. Tubulovesicular networks are structures (TVNs) invaginated from regions of PVM into the erythrocyte cytosol. It has been theorised that TVN facilitates the exchange of solutes between the erythrocyte cytosol and the PVM [18]. TVN has been shown to be blocked by DL-threo-1-phenyl-2-palmitoylamino-3-morpholino-1-propanol (PPMP) [19].

4.2.3 The Parasite Plasma Membrane (PPM)

The substantial ion gradients, the flux of the solutes, and the disposal of metabolic waste across the PPM were thought to be maintained by a range of channels and transporters. H^+ thought to extruded and a substantial inwardly negative membrane potential generated via a V-type H^+-ATPase in the PPM. This current approach was associated with the influx of K^+ via Ba^{2+} and Cs-sensitive K^+ channels [16]. A second H^+-pump was believed to be an H^+-pumping pyrophosphatase and in present PPM [20]. The parasite requires nutrients to maintain its high growth rate and replication, among these nutrients a source of hexon sugar such as glucose or fructose, a purine source, and certain essential vitamins [16]. Pantothenate is known to transport across the PPM via a low-affinity H^+ transporter [21].

4.3 The Emergence of Resistance and Antimalarial Therapy Approach

Identifying the species of the *Plasmodium* infection, the seriousness of signs and symptoms, pre-infection exposure if there is any, the clinical status of the patient and drug susceptibility, and where the infection was acquired all are essential factors to be considered before any antimalarial treatment can be considered to reduce the malaria-associated morbidity and mortality [22–24].

Treating malaria has become the most significant challenge despite all the advances in technology and innovations. The main reason for the failure of current conventional therapy is the development of multi-drug resistance and non-specific targeting to the intracellular parasite, which results in a high dose of therapeutic agents and their related toxicities. The *P. falciparum* strain has developed a sophisticated mechanism for drug resistance [22]. The extensive use of a mono antimalarial treatment may cause a phenomenon known as 'recrudescence', in which parasitaemia falls below the detectable levels and then later increases to a latent parasitaemia, generating a treatment failure, requiring high doses of therapeutic agents which may lead to toxicity and adverse effects.

The parasite's ability to survive and multiply despite the administration of equal or higher doses of the drug within the limits of the recommended dose is termed as parasite resistance. Through the years, a complex mechanism of drug resistance has been developed by the *Plasmodium* strains as a consequence of their genetic diversity, demonstrated by *Plasmodium*'s ability to elude the unfavourable conditions imposed by drug therapy. Hence, the vast majority of widely used antimalarial medicines have lost their effectiveness over the time. A good example is of chloroquine (CQ) resistance. The parasite digests the haemoglobin to convert into heme and peptides. Heme is toxic to the parasite, hence converted into hemozoin pigment by polymerisation pathway. CQ accumulates in the parasite's digestive vacuole and intersects the detoxification pathway, leading to heme accumulation, which kills the parasite [25]. However, CQ resistance emerged in late 1950. As per our knowledge, the mechanism of CQ has not been understood; theories supporting the reduction of CQ in the digestive vacuole were debated. Many studies suggested a strong association between *P. falciparum* CQ transporter gene (pfcrt) and the *P. falciparum* multidrug resistance gene (pfmdr1) and CQ resistance [26–28]. The genetic mutation in the *pfcrt* gene results in the substitution of amino acid lysine with threonine, leading to active efflux mechanism that facilitates the transport of CQ out of the digestive vacuole [25]. The *P. falciparum* resistance strain under continued drug exposure becomes dormant over the period of time. The P-glycoprotein homologous 1 (Pgh1) was implicated in both CQ and mefloquine (MQ) resistance [22].

At the border area between Thailand and Cambodia, the *P. falciparum* resistance to CQ was reported first in the 1950s [29]. It took almost 20 years for CQ-resistant *P. falciparum* to reach Africa, and then inevitably it has spread across the continent making this drug useless for the treatment of malaria. Resistance to the combination of sulfadoxine/pyrimethamine (SP) was reported for the first time in the same area in 1967, the same year as its introduction in Thailand. Finally, resistance to mefloquine was reported in 1982 for *P. falciparum* isolates from the border between Thailand and Myanmar, only five years after its introduction as a first-line drug for the treatment of strains resistant to CQ and SP [30].

A study conducted in 2008 in Thailand indicated a decreased sensitivity of *P. falciparum* to artemisinin [31]. After this first report, resistance to artemisinin has been spreading throughout the Greater Mekong Subregion (GMS), which includes Myanmar, Laos, Thailand, Cambodia, Vietnam, and the Chinese Province of Yunnan, and it is now well established in Thailand, Eastern Myanmar, and Southern Vietnam, whilst it is emerging in northeastern Cambodia and Southern Laos. The mean half-life for parasite clearance increased from 2.5 hours in 2001 to 3.7 in 2010, and 5.5 hours in western Cambodia in 2010 [32–35]. With the recent discovery of this phenomenon, *P. falciparum* resistance is now defined by a parasite clearance half-life of >5 hours [32]. Recrudescent infections were significantly correlated with resistance-associated with parasite K13 mutation gene; which is responsible for regulating the unfolded protein response pathway that may antagonise the artemisinin's pro-oxidant activity [36]. The artemisinins resistance is incredibly worrying, based on the WHO report [1], the only possibility to avoid the deaths of millions of children is the elimination of *P. falciparum* in the whole GMS, requiring an effort that is unprecedented in the history of the fight against malaria. Earlier, the WHO, in collaboration with several stakeholders, launched in January 2011 the Global Plan for Artemisinin Resistance Containment (GPARC), an ambitious project aimed to preserve the efficacy of ACTs for *P. falciparum* malaria treatment by containing or eliminating artemisinin resistance where it already exists and preventing artemisinin resistance where it has not yet appeared [37]. The vital recommendations presented in the GPARC document are: (i) stop the spread of resistant parasites; (ii) increase monitoring and surveillance to evaluate the threat of artemisinin resistance; (iii) improve access to diagnostics and rational treatment with ACT (iv) to invest in research related to artemisinin resistance; and motivate action and mobilise resources. Moreover, in 2014, the WHO launched the Emergency Response to Artemisinin Resistance (ERAR) in the GMS with the support of the Australian Department of Foreign Affairs and Trade, and the Bill & Melinda Gates Foundation. The project was implemented by the WHO Global Malaria Programme [5].

The development of resistance can be avoided by combining antimalarial drugs with synergistic action, ensuring a very high cure rate [38]. New strategies for intracellular antimalarial delivery would prevent the mechanism of drug resistance in malaria therapy. By encapsulating the drug in the nanosystem, CQ transporters can be avoided to pass through the digestive vacuole membrane by different mechanisms [22].

Another critical aspect to be considered in malaria is the route of administration. For uncomplicated malaria, the oral route should be the first choice of drug administration. Parenteral therapy would be favourable in severe or complicated malaria, and intravenous administration is mandatory in the management of cerebral malaria [39]. The backbone of cerebral malaria therapy is the use of either quinine (QN) or artemisinin, both of which are effective antimalarials by the parenteral route. Though QN can cause high toxicity when administered intravenously and artemisinin derivatives are lipophilic and present short plasma half-lives upon parenteral administration [22, 40, 41].

When developing a new antimalarial therapy, the parasite is inside the RBCs should be the focus, a high concentration of the drug in the intracellular parasitophorous vacuole is desirable for an optimum effect [22]. For the drug to reach the intra-parasitic targets of the RBC resident parasite, it has to bypass various barriers such as the host RBCM, the PVM, the PPM, tubulovesicular membrane (TVM) and possibly a further organelle membrane (e.g. a food vacuole membrane [FVM] or a mitochondrial membrane [MM] or endoplasmic reticulum [ER], depending on the site of action of the drug [42]). It is essential to know how solutes and macromolecules move between the intracellular parasite and the external medium. Usually, solutes taken up by the intracellular parasite enter the erythrocyte through RBCM. From there, they move into the parasite or are carried successively across the PVM and PPM by endocytosis. However, mature erythrocytes do not show endocytosis while *P. falciparum* parasitised RBCs (pRBCs) are capable of endocytosis [43]. The increased permeability of pRBCs is due to remodelling after parasite infection and formation of NPPs, TVNs, and other transport pathways. These pathways facilitate the efflux of waste and the influx of essential nutrients for parasite development and proliferation [12, 16]. These pathways can be exploited as potential targets for a selective antimalarial drugs delivery system.

4.4 Nanocarriers for Antimalarial Drug Delivery

The terms 'NanoSystems' or 'nanocarriers' have been used to denote all the drug carrier systems displaying sizes <1000 nm. Due to their reduced size, nanoparticles (NPs) have significant physicochemical properties and differ from bulk materials of the same composition [44, 45]. Moreover, the use of nanocarrier delivery systems in biomedicine has some advantages over a conventional system. They can be used to improve the pharmacokinetic profile of poorly water-soluble drugs [46]. Nanocarriers can enhance therapeutic responses, improve biological stability and reduce toxicity by enhanced intracellular penetration and distribution, leading to dose reduction [45, 47].

The purpose of using nanocarriers as drug delivery systems is to prevent drug degradation [48], improve target selectivity [49], reduce administration frequency and treatment duration and to improve the pharmacokinetics of the drug [50]. Many efforts have been made to implement nanotechnologies in the context of malaria [51, 52]. The most important aim of a nanocarrier is its ability to remain in circulation in the bloodstream for a prolonged period [53], which may improve the interaction with pRBCs and parasite membrane in case of malaria infection [54]. Additionally, nanocarriers would provide for the protection of unstable drugs and ability to be surface-modified by conjugation of specific ligands with an increase in cell-adhesion properties [55]. These benefits of colloidal nanocarriers can be extended to the treatment of cerebral malaria also that fit intravenous administration [56–58]. Advantages of nanoparticles in antimalarial drug delivery are illustrated in the schematic diagram given in Figure 4.2.

Thus, there is a need to design drug delivery systems with desirable pharmacokinetics and efficient targeting, invoking minimum immune response, thereby enhancing the efficacy of antimalarial treatment and reduction in drug toxicity. This will improve patient compliance and help with medication adherence. A variety of nanocarriers has been used for encapsulation of antimalarial drugs including liposomes, nano-capsules, nanoparticles, solid lipid nanoparticles (SLNs), nano-emulsions (NEs) as illustrated in Figure 4.3. Some of the nanocarrier systems are described below:

4.4.1 Liposomes

Liposomes are vesicles with an aqueous core surrounded by one or several phospholipids bilayers that can be used for sustained release of drugs. Liposomes can be used to encapsulate both hydrophobic and hydrophilic drugs. The amphiphilic phospholipid molecules form a closed spherical bilayer to shield their hydrophobic groups from the aqueous environment but maintaining interface with the aqueous phase via the hydrophilic head groups. The resulting closed sphere encapsulates the aqueous soluble drugs within the central aqueous compartment and the lipid-soluble drugs in the bilayer membrane. Liposomal drug delivery system is less toxic, biodegradable, and can protect the drug from chemical degradation and site-specific targeting can be achieved [57]. CQ had a better efficacy, and the resistance problem was addressed

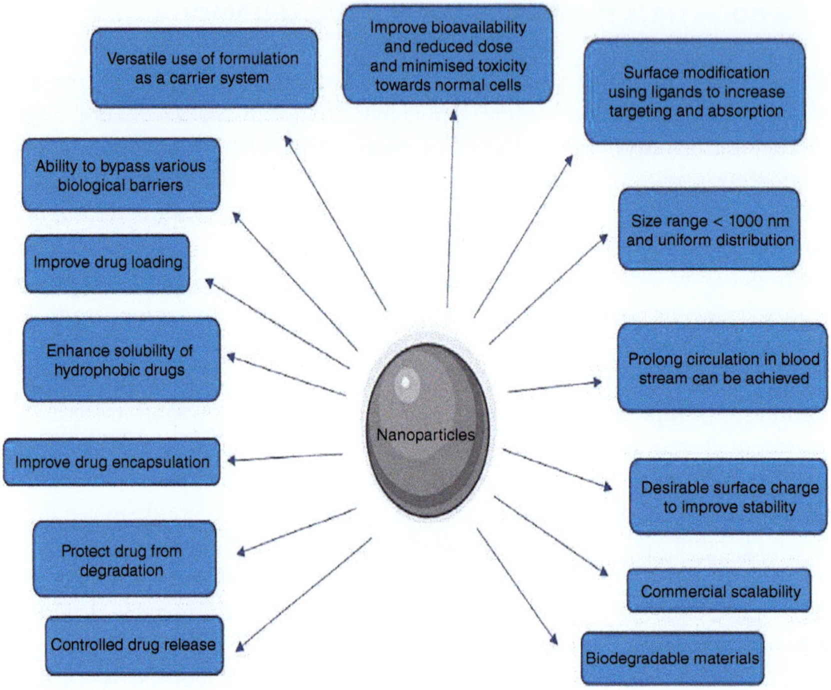

Figure 4.2 Schematic diagram indicating advantages of nanoparticles in antimalarial drug delivery.

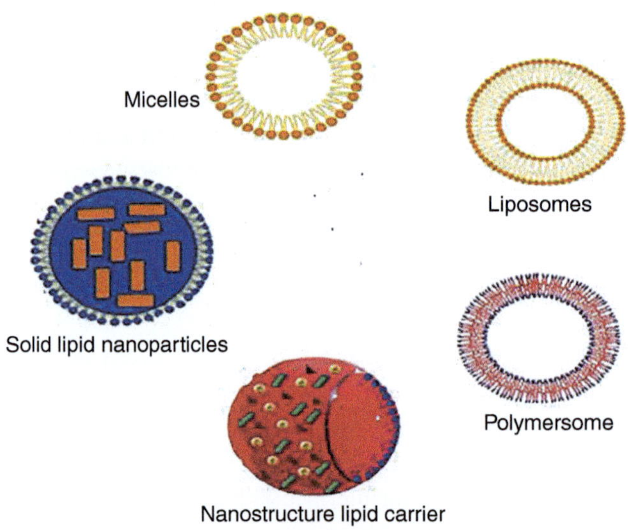

Figure 4.3 Illustration showing various types of nanocarriers used in drug delivery.

by encapsulating it in egg phosphatidylcholine and cholestrol (EPC-CHOL) liposomes [59]. Artesunate's rapid onset and quick elimination both were addressed by incorporating it in EPC-CHOL, fabricating the artesunate at pH 5 in liposomal drug delivery system solved its aqueous stability problem [60]. Moreover, using distearoyl phosphatidylcholine and cholestrol (DSPC-CHOL) to encapsulate CQ in liposomes increased its therapeutic efficacy and bioavailability [11, 61].

4.4.2 Solid Lipid Nanoparticles (SLNs)

SLNs are colloidal carriers of highly purified triglycerides, complex glyceride mixture, hard fat, and with or without wax. More stable than liposomes, they can be used to encapsulate both hydrophilic and lipophilic drugs. SLNs are naturally stable and prevent drugs from degradation [59]. Primaquine showed a 20% increase in efficacy when it was loaded in SLN [62]. Similarly, the efficacy of quinine dihydrochloride was improved by encapsulating it in SLN [63]. Dihydroartemisinin (DHA) poor solubility was reduced when it was loaded to SLN. DHA–SLN antimalarial efficacy was evaluated, and it was increased by 24.12% as compared to free DHA [64].

4.4.3 Nanostructured Lipid Carriers (NLCs)

Nanostructured lipid carriers (NLCs) are second-generation lipid nanoparticles, in which both liquid and solid lipids are available in the lipid phase. NLCs have an amorphous structure, and they have a better drug loading capacity, physicochemical stability as compared to SLNs [65]. Studies showed that better antimalarial activity against *P. falciparum* was achieved when artemether (ARM) was co-loaded with lumefantrine in the form of NLCs [66, 67]. Also, NLCs provide sustained delivery, thus maintaining drug levels for a prolonged period which helps combat recrudescence commonly associated with antimalarial drugs. Joshi et al. [46, 68] have reported NLCs (Nanoject) for the intravenous delivery of ARM employing microemulsion (ME) template technique, with encapsulation efficiency of $30 \pm 2\%$ and sustained release up to 24 hours [46]. Nanoject had lower haemolytic potential (~13%) as compared with all the formulation components when studied individually. Artemether loaded spherical NLCs were prepared using thin film hydration method comprising of glyceryl trimyristrate as solid lipid and soyabean oil as liquid lipid [69]. Infected mice treated with artemether-loaded lipid nanoparticles at 5 mg/kg body weight showed - increase in the survival period as compared with those treated with the free drug at the same dose.

4.4.4 Nano-emulsions (NEs)

The NEs, microemulsions (ME), and self-micro emulsifying drug delivery systems (SMEDDS) all have been investigated for delivery of various antimalarial drugs. NEs are of low cost and available as oral dosage forms. SMEDDS can be used to fill in conventional hard gelatine capsules and thus improve the bioavailability of poorly water-soluble drugs.

Primaquine is used especially for the management of relapsing malaria. Primaquine NE for liver targeting has been reported [70], primaquine lipid NE showed about 94% suppression of parasitaemia and high survival time (40–41 days). It was found to be effective at a lower dose level as compared with the plain drug solution.

Microemulsion preconcentrate for ARM exhibited 2.6-fold higher antimalarial activity than the marketed formulation Larither® [68]. Nano-size of the microemulsion, instantaneous dissolution of the drug, quick absorption, enhancement in bioavailability, protection of ARM from the acidic microenvironment of the stomach, and antimalarial effect of the excipients have been listed as possible attributes responsible for its higher activity.

4.4.5 Polymeric Nanoparticles

Polymeric nanoparticles are formulated from biodegradable and biocompatible polymers. Polymers used as nanocarriers are synthetic polymers such as polyacrylamide, polylactic glycolic acid (PLGA) and natural polymers such as albumin, chitosan, gelatin, lecithin which are widely used but have a disadvantage of poor batch-to-batch reproducibility [59]. Ideal nanoparticle polymeric carriers are biocompatible, biodegradable, non-toxic, non-immunogenic, inexpensive, water-soluble, and easy to synthesis. Methods used to formulate polymeric nanoparticles are nanoprecipitation, ionic gelation, emulsion cross-linking, spray-drying, and salting-out method [71]. Encapsulating curcumin in chitosan nanoparticles increased its cellular uptake and anti-plasmodial activity. Additionally, curcumin–chitosan nanoparticles had slower degradation when compared with curcumin alone in the mouse plasma [72]. Monensin antimalarial activity was 10 times increased when it was encapsulated in PLGA nanoparticles. Monensin–PLGA nanoparticles reported no hemolytic effect and showed biphasic drug release; the initial drug release phase was fast followed by subsequent sustained release phase [73]. Artemether loaded human serum albumin nanoparticles showed two-fold higher drug concentrations in the RBCs with antimalarial activity at 50% of therapeutic doses in Plasmodium bergei infected mice [58].

4.5 Targeted Antimalarial Drug Delivery Systems

Targeted nanocarriers can deliver one or more therapeutics together to the intracellular location, which will help overcome the issues of drug resistance and side effects [74]. Nanoparticulate drug delivery systems for active and passive targeting [75] to the infected erythrocytes and the hepatocytes are being actively explored.

Surface modification of nanocarriers using ligands can enhance targeting, absorption, and bioavailability [52, 71], while polyethylene glycol (PEG) will improve circulation of the nanocarriers in the bloodstream, allowing them to withstand physiological stress and avoid opsonisation [76].

4.5.1 Passive Drug Targeting with Conventional Nanocarriers

Passive targeting makes use of physicochemical factors of nanocarrier or pathophysiological and anatomic features of the diseased site for the accumulation of the drug-loaded carrier at a specific body site. Macrophages are a simple target due to their phagocytic properties. In contrast, cells that are deprived of phagocytic activity are much more difficult to target. However, conventional nanocarriers given parenterally are rapidly taken up by mononuclear phagocyte system (MPS) cells [77], delivering the drug inside macrophages. Thus, exposure of phagocytes to nanocarrier overload could lead to an initial blockage of the phagocytic uptake that is resolved within 24–48 hours, followed by a subsequent twofold rise in the macrophage capacity. This could reduce the rapid action of an antimalarial drug entrapped in a nanocarrier but makes an interesting strategy to generate a depot that releases slowly into the blood, thereby altering the pharmacokinetic profile of a short half-life antimalarial drug. On the other hand, the use of conventional nanocarriers for treating *P. vivax* infections in which hypnozoites are the dormant forms of the parasite in the hepatocytes, aligned with Kupffer cells, maybe an interesting strategy.

RBCs are regarded as inactive phagocytically and endocytically. The infected RBCs undergo morphological changes which selectively enhance their permeability to a wide range of molecules <200 nm in size [78]. Passive targeting is achieved using conventional nanocarriers such as; SLNs [79], NLCs [46], liposomes [80], human serum albumin [58] and polymeric nanoparticles [52], or surface-modified long-circulating nanocarriers, e.g. PEGylated nanocarriers [47]. PEGylation or surface engineering with hydrophilic polymers of nanocarriers results in prolonged drug half-life and the possibility of increased contact with RBCs [81]. It would also allow regulation of the biodistribution and altered pharmacokinetics of the drug. Mechanisms include reduced protein adsorption, reduced opsonisation coupled with complement activation. Long circulating nanocarriers improve the bioavailability of the drugs and reduce the frequency of dosing, due to enhanced selectivity.

In Table 4.1, some of the nanosystems that have been explored for improved antimalarial properties with passive targeting approach have been summarised. Primaquine dendrimers reduced the haemolytic properties of primaquine, with reduced toxicity and increased efficacy [87]. Primaquine nanoemulsion suppressed 94% of parasitaemia and resulted in high survival rate of infected mice [70]. ARM had a quick onset action, high survival rate, less haemolytic potential, and 24 hours sustained release when it was encapsulated in NLCs [46]. Chitosan–CQ nanoparticles increased parasite inhibition and protected the lymphocytes, RBCs, and serum against infection by increasing the antioxidant status and decreasing free radical generation, lipid and protein damage [86]. Primaquine and CQ dendrimers had long circulating time and reduced IC_{50} to threefold and fourfold of primaquine and CQ, respectively [88]. A potentially better therapeutic efficacy was shown when ARM was loaded into human serum albumin nanoparticles [56, 58].

4.5.2 Active Drug Targeting with Surface-Modified Nanocarrier

Active targeting has been attained using nanocarriers surface-modified with specific ligands such as carbohydrates, proteins, peptides, antibodies, or vitamins

Table 4.1 List of various passive-targeting nanocarrier-based drug delivery systems for malaria and their key features and advantages.

Drug delivery system	Method of preparation	Mean particle size (nm)	Advantages	References
Artemether nanolipid carrier (Nanoject)	Microemulsion template technique	60–90	Low haemolytic potential, Sustained release up to 24 h, quick onset of action, high survival rate	[46]
Artemether lipid nanoparticles	Thin film hydration followed by ultrasonic probe technique	120–250	An increase in the infected mice survival period observed	[69]
Artemisinin–curcumin-loaded PEGylated liposomes	Film hydration method	130–160	Parasitaemia reduced by 60% after only 3 d	[82]
Heparin-coated primaquine liposomes	Film hydration method	150–200	High antimalarial activity independent of the presence of primaquine thus showing targeting potential of heparin towards pRBCs	[80]
Human antiglycophorin A conjugated immunoliposomes of chloroquine	Film hydration method and covalent conjugation of half antibodies	~200	Specific-targeting to the pRBCs; reduction of Chloroquine $IC_{50} \geq 10$ times	[51]
Primaquine nanoemulsion	High-speed stirring and high-speed homogeniser technique	10–200	94% suppression of parasitaemia and high survival time (40–41 d) at a low dose of 1.5 mg/kg/day	[70]
Primaquine microemulsion	Hydration of lipid thin film, followed by vortexing and water bath sonication	183–225	Enhanced primaquine concentration in liver	[83]
Artemether microemulsion (NanOsorb-ARM)	Microemulsion preconcentrate	~183	2.6-fold higher activity than Larither, quick dissolution of ARM leading to rapid absorption and increased bioavailability, drug protection from the acidic microenvironment of stomach	[68]
Curcumin SMEDDS	Continuous agitation method	30–40	90–95% of curcumin solubility, increased survival rate, delay	[84]

Human serum albumin nanoparticles	Precipitation followed by high-pressure homogenisation	66.1	The use of human serum albumin as a biodegradable, endogeneous drug carrier for pRBC targeting	[58, 85]
Chloroquine chitosan nanoparticles	Ionotropic gelation	150–300	Increased parasite inhibition protected the lymphocytes, serum and RBC against *P. berghei* infection by decreasing free radical generation, lipid and protein damage, an increase in the antioxidant status	[86]
Poly amidoamine (PAAs) nanoparticles	Dropwise addition of drug solution followed by freeze-drying	~7	Preferential binding to pRBCs, low toxicity, high biodegradability	[52]
Primaquine dendrimers	Equilibrium dialysis	>2.4	Stable systems, high drug entrapment, reduced hemolytic properties of selective primaquine delivery to liver parenchyma cells, reduced toxicity and increased efficacy	[87]
Primaquine and chloroquine dendrimers	Equilibrium dialysis	170–500	Specific targeting to pRBCs; IC_{50} of CQ and PQ reduced three- and fourfold; long-circulating	[88]
Artemisone pheroids	Pheroid technology	3.81 μm	Increased C_{max}, delayed T_{max}, increased relative absorption	[89]
Streptomyces spp. mediated gold nanoparticles	Incubation method	5–50	Up-regulation of TGF-β and down-regulation of TNF-α in tissue and serum levels	[90]
Eclipta prostrata silver nanoparticles	Incubation method	35–60	Mosquito larvicidal activity	[91]
Resealed erythrocytes	Hypotonic swelling, isotonic resealing, and reannealing		Stable, shock resistant cells, slow release of primaquine	[92]

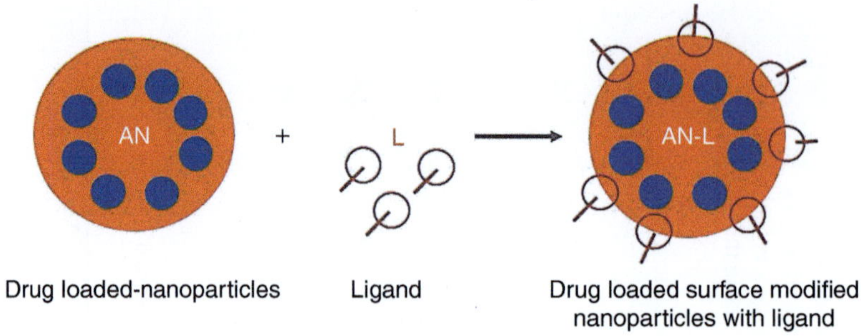

Figure 4.4 An illustration of the active-targeting concept. AN is a drug-loaded nanoparticle. L is the surface ligand. AN-L is drug-loaded surface-modified nanoparticle with ligand.

[93–95]. Active targeting of nanoparticles as illustrated in Figure 4.4 is achieved by conjugating a cell-specific ligand on the surface of the nanocarrier; which will allow the drug to accumulate in the targeted infected cell or tissue [96]. This approach might be successful if the receptors for surface-bound ligands are exclusively expressed on the infected cells or, their expression is significantly higher in the infected cells as compared to normal cells. In the event of malaria, RBCs and hepatocytes in the liver are the primary target sites for drug delivery. The identification of new targets of *Plasmodium* or infected cell can be employed in improving existing drug delivery systems using ligands to deliver the drug to the targeted sites efficiently. For the success of cell recognition, adequate ligand percentage exposed to the nanoparticles plays a vital role [47, 93, 96].

The benefits of such a strategy may have an important role in malaria treatment, especially for parenteral administration in the management of cerebral malaria [57]. Although this approach has been widely used for anticancer drugs, few attempts using active targeting strategy in an experimental malaria treatment with colloidal nanocarriers have been studied. The active targeting approach was explored using immuno-liposomes of lumefantrine conjugated with thiolated antibodies rosetting *P. falciparum* targeting [57] and immuno-liposomes of lumefantrine targeted with pRBC-specific monoclonal antibody BM1234 [97]. Also, using heparin functionalised liposomes for targeted drug delivery, pRBCs has shown better affinity vs uninfected red blood cell (uRBCs) due to pRBCs binding molecules known as glycosaminoglycans (GAGs). Heparin and heparin sulfate (HS) or HS-like molecule is one of many GAGs exposed on the surface of pRBC and is responsible for cluster formation between pRBCs and uRBCs called rosettes. GAGs reportedly can disrupt rosettes, block sporozoite adhesion to hepatic cells, and inhibit pRBC sequestration [80, 98]. However, as heparin has anticoagulant properties, high risk of antigen reaction with the antibody limits its use, though that could be addressed by using a non-anticoagulation concentration of heparin. At 1 μg/ml heparin concentration would improve the encapsulated primaquine liposomes activity to threefold. The data of that study indicated a dual effect of heparin as an antimalarial and as a targeting ligand of drug-loaded nanoparticles. Higher antimalarial and targeting activities can be achieved using a higher concentration of heparin but, not at the cost of haemorrhage and antigenic risks [80].

There is a need to investigate drug delivery vectors approach for preferential targeting to malaria-infected RBCs. Specific targeting would overcome the problem of drug resistance [11], reduce side effects, and contribute to lower drug IC_{50} [99].

4.6 Conclusion: Moving Towards the Future

The policy for the first-line treatment of malaria is a critical factor in determining malaria mortality. The choice of treatment must not be decided only by its efficacy, but also affordability by individuals to sustain its routine use. There are no cutoff points or firm benchmarks recommended for cost-effective interventions, treatments, and diagnosis of malaria; but there are some guidelines. Based on the sub-Saharan African and in Asia per capita health expenditure, the Commission on Macroeconomics and Health (CMH) recommended the cost should be three times less gross domestic product (GDP) per capita for each Disability-Adjusted Life-Year (DALY). The WHO built on this principle defining cost-effective interventions, in which each DALY avoided costs between one and three times GDP per capita; while very cost-effective interventions are those cost less than GDP per capita to avoid each additional DALY [100–102]. For nano-based antimalarial drugs, they would need to comply with cost-effectiveness as they will be deployed in low-income countries. Incidentally, using a targeted drug delivery system will contribute to reducing the cost of their development. Administration of drugs specifically to their target cells is an efficient tool to increase the bioavailability, reduce the dose, lower toxicity, and avoid drug resistance which is a major concern in case of malaria. Implementing a new drug delivery method is cheaper than processes leading to drug discovery. In addition, if the carrier system is well designed, it can be adapted to several drugs. At present, it is worth presenting the aspect of nanocarrier systems as a potential targeted delivery tool to enable a better understanding of the recent and upcoming approach to explore potential future applications in malaria prevention, treatment, and selectivity drug delivery.

Acknowledgements

Mr Donatas Gricius is gratefully acknowledged for the design and preparation of illustrations in this chapter.

References

1 WHO (2021). World Malaria Report 2021 [Online]. https://www.who.int/newsroom/fact-sheets/detail/malaria (accessed 28 April 2022).

2 Alonso, P. and Noor, A.M. (2017). The global fight against malaria is at crossroads. *The Lancet* 390: 2532–2534.

3 Baird, J.K. (2013). Evidence and implications of mortality associated with acute *Plasmodium vivax* malaria. *Clinical Microbiology Reviews* 26: 36–57.

4 Snow, R.W. (2015). Global malaria eradication and the importance of *Plasmodium falciparum* epidemiology in Africa. *BMC Medicine* 13: 23.

5 WHO (2014). World Malaria Report 2014 [Online] https://www.who.int/publications/i/item/9789241564830 (accessed 28th April 2022).

6 Gething, P.W., Elyazar, I.R., Moyes, C.L. et al. (2012). A long neglected world malaria map: *Plasmodium vivax* endemicity in 2010. *PLoS Neglected Tropical Diseases* 6: e1814.

7 Culleton, R., Ndounga, M., Zeyrek, F.Y. et al. (2009). Evidence for the transmission of *Plasmodium vivax* in the Republic of the Congo, West Central Africa. *The Journal of Infectious Diseases* 200: 1465–1469.

8 Howes, R.E., Reiner, R.C. Jr., Battle, K.E. et al. (2015). *Plasmodium vivax* transmission in Africa. *PLoS Neglected Tropical Diseases* 9: e0004222.

9 Gneme, A., Guelbeogo, W.M., Riehle, M.M. et al. (2013). *Plasmodium* species occurrence, temporal distribution and interaction in a child-aged population in rural Burkina Faso. *Malaria Journal* 12: 67.

10 Strydom, K.A., Ismail, F., and Frean, J. (2014). *Plasmodium ovale*: a case of not-so-benign tertian malaria. *Malaria Journal* 13: 85.

11 Aditya, N.P., Vathsala, P.G., Vieira, V. et al. (2013). Advances in nanomedicines for malaria treatment. *Advances in Colloid and Interface Science* 201, 202: 1–17.

12 Kirk, K. (2001). Membrane transport in the malaria-infected erythrocyte. *Physiological Reviews* 81: 495–537.

13 Kirk, K., Horner, H.A., Elford, B.C. et al. (1994). Transport of diverse substrates into malaria-infected erythrocytes via a pathway showing functional characteristics of a chloride channel. *Journal of Biological Chemistry* 269: 3339–3347.

14 Saliba, K.J., Horner, H.A., and Kirk, K. (1998). Transport and metabolism of the essential vitamin pantothenic acid in human erythrocytes infected with the malaria parasite *Plasmodium falciparum*. *Journal of Biological Chemistry* 273: 10190–10195.

15 Baumeister, S., Endermann, T., Charpian, S. et al. (2003). A biotin derivative blocks parasite induced novel permeation pathways in *Plasmodium falciparum*-infected erythrocytes. *Molecular and Biochemical Parasitology* 132: 35–45.

16 Kirk, K. (2004). Channels and transporters as drug targets in the *Plasmodium*-infected erythrocyte. *Acta Tropica* 89: 285–298.

17 Duranton, C., Tanneur, V., Lang, C. et al. (2008). A high specificity and affinity interaction with serum albumin stimulates an anion conductance in malaria-infected erythrocytes. *Cellular Physiology and Biochemistry* 22: 395–404.

18 Lauer, S.A., Rathod, P.K., Ghori, N., and Haldar, K. (1997). A membrane network for nutrient import in red cells infected with the malaria parasite. *Science* 276: 1122–1125.

19 Jain, S.A., Basu, H., Prabhu, P.S. et al. (2014). Parasite impairment by targeting *Plasmodium*-infected RBCs using glyceryl-dilaurate nanostructured lipid carriers. *Biomaterials* 35: 6636–6645.

20 Saliba, K.J., Allen, R.J., Zissis, S. et al. (2003). Acidification of the malaria parasite's digestive vacuole by a H^+-ATPase and a H^+-pyrophosphatase. *Journal of Biological Chemistry* 278: 5605–5612.

21 Saliba, K.J. and Kirk, K. (2001). H^+-coupled pantothenate transport in the intracellular malaria parasite. *Journal of Biological Chemistry* 276: 18115–18121.

22 Santos-Magalhães, N.S. and Mosqueira, V.C. (2010). Nanotechnology applied to the treatment of malaria. *Advanced Drug Delivery Reviews* 62: 560–575.

23 Barnes, T.J. and Prestidge, C.A. (2000). PEO–PPO–PEO block copolymers at the emulsion droplet–water interface. *Langmuir* 16: 4116–4121.

24 Redhead, H.M., Davis, S.S., and Illum, L. (2001). Drug delivery in poly(lactide-*co*-glycolide) nanoparticles surface modified with poloxamer 407 and poloxamine 908: in vitro characterisation and in vivo evaluation. *Journal of Controlled Release* 70: 353–363.

25 Martin, R.E. and Kirk, K. (2004). The malaria parasite's chloroquine resistance transporter is a member of the drug/metabolite transporter superfamily. *Molecular Biology and Evolution* 21: 1938–1949.

26 Baro, N.K., Callaghan, P.S., and Roepe, P.D. (2013). Function of resistance conferring *Plasmodium falciparum* chloroquine resistance transporter isoforms. *Biochemistry* 52: 4242–4249.

27 Ecker, A., Lehane, A.M., Clain, J., and Fidock, D.A. (2012). PfCRT and its role in antimalarial drug resistance. *Trends in Parasitology* 28: 504–514.

28 Fidock, D.A., Nomura, T., Talley, A.K. et al. (2000). Mutations in the *P. falciparum* digestive vacuole transmembrane protein PfCRT and evidence for their role in chloroquine resistance. *Molecular Cell* 6: 861–871.

29 Wellems, T.E. and Plowe, C.V. (2001). Chloroquine-resistant malaria. *The Journal of Infectious Diseases* 184: 770–776.

30 Medicines for Malaria Venture. 2019. History of antimalarials [Online]. https://www.mmv.org/malaria-medicines/history-antimalarials (accessed 22 October 2021).

31 Dondorp, A.M., Nosten, F., Yi, P. et al. (2009). Artemisinin resistance in *Plasmodium falciparum* malaria. *The New England Journal of Medicine* 361: 455–467.

32 Ashley, E.A., Dhorda, M., Fairhurst, R.M. et al. (2014). Spread of artemisinin resistance in *Plasmodium falciparum* malaria. *New England Journal of Medicine* 371: 411–423.

33 Gueye, C.S., Newby, G., Hwang, J. et al. (2014). The challenge of artemisinin resistance can only be met by eliminating *Plasmodium falciparum* malaria across the Greater Mekong subregion. *Malaria Journal* 13: 286.

34 Severini, C. and Menegon, M. (2015). Resistance to antimalarial drugs: an endless world war against *Plasmodium* that we risk losing. *Journal of Global Antimicrobial Resistance* 3: 58–63.

35 Zaw, M.T., Emran, N.A., and Lin, Z. (2018). Updates on k13 mutant alleles for artemisinin resistance in *Plasmodium falciparum*. *Journal of Microbiology, Immunology and Infection* 51: 159–165.

36 Fairhurst, R.M. and Dondorp, A.M. (2016). Artemisinin-resistant *Plasmodium falciparum* malaria. *Microbiology Spectrum* 4.

37 WHO (2011). Global plan for artemisinin resistance containment – GPARC (archived) [Online]. https://www.who.int/malaria/publications/atoz/9789241500838/en/ (accessed 22 October 2021).

38 Ittarat, W., Pickard, A.L., Rattanasinganchan, P. et al. (2003). Recrudescence in artesunate-treated patients with falciparum malaria is dependent on parasite burden not on parasite factors. *The American Journal of Tropical Medicine and Hygiene* 68: 147–152.

39 WHO (2012). *Management of Severe Malaria: A Practical Handbook*. World Health Organization.

40 Newton, C.R. and Krishna, S. (1998). Severe falciparum malaria in children: current understanding of pathophysiology and supportive treatment. *Pharmacology & Therapeutics* 79: 1–53.

41 Mishra, S.K. and Newton, C.R. (2009). Diagnosis and management of the neurological complications of falciparum malaria. *Nature Reviews Neurology* 5: 189.

42 Biagini, G.A., Ward, S.A., and Bray, P.G. (2005). Malaria parasite transporters as a drug-delivery strategy. *Trends in Parasitology* 21: 299–301.

43 Kutner, S., Baruch, D., Ginsburg, H., and Cabantchik, Z. (1982). Alterations in membrane permeability of malaria-infected human erythrocytes are related to the growth stage of the parasite. *Biochimica Et Biophysica Acta (BBA)-Biomembranes* 687: 113–117.

44 Kura, A.U., Fakurazi, S., Hussein, M.Z., and Arulselvan, P. (2014). Nanotechnology in drug delivery: the need for more cell culture based studies in screening. *Chemistry Central Journal* 8: 46.

45 Suri, S.S., Fenniri, H., and Singh, B. (2007). Nanotechnology-based drug delivery systems. *Journal of Occupational Medicine and Toxicology* 2: 16.

46 Joshi, M., Pathak, S., Sharma, S., and Patravale, V. (2008). Design and in vivo pharmacodynamic evaluation of nanostructured lipid carriers for parenteral delivery of artemether: Nanoject. *International Journal of Pharmaceutics* 364: 119–126.

47 Kouchakzadeh, H., Shojaosadati, S.A., Maghsoudi, A., and Vasheghani Farahani, E. (2010). Optimization of PEGylation conditions for BSA nanoparticles using response surface methodology. *AAPS PharmSciTech* 11: 1206–1211.

48 Vishwakarma, N., Jain, A., Sharma, R. et al. (2019). Lipid-based nanocarriers for lymphatic transportation. *AAPS PharmSciTech* 20: 83.

49 Choi, Y., Lim, S., Yoon, H.Y. et al. (2019). Tumor-targeting glycol chitosan nanocarriers: overcoming the challenges posed by chemotherapeutics. *Expert Opinion on Drug Delivery* 16: 835–846.

50 Trousil, J., Pavliš, O., Kubíčková, P. et al. (2020). Antitubercular nanocarrier monotherapy: study of in vivo efficacy and pharmacokinetics for rifampicin. *Journal of Controlled Release* 321: 312–323.

51 Urbán, P., Estelrich, J., Cortes, A., and Fernandez-Busquets, X. (2011). A nanovector with complete discrimination for targeted delivery to *Plasmodium falciparum*-infected versus non-infected red blood cells in vitro. *Journal of Controlled Release* 151: 202–211.

52 Urbán, P., Valle-Delgado, J.J., Mauro, N. et al. (2014). Use of poly(amidoamine) drug conjugates for the delivery of antimalarials to *Plasmodium*. *Journal of Controlled Release* 177: 84–95.

53 Peng, S., Ouyang, B., Men, Y. et al. (2020). Biodegradable zwitterionic polymer membrane coating endowing nanoparticles with ultra-long circulation and enhanced tumor photothermal therapy. *Biomaterials* 231: 119680.

54 Mosqueira, V.C.F., Loiseau, P.M., Bories, C. et al. (2004). Efficacy and pharmacokinetics of intravenous nanocapsule formulations of halofantrine in Plasmodiim berghei–infected mice. *Antimicrobial Agents and Chemotherapy* 48 (4): 1222–1228.

55 Zhang, M., Zang, X., Wang, M. et al. (2019). Exosome-based nanocarriers as bio-inspired and versatile vehicles for drug delivery: recent advances and challenges. *Journal of Materials Chemistry B* 7: 2421–2433.

56 Boateng-Marfo, Y., Dong, Y., Loh, Z.H. et al. (2018). Intravenous human serum albumin (HSA)-bound artemether nanoparticles for treatment of severe malaria. *Colloids and Surfaces A: Physicochemical and Engineering Aspects* 536: 20–29.

57 Moles, E., Moll, K., Ch'ng, J.H. et al. (2016). Development of drug-loaded immunoliposomes for the selective targeting and elimination of rosetting *Plasmodium falciparum*-infected red blood cells. *Journal of Controlled Release* 241: 57–67.

58 Sidhaye, A.A., Bhuran, K.C., Zambare, S. et al. (2016). Bio-inspired artemether-loaded human serum albumin nanoparticles for effective control of malaria-infected erythrocytes. *Nanomedicine* 11: 2809–2828.

59 Baruah, U.K., Gowthamarajan, K., Vanka, R. et al. (2017). Malaria treatment using novel nano-based drug delivery systems. *Journal of Drug Targeting* 25: 567–581.

60 Gabriels, M. and Plaizier-Vercammen, J. (2003). Physical and chemical evaluation of liposomes, containing artesunate. *Journal of Pharmaceutical and Biomedical Analysis* 31: 655–667.

61 Peeters, P.A., Brunink, B.G., Eling, W.M., and Cromelin, D.J. (1989). Therapeutic effect of chloroquine (CQ)-containing immunoliposomes in rats infected with Plasmodium berghei parasitized mouse red blood cells: comparison with combinations of antibodies and CQ or liposomal CQ. *Biochimica Et Biophysica Acta (BBA)-Biomembranes* 981: 269–276.

62 Omwoyo, W.N., Ogutu, B., Oloo, F. et al. (2014). Preparation, characterization, and optimization of primaquine-loaded solid lipid nanoparticles. *International Journal of Nanomedicine* 9: 3865.

63 Gupta, Y., Jain, A., and Jain, S.K. (2007). Transferrin-conjugated solid lipid nanoparticles for enhanced delivery of quinine dihydrochloride to the brain. *Journal of Pharmacy and Pharmacology* 59: 935–940.

64 Omwoyo, W.N., Melariri, P., Gathirwa, J.W. et al. (2016). Development, characterization and antimalarial efficacy of dihydroartemisinin loaded solid lipid nanoparticles. *Nanomedicine: Nanotechnology, Biology and Medicine* 12: 801–809.

65 Müller, R.H., Radtke, M., and Wissing, S.A. (2002). Solid lipid nanoparticles (SLN) and nanostructured lipid carriers (NLC) in cosmetic and dermatological preparations. *Advanced Drug Delivery Reviews* 54: S131–S155.

66 Parashar, D., Aditya, N.P., and Murthy, R.S.R. (2016). Development of artemether and lumefantrine co-loaded nanostructured lipid carriers: physicochemical characterization and in vivo antimalarial activity. *Drug Delivery* 23: 123–129.

67 Prabhu, P., Suryavanshi, S., Pathak, S. et al. (2016). Nanostructured lipid carriers of artemether–lumefantrine combination for intravenous therapy of cerebral malaria. *International Journal of Pharmaceutics* 513: 504–517.

68 Joshi, M., Pathak, S., Sharma, S., and Patravale, V. (2008). Solid microemulsion preconcentrate (NanOsorb) of artemether for effective treatment of malaria. *International Journal of Pharmaceutics* 362: 172–178.

69 Aditya, N., Patankar, S., Madhusudhan, B. et al. (2010). Arthemeter-loaded lipid nanoparticles produced by modified thin-film hydration: pharmacokinetics, toxicological and in vivo anti-malarial activity. *European Journal of Pharmaceutical Sciences* 40: 448–455.

70 Singh, K.K. and Vingkar, S.K. (2008). Formulation, antimalarial activity and biodistribution of oral lipid nanoemulsion of primaquine. *International Journal of Pharmaceutics* 347: 136–143.

71 Jawahar, N. and Meyyanathan, S. (2012). Polymeric nanoparticles for drug delivery and targeting: a comprehensive review. *International Journal of Health & Allied Sciences* 1: 217.

72 Akhtar, F., Rizvi, M.M.A., and Kar, S.K. (2012). Oral delivery of curcumin bound to chitosan nanoparticles cured *Plasmodium yoelii* infected mice. *Biotechnology Advances* 30: 310–320.

73 Surolia, R., Pachauri, M., and Ghosh, P.C. (2012). Preparation and characterization of monensin loaded PLGA nanoparticles: in vitro anti-malarial activity against *Plasmodium falciparum*. *Journal of Biomedical Nanotechnology* 8: 172–181.

74 Sahoo, S.K., Jain, T.K., Reddy, M.K., and Labhasetwar, V. (2008). Nano-sized carriers for drug delivery. In: *NanoBioTechnology*. Springer; Berlin/Heidelberg, Germany. pp. 329–348.

75 Puttappa, N., Kumar, R.S., Kuppusamy, G., and Radhakrishnan, A. (2019). Nano-facilitated drug delivery strategies in the treatment of *Plasmodium* infection. *Acta Tropica* 195: 103–114.

76 Owens, D.E. and Peppas, N.A. (2006). Opsonization, biodistribution, and pharmacokinetics of polymeric nanoparticles. *International Journal of Pharmaceutics* 307: 93–102.

77 Cabral, H. and Kataoka, K. (2020). Erythrocyte depletion lifts nanoparticle half-lives. *Nature Biomedical Engineering* 4: 670–671.

78 Rothen-Rutishauser, B.M., Schürch, S., Haenni, B. et al. (2006). Interaction of fine particles and nanoparticles with red blood cells visualized with advanced microscopic techniques. *Environmental Science & Technology* 40: 4353–4359.

79 Nayak, A.P., Tiyaboonchai, W., Patankar, S. et al. (2010). Curcuminoids-loaded lipid nanoparticles: novel approach towards malaria treatment. *Colloids and Surfaces B: Biointerfaces* 81: 263–273.

80 Marques, J., Moles, E., Urbán, P. et al. (2014). Application of heparin as a dual agent with antimalarial and liposome targeting activities toward *Plasmodium*-infected red blood cells. *Nanomedicine: Nanotechnology, Biology and Medicine* 10: 1719–1728.

81 Hussain, Z., Khan, S., Imran, M. et al. (2019). PEGylation: a promising strategy to overcome challenges to cancer-targeted nanomedicines: a review of challenges to clinical transition and promising resolution. *Drug Delivery and Translational Research* 9: 721–734.

82 Isacchi, B., Bergonzi, M.C., Grazioso, M. et al. (2012). Artemisinin and artemisinin plus curcumin liposomal formulations: enhanced antimalarial efficacy against *Plasmodium berghei*-infected mice. *European Journal of Pharmaceutics and Biopharmaceutics* 80: 528–534.

83 Dierling, A.M. and Cui, Z. (2005). Targeting primaquine into liver using chylomicron emulsions for potential vivax malaria therapy. *International Journal of Pharmaceutics* 303: 143–152.

84 Memvanga, P.B., Coco, R., and Préat, V. (2013). An oral malaria therapy: curcumin-loaded lipid-based drug delivery systems combined with β-arteether. *Journal of Controlled Release* 172: 904–913.

85 Ibrahim, N., Ibrahim, H., Dormoi, J. et al. (2014). Albumin-bound nanoparticles of practically water-insoluble antimalarial lead greatly enhance its efficacy. *International Journal of Pharmaceutics* 464: 214–224.

86 Tripathy, S., Das, S., Chakraborty, S.P. et al. (2012). Synthesis, characterization of chitosan–tripolyphosphate conjugated chloroquine nanoparticle and its in vivo anti-malarial efficacy against rodent parasite: a dose and duration dependent approach. *International Journal of Pharmaceutics* 434: 292–305.

87 Bhadra, D., Yadav, A., Bhadra, S., and Jain, N. (2005). Glycodendrimeric nanoparticulate carriers of primaquine phosphate for liver targeting. *International Journal of Pharmaceutics* 295: 221–233.

88 Movellan, J., Urbán, P., Moles, E. et al. (2014). Amphiphilic dendritic derivatives as nanocarriers for the targeted delivery of antimalarial drugs. *Biomaterials* 35: 7940–7950.

89 Steyn, J.D., Wiesner, L., Du Plessis, L.H. et al. (2011). Absorption of the novel artemisinin derivatives artemisone and artemiside: potential application of Pheroid™ technology. *International Journal of Pharmaceutics* 414: 260–266.

90 Karthik, L., Kumar, G., Keswani, T. et al. (2013). Marine actinobacterial mediated gold nanoparticles synthesis and their antimalarial activity. *Nanomedicine: Nanotechnology, Biology and Medicine* 9: 951–960.

91 Rajakumar, G. and Rahuman, A.A. (2011). Larvicidal activity of synthesized silver nanoparticles using *Eclipta prostrata* leaf extract against filariasis and malaria vectors. *Acta Tropica* 118: 196–203.

92 Talwar, N. and Jain, N. (1992). Erythrocytes as carriers of primaquine-preparation: characterization and evaluation. *Journal of Controlled Release* 20: 133–141.

93 Dubey, R.D., Alam, N., Saneja, A. et al. (2015). Development and evaluation of folate functionalized albumin nanoparticles for targeted delivery of gemcitabine. *International Journal of Pharmaceutics* 492: 80–91.

94 Jaimes-Aguirre, L., Morales-Avila, E., Ocampo-García, B.E. et al. (2017). Biodegradable poly(D,L-lactide-co-glycolide)/poly(L-γ-glutamic acid) nanoparticles conjugated to folic acid for targeted delivery of doxorubicin. *Materials Science and Engineering: C* 76: 743–751.

95 Rollett, A., Reiter, T., Nogueira, P. et al. (2012). Folic acid-functionalized human serum albumin nanocapsules for targeted drug delivery to chronically activated macrophages. *International Journal of Pharmaceutics* 427: 460–466.

96 Torchilin, V.P. (2006). Multifunctional nanocarriers. *Advanced Drug Delivery Reviews* 58: 1532–1555.

97 Urbán, P., Estelrich, J., Adeva, A. et al. (2011). Study of the efficacy of antimalarial drugs delivered inside targeted immunoliposomal nanovectors. *Nanoscale Research Letters* 6: 620.

98 Juillerat, A., Igonet, S., Vigan-Womas, I. et al. (2010). Biochemical and biophysical characterisation of DBL1α1-varO, the rosetting domain of PfEMP1 from the VarO line of *Plasmodium falciparum*. *Molecular and Biochemical Parasitology* 170: 84–92.

99 Fernàndez-Busquets, X. (2016). *Novel Strategies for Plasmodium-Targeted Drug Delivery*. Taylor & Francis.

100 Apouey, B., Picone, G. & Wilde, J. (2018). *The Economics of Malaria Prevention*. In: Oxford Research Encyclopedia of Economics and Finance. Editor: Andrew Jones. Oxford University Press, New York. [https://bit.ly/3EvP705].

101 Gelband, H., Panosian, C.B., and Arrow, K.J. (2004). *Saving Lives, Buying Time: Economics of Malaria Drugs in an Age of Resistance*. National Academies Press.

102 Lubell, Y., Riewpaiboon, A., Dondorp, A.M. et al. (2011). Cost-effectiveness of parenteral artesunate for treating children with severe malaria in sub-Saharan Africa. *Bulletin of the World Health Organization* 89: 504–512.

5

The Imminent Threat of Antimalarial Drug Resistance

Bharti Singal[1] *and Jyoti Chhibber-Goel*[2]

[1] *Nanyang Technological University, School of Biological Sciences, 60 Nanyang Dr, 637551, Singapore*
[2] *International Centre for Genetic Engineering and Biotechnology, Molecular Medicine, Aruna Asaf Ali Marg, Vasant Kunj, New Delhi 110067, India*

5.1 Introduction

Plasmodium spp. of the genus *Apicomplexa* causes malaria. *Plasmodium* spp. have a complex, two-stage life cycle – with an insect vector (mosquito) sexual stage and a vertebrate host (mammals) asexual stage. The female *Anopheles* mosquito injects sporozoites into the vertebrate host during the process of blood feeding. The injected sporozoites transmigrate to the liver where they attack and infect the hepatocytes, thereby replicating into schizonts. After one week of development, hepatic schizonts release thousands of merozoites from every infected hepatocyte into the bloodstream. Similarly, upon invasion of the red blood cells (RBCs), sporozoites form mature schizonts via asexual reproduction, thereby repeating the cycle to invade new RBCs. Several of the blood-stage parasites differentiate into the male and female gametocytes, which upon ingestion by the mosquito are programmed to produce gametes. The gametes fuse in the mosquito midgut thereby producing a zygote, subsequently transforming into an oocyst. The life cycle of the *Plasmodium* parasite is completed when sporozoites released from the ruptured oocyst migrate to the salivary glands of the mosquitoes. The sporozoites are then introduced into a new host (Figure 5.1) [1].

The *Plasmodium* spp. known to infect humans are: *P. falciparum, P. vivax, P. malariae, P. ovale*, and *P. knowlesi* [2]. Malaria in humans is mainly caused by *P. falciparum* and *P. vivax. P. falciparum* malaria is relatively fatal when compared with *P. vivax* malaria. However, in *P. vivax*, but not *P. falciparum*, several liver parasites remain quiescent (hypnozoites), resuming replication and infection after several weeks, months, or even years of relapse [3, 4]. Repeated infections in

Bharti Singal and Jyoti Chhibber-Goel contributed equally.

Drug Development for Malaria: Novel Approaches for Prevention and Treatment, First Edition.
Edited by Pravin Kendrekar.

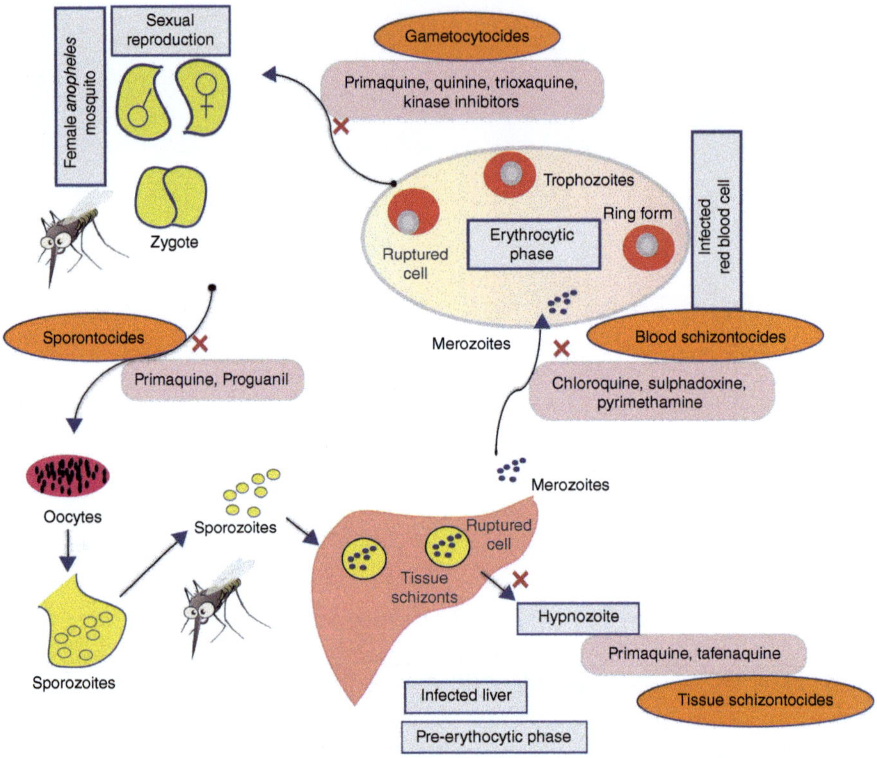

Figure 5.1 *Plasmodium* life cycle and stage-specific antimalarial drugs. *Plasmodium* life cycle in the human and female *Anopheles* mosquito host. The category of antimalarial drugs targeting the specific stages of the *Plasmodium* cycle in orange (gametocytocides, sporontocides, tissue schizonticides, and blood schizonticides) and the antimalarial are in pink are shown.

individuals from malaria endemic regions bestow partial immunity that quickly weakens without exposure, thereby resulting in individuals becoming asymptomatic carriers [5]. Relapse infections, asymptomatic carriers, and evolution of antimalarial drug resistance, complicated malaria treatment control and hamper the disease elimination goals. Additionally, socioeconomic factors – schooling, employment, income and affordability, distribution facilities, volume of production, counterfeit or low-quality products, noncompliance with patients, improper use of monotherapies, and contraindications hamper efforts and add to the burden of the disease [6, 7].

The Greater Mekong Subregion is the cradle for the emergence of antimalarial resistance toward chloroquine (CQ), sulfadoxine–pyrimethamine (SP), artemisinin (ART), piperaquine (PPQ), as well as mefloquine (MFQ) [8–11]. Drug resistance can be attributed to either the removal or sequestration of the drug, mutation or the amplification of the drug target(s) as well as the stress-response-based survival mechanisms. In this chapter, we will focus on the proclivity of *Plasmodium* parasites toward drug resistance with a focus on the CQ, SP, and ART resistance. Understanding the evolution of antimalarial drug resistance is critical to prolonging current antimalarial drug effectiveness and optimizing the pipeline of future medicines. Thus, drug development in malaria using modern molecular biology tools is heavily reliant on best possible ways to avoid the rather inescapable, inevitable mutations, which occur in malaria parasites. A deep molecular understanding of drug resistance at the level of interacting crucial proteins is clearly essential – both from a basic mechanistic perspective and from the view of providing insights into drug resistance.

5.2 Antimalarial Drugs: An Overview

Antimalarial drugs are categorized according to their antimalarial activity and the stage of the *Plasmodium* spp. inhibition (Figure 5.1). The drug development in malaria focuses on symptomatic blood stages of the *Plasmodium* species. This is majorly because of the ease to conduct research experiments. These drugs are (i) tissue schizonticides – (for causal prophylaxis or preventing relapse) – pyrimethamine and primaquine; (ii) blood schizonticides – CQ, quinine, MFQ, halofantrine, pyrimethamine, sulfadoxine, sulfones, tetracyclines, etc.; (iii) gametocytocides – CQ (against *P. vivax* and *P. malariae*) and primaquine (against all *Plasmodia*); (iv) sporontocides – primaquine and chloroguanide. In terms of their chemical structures and mode of action, antimalarials are also categorized into – (i) *aryl aminoalcohol compounds* (*quinolines*): quinine, quinidine, CQ, amodiaquine, MFQ, halofantrine, lumefantrine, PPQ, tafenoquine. (ii) *Antifolate compounds* (*"antifols"*): pyrimethamine, proguanil, chlorproguanil, trimethoprim. (iii) *ART compounds* (ART, dihydroART [DHA], artemether, artesunate) [12] (Figure 5.2). These drugs are extensively used for the treatment of malaria. The mechanism of action of the quinolines class of drugs involves the inhibition of heme polymerization during the intraerythrocytic stage. CQ is given in the complicated cases of malaria caused by *P. vivax*, as a phosphate salt. The other class of drugs, antifolates, target the folate biosynthesis pathway and thus inhibit the synthesis of folate cofactors. This leads to disruption in nucleotide synthesis and amino acid metabolism. Atovaquone, an antimalarial inhibits the electron transport chain of the mitochondria and changes the polarization state of the membrane. ART analogous derived from natural compound, ART, targets the ring stage of the *Plasmodium* life cycle and helps in controlling transmission of the gametes. The clear evidence about molecular targets of ART is not much clear; however, whole genome sequencing results show presence of mutations in Kelch propeller domain in drug-resistant forms. Another study has recently reported ART as the inhibitor of *P. falciparum* phosphatidylinositol-3-kinase, *Pf*PI3K [13].

(a)

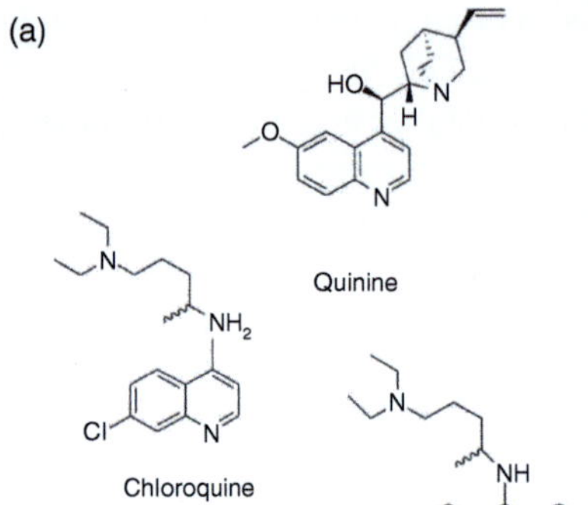

Commercial name (manufacturer)	Drug
Coartem® Dispersible (Novartis)	Artemether–Lumefantrine
Artesun® (Guilin Pharmaceutical)	Artesunate
ASMQ (Cipla)	Artesunate–Mefloquine
Krintafel (GlaxoSmithKline)	Tafenoquine
Eurartesim® (Alfasigma/Pierre Fabre)	Dihydroartemisinin–Piperaquine
Pyramax® Granules (Shin Poong)	Pyronaridine–Artesunate
ASAQ Winthrop® (Sanofi)	Artesunate–Amodiaquine
Malarone® (GlaxoSmithKline)	Atovaquone/Proguanil
SPAQ-CO™ (Guilin Pharmaceutical)	Pyrimethamine/Sulfadoxine–Amodiaquine

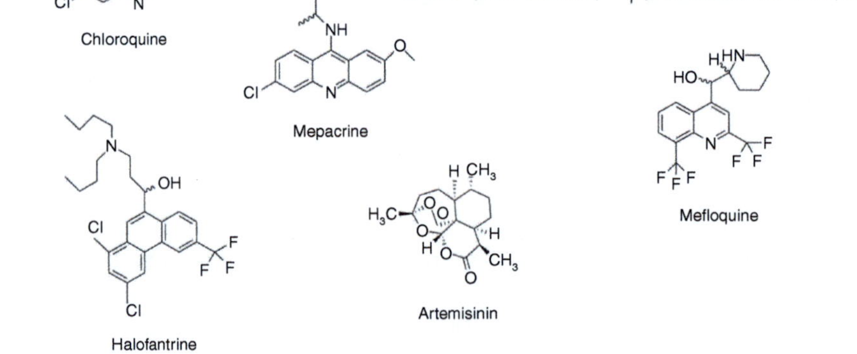

(b)

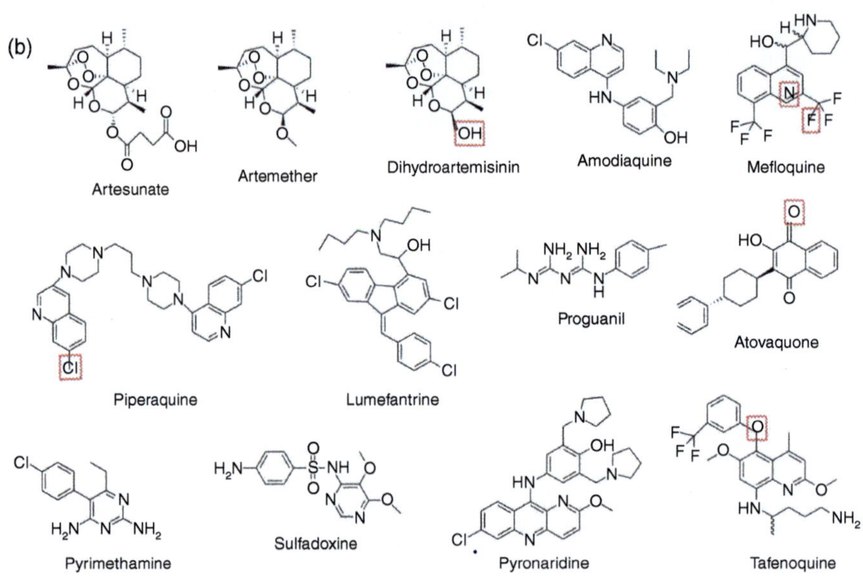

Figure 5.2 Antimalarial drugs.

5.3 The Evolution of CQ Resistance

Quinine is the active compound that is found in the tree bark of cinchona. For the natives of South America, the indigenous people of Peru and tropical parts of the Andes, the medicinal properties of this wonder tree-bark extract were long known and used to treat fever and chills [14]. Its appearance in the seventeenth century in Europe later contributed to its use for the treatment of malaria. The pure compound quinine was isolated in 1820 by Caventou and Pelletier and later synthesized chemically in 1944 by Woodword and von Doering [15–17]. Simultaneously in 1934, the quest for quinine alternatives by Hans Andersag and coworkers led to the discovery of CQ [18]. However, at the time CQ (Resochin) was marked toxic for human use by Bayer. CQ derivative – 3-methyl-chloroquine (MCQ) (Sontochin), came into use during World War II [19]. After witnessing the unambiguous effectiveness of the medication as an antimalarial, the drug made its way to the United States where it was further tested and approved for clinical antimalarial trials. By 1947, CQ gradually became a part of prophylactic malaria therapy. Due to its affordability, ease of use, and antimalarial efficacy, CQ was extensively used as an important malarial treatment. Resistance to CQ posed a challenge as malaria-related mortality increased in many countries and led to CQ removal from the malaria control regime in a number of countries. Resistance to its fixation levels in malaria endemic countries took three decades from the first incidence of CQ resistance in 1957. The introduction of other antimalarial agents resulted in the replacement of CQ from the first-line treatment for malaria. As per FDA regulations, CQ is approved for the treatment and prophylaxis of uncomplicated malaria in Mexico, areas of Central America to the West of the Panama canal, the Caribbean, East Asia, and the few Middle Eastern countries [20, 21]. The CQ-prone strains of *Plasmodium* parasites are also prevalent in these countries. The evolution of CQ is interesting as from the first incidences of CQ-resistant in *P. falciparum* parasites that led to the discontinuation of CQ, the latest reports where parasites show susceptibility to CQ can bring back the use of the most affordable and highly efficient drug for malaria treatment.

5.3.1 Mechanism of Action of CQ

The CQ and MCQ belong to the four amino quinolines class of antimalarials. CQ is given orally as CQ phosphate or injected intramuscular as CQ hydrochloride. The drug is not only effective against *Plasmodium* spp. but also several other parasitic worms and amoeba and is used in the treatment of rheumatoid arthritis and lupus. Among the several theories put forward to explain the structure–activity relationships and biological effects of the CQ, it is suggested that binding of heme moiety to CQ increases the accumulation of CQ in food vacuole, which interferes with the hemoglobin metabolism in the parasite. In brief, the malaria parasite endocytosed the cytosol of the host cell as it grows within the erythrocyte. The endocytosed material is deposited in the lysosome-like acidic "digestive vacuole" (DV) of the parasite [22]. The hemoglobin is digested inside these vacuoles, the

Figure 5.3 Structural characterization of chloroquine mutations and their proposed mechanism of action. (a) Chloroquine mechanism of action is shown. CQ inhibits the formation of hemozoin from heme and thus free heme increases. Mutation in CRT results in decreased CQ accumulation. (b) Predicted structure of chloroquine sensitive *Pf*CRT. The *Pf*CRT is predicted to have 10 transmembrane (TM1-10) domains connected by loops (L2-10) with both L1/N- and L11/C-termini in the cytosolic side of the membrane of DV. The mutations corresponding to chloroquine-resistance are listed as per their presence in respective TMs and Ls. (c) Mapped points of mutation in chloroquine resistant *Pf*CRT 7G8 isoform (PDB ID: 6UKJ). The left panel shows the overall structure of *Pf*CRT 7G8 isoform with 10 transmembrane domains (blue). The residues mutated in 7G8 isoform in comparison to CQ sensitive isoform are shown in yellow and the point of mutations generally observed in other resistant isoforms are shown in red. The right panel shows the zoomed-out spatial distribution of all the point mutations.

peptide components formed are exported out, whereas the ferriprotoporphyrin IX (FPIX) stays in the vacuole as heme [22, 23]. Heme is a toxic by-product of the hemoglobin metabolism and can eventually kill the parasites by its own mechanism Figure 5.3a. However, this heme forms inert crystalline substances by associating as dimers of β-hematin [24]. This crystalline substance is called Hemozoin. Hemozoin is essential for malarial parasites as a food source. CQ contains a side chain of diethylamine nitrogen with a pK_a of 10.2 and the quinoline ring heteroatom nitrogen with a pK_a of 8.1 [25]. These properties make CQ a weak base. This unprotonated CQ can easily penetrate the membrane and distribute around the cell compartments, which gets accumulated inside the DV of the parasite after conversion into double-protonated, membrane-impermeable form. When CQ interacts with heme, it forms a drug–hemozoin complex to cap the polymerizing chain and further leads to accumulation of free heme in the food vacuole [26, 27], thereby hindering hemoglobin metabolism in the parasite, resulting in subsequent parasitic death (Figure 5.3a) [28, 29].

5.3.2 Basis of CQ Resistance

The CQ-resistant parasite accumulates far less concentration of CQ and thus enables the parasite to detoxify the toxic by-products of hemoglobin metabolism. In previous studies, the removal of CQ from the DV and thus resistance to CQ were explained as an attribute of mutant parasites. The resistance was mapped to various mutations in the *P. falciparum* CQ resistance transporter gene present on chromosome 7 [30, 31]. This gene is highly interrupted and has 13 exons encoding 424 amino acids [32]. This encodes a 49 kDa CRT protein, which is a transmembrane protein with 10 transmembrane domains Figure 5.3b. The localization experiments of *Pf*CRT were done by immunofluorescence, and immunoelectron microscopy suggested the presence of *Pf*CRT to the DV membrane [32, 33]. The mutations of the basic and hydrophobic amino acid residues in this protein are associated with the CQ resistance phenotypes as studied in cultured isolates across the globe (Figure 5.3c). CRT is identified to have a role in drug/metabolite transport [34]. Research has shown that when nonprotonated CQ enters the food vacuole, it changes to diprotonated

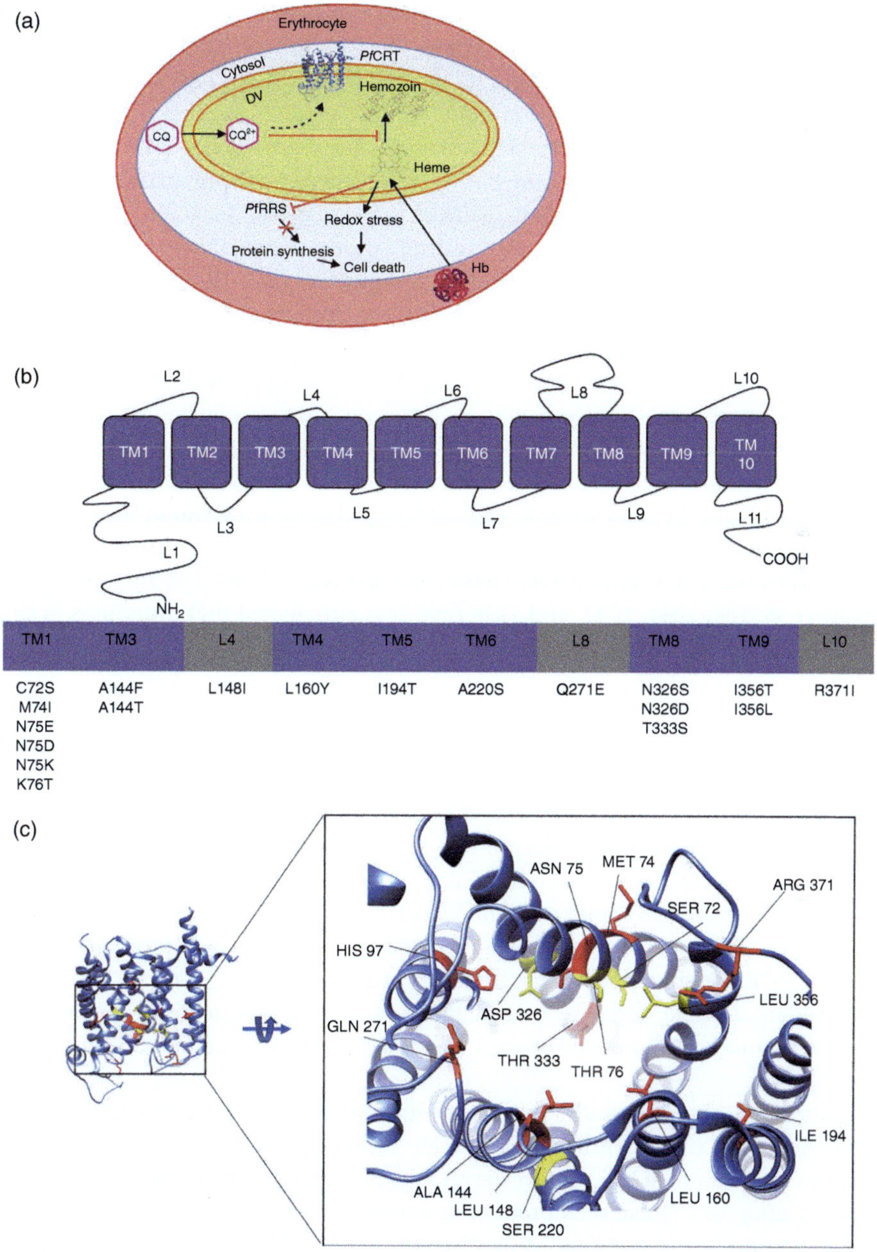
(a)
Erythrocyte
Cytosol
PfCRT
DV
Hemozoin
CQ
CQ2+
Heme
PfRRS
Redox stress
Protein synthesis
Cell death
Hb
(b)
L2
L4
L6
L8
L10
TM1
TM2
TM3
TM4
TM5
TM6
TM7
TM8
TM9
TM 10
L3
L5
L7
L9
L11
L1
COOH
NH2
TM1
TM3
L4
TM4
TM5
TM6
L8
TM8
TM9
L10
C72S
M74I
N75E
N75D
N75K
K76T
A144F
A144T
L148I
L160Y
I194T
A220S
Q271E
N326S
N326D
T333S
I356T
I356L
R371I
(c)
ASN 75
MET 74
ARG 371
SER 72
HIS 97
LEU 356
ASP 326
GLN 271
THR 333
THR 76
ILE 194
ALA 144
LEU 148
SER 220
LEU 160

form, and thus its efflux is prevented through the positively charged CRT at the critical K76 site. Most of the mutations reported in CRT are found in the barrel of the transporter predicted to have a role in substrate selectivity [34]. Till now, how *Pf*CRT maintains the critical concentration in DV remains unclear. However, change in the pH of the DV in the CQ-resistant parasites and transport of CQ out of DV explain the role of *Pf*CRT in CQ resistance [28]. Both mechanisms tend to prevent accumulation of CQ inside the food vacuole of the parasite.

Multidrug resistance to antimalarial drugs occurs when the parasite becomes resistant to a broad range of structurally different drugs [35]. The protein associated with this phenomenon is named as multidrug resistance (mdr) transporter or P-glycoprotein 1 (Pgp1). The homolog of this mammalian protein is encoded by *mdr1* gene in *P. falciparum* [36]. It belongs to the family of ABC transporters. Its molecular weight is ~162 kDa, and it possesses two domains having six transmembrane segments each of which is linked to a nucleotide binding fold by a linker region [37]. Unlike its mammalian homolog, *Pf*MDR1 (*Pf*PGP1) is reported to pump drugs into the food vacuole and aid in regulating intracellular drug concentration. It gets phosphorylated by a calcium-dependent protein kinase and also binds ATP [38]. The polymorphism has been observed in *Pfmdr1* coding residues at position 86, 184, 1034, 1042, and 1246 [39]. It is anticipated that mutations in this protein add to the resistance associated with CRT protein [40].

5.3.3 Prevalence of CQ Resistance

The excessive use of CQ made it the most widely used synthetic antimalarial in the 1960s and 1970s. The emergence of CQ drug-resistant *P. falciparum* was first reported in Thailand–Cambodia border in 1957 [41]. Eventually the resistance spread through various countries of Asia including Southeast Asia. Soon, CQ resistance appeared in Venezuela and Colombia [42]. Around the mid-1970s, the emergence of CQ drug resistance was reported in Port Moresby, Papua New Guinea [43]. In 1978, the first report came from Kenya and Tanzania, which further spread into Sudan, Zambia, Uganda, and Malawi [44, 45]. The increase in incidence of drug resistance to CQ in sub-Saharan Africa led to an increase in mortality due to malaria [46].

Interestingly, recent studies conducted to observe prevalence of CQ resistance genotypes after its discontinuation provide evidence of decrease in frequency of *Pfcrt* K76T mutants in Uganda, western Kenya, Rwanda, and Mozambique [47, 48]. The cessation of CQ use thus brought re-emergence of CQ-sensitive *P. falciparum* depending upon the duration of its discontinuation [49]. In addition to decrease in *Pfcrt* K76T allele frequency, discontinuation of CQ has also been associated with less than 10% prevalence of *Pfmdr1* 86Y alleles in Western Kenya, Rwanda, and Mozambique [49]. Certain other reports stated that the prevalence of mutant *Pfcrt* and *Pfmdr1* alleles was sustained in Thailand above 85% after 10 years of cessation of CQ [49]. This was also true for the study conducted in India, where the prevalence of *Pfcrt* K76T remained 84.2% [50] (Figure 5.3b,c).

5.3.4 WHO Guidelines to Use CQ

After World War II, CQ and DDT were considered as the arsenal to eradicate malaria globally. However, the subsequent resistance to both challenged every ambitious plan. As per the current policies in the WHO regions (updated on December 2018) [51], CQ is recommended in the regions mentioned as follows:

1. **Africa:** In Algeria, Ethiopia, and South Africa, CQ is used for the treatment of malaria due to *P. falciparum* during pregnancy with quinine and/or clindamycin and for prevention with primaquine.
2. **America:** In South American countries including Argentina, Belize, Bolivia, Brazil, Colombia, Costa Rica, Dominican Republic, Ecuador, El Salvador, French Guiana, Guatemala, Guyana, Haiti, Honduras, Mexico, Nicaragua, Panama, Paraguay, Peru, Suriname, and Venezuela, CQ is used along with primaquine for the treatment of malaria due to *P. vivax*. The *P. falciparum* malaria treatment varies in these countries and often uses CQ with primaquine for uncomplicated and confirmed cases or treatment of *vivax* during pregnancy.
3. **Europe:** The policies suggest usage of CQ with primaquine (14d) for the treatment of *P. vivax* in Armenia, Azerbaijan, Georgia, Tajikistan, Turkey, and Turkmenistan.
4. **South-East Asia:** The countries, namely Bangladesh, Bhutan, DPR Korea, India, Indonesia, Maldives, Myanmar, Nepal, Sri Lanka, Thailand, and Timor Leste, treat malaria due to *P. vivax* by the combination of CQ and primaquine.
5. **Eastern Mediterranean:** Similar to South-East Asian countries, the antimalarial combination of CQ and primaquine is used in Afghanistan, Djibouti, Egypt, Iran (Islamic republic), Oman, Pakistan, Syrian Arab Republic, and Yemen to treat *P. vivax*.
6. **Western Pacific:** In China and Vietnam, CQ and primaquine are given for the treatment of *P. vivax*, whereas in the Philippines, Malaysia, and Lao PDR, it is combined with artemether–lumefantrine.

5.4 Impact of Sulfadoxine–Pyrimethamine Resistance

The two drugs, pyrimethamine (Pyr) and sulfadoxine (Sdx), were developed in the second half of the nineteenth century. Proguanil was the first anti-folate drug, which was reported in 1945 [52], and its success in treating malaria led to the study of its chemical class, which resulted in discovery of Pyr [53]. In the 1950s, Pyr was developed by two scientists Gertrude Elion and George Hitchings, and their contributions to medicine were awarded in the year 1988 for "their discoveries of important principles for drug treatment" along with Sir James W. Black. Since the introduction of Pyr as an antimalarial treatment, drug resistance appeared very quickly in the year 1953, which led to the addition of Sdx in the therapy. Sdx, which was already known to show resistance in 1957, still made it to the combination therapy, i.e. together with Pyr.

Sdx belongs to the class of sulfonamide and has different mechanisms of action than Pyr. The combination of these two drugs appeared promising at first in the year 1967 when they were recommended in the settings where *Plasmodium* species were already resistant to CQ [54]. However, within two years of its first usage, the first report of SP resistance came in 1970s. The treatment was first approved in 1981 in the United States to surmount the emergence of Pyr resistance due to its usage as a monotherapy. This drug combination is sold under the name Fansidar and targets folate biosynthesis pathway of the parasite. This therapy was able to target the liver and blood stages of malaria. Until the 1990s, the resistance of SP stayed low in Africa but unfortunately eventually started spreading rapidly.

5.4.1 Mechanism of Action of SP

The viability of the malarial parasite critically depends on the functioning of folate metabolic pathway. It has been targeted for over a century in the prophylaxis and treatment of malaria. The two drugs in the therapy act synergistically in order to block the folate biosynthesis pathway. PYR acts on dihydrofolate reductase (DHFR), and Sdx inhibits dihydropteroate synthetase (DHPS) (Figure 5.4a). In addition to these two, proguanil and dapsone also fall into the category of antifolates. As understood from other organisms, the main folate pathway utilizes guanosine-5′-triphosphate (GTP) for the formation of basic folate structure, i.e. dihydrofolate (DHF) and later get fully reduced following series of reactions into tetrahydrofolate (THF). The pool of THF and DHF is thus maintained by a folate pathway in which biosynthesis of folate is carried out by successive five enzymatic reactions and interconversion of folate to other forms that carry out C1 transfer reactions, other four enzymes are required. One of the enzymes of this critically important pathway, DHFR, is the target of PYR and was cloned and analyzed in 1987 [55]. It was reported as one of the domains of a bifunctional protein from *P. falciparum* dihydrofolate reductase-thymidylate synthase (DHFR-TS). DHFR has a crucial role in the biosynthesis of DNA and proteins as it aids in production of tetrahydrofolate, which acts as a cofactor in transferring C1 units for the biosynthesis of nucleic acids [56, 57]. All other genes encoding enzymes related to folate biosynthesis pathway were gradually identified while the *P. falciparum* genome sequencing project was still underway with an exception of a few [56].

Figure 5.4 The sulfadoxine–pyrimethamine drug targets and the structural analysis of the SP resistance mutations. (a) Sulfadoxine (Sdx) and Pyrimethamine (Pyr) act synergistically where Pyr acts on dihydrofolate reductase (DHFR) and Sdx inhibits dihydropteroate synthetase (DHPS). (b) The domain representation of the bi-functional DHFR-TS and HPPK-DHPS protein from *P. falciparum* and *P. vivax* with the Pyr and Sdx resistance mutations marked. The three-dimensional crystal structure of the (c) *Pf*DHPS, (d) *Pv*DHPS, (e) *Pf*DHFR, and (f) *Pv*DHFR with the spatial distribution of the drug resistance mutations (in red) with respect to the bound substrates/drugs (in green) is shown. XTZ, HH2, PAB, CP6, CP7. The percentage prevalence of the different mutations observed in the (g) DHFR enzyme and (h) DHPS enzyme for *P. falciparum* and *P. vivax* are shown.

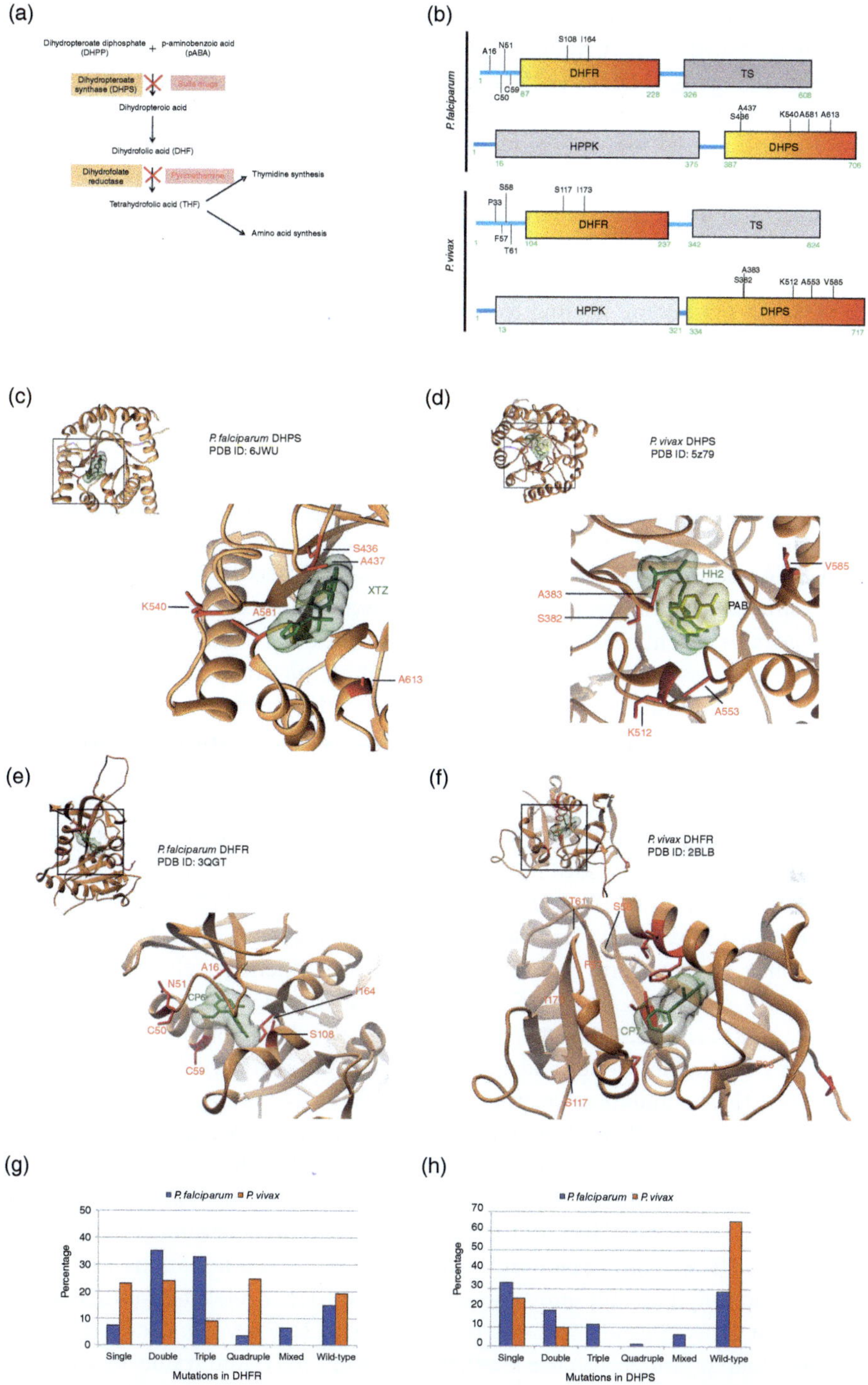
(a)
Dihydropteroate diphosphate (DHPP)
+
p-aminobenzoic acid (pABA)
Dihydropteroate synthase (DHPS)
Dihydropteroic acid
Dihydrofolic acid (DHF)
Dihydrofolate reductase
Thymidine synthesis
Tetrahydrofolic acid (THF)
Amino acid synthesis
(b)
P. falciparum
A16
N51
C59
C50
S108 I164
DHFR
TS
1
87
228
326
608
A437
S436
K540 A581 A613
HPPK
DHPS
15
375
387
706
P. vivax
S58
P33
F57
T61
S117 I173
DHFR
TS
1
104
237
342
824
A383
S382
K512 A553 V585
HPPK
DHPS
13
321
334
717
(c)
P. falciparum DHPS
PDB ID: 6JWU
S436
A437
XTZ
K540
A581
A613
(d)
P. vivax DHPS
PDB ID: 5z79
V585
HH2
A383
PAB
S382
A553
K512
(e)
P. falciparum DHFR
PDB ID: 3QGT
A16
N51
I164
C50
S108
C59
(f)
P. vivax DHFR
PDB ID: 2BLB
T61
S117
(g)
P. falciparum
P. vivax
Percentage
50
40
30
20
10
0
Single
Double
Triple
Quadruple
Mixed
Wild-type
Mutations in DHFR
(h)
P. falciparum
P. vivax
Percentage
70
60
50
40
30
20
10
0
Single
Double
Triple
Quadruple
Mixed
Wild-type
Mutations in DHPS

On the other hand, *P. falciparum* exhibits another bifunctional protein that contains 7,8-dihydro-6-hydroxymethylpterin pyrophosphokinase (PPPK) and C-terminal region homologous to DHPS [58]. DHPS is coded by *Pf*dhps gene, which catalyzes the synthesis of DHF in the parasite [58]. DHF is required as a precursor for pyrimidine synthesis, which in turn is required in RNA and DNA biosynthesis. Sdx belongs to the class of sulfa drugs known to inhibit folate synthesis, and Sdx thus acts as a competitive inhibitor of DHPS as it is analogous to *p*-aminobenzoic acid (PABA) [59]. The synergistic mechanism of action of these two drugs affects the pool of tetrahydrofolate and thus interferes with the synthesis of deoxythymidine monophosphate (dTMP) and pyrimidine leading to parasite death [59]. It has been reported that resistance to even one of these two drastically reduces the efficiency of other [59].

5.4.2 SP Resistance

The treatment failure in the absence of CQ led to the usage of SP combination as the first-line drug to treat malaria [60]. However, the SP-resistant mutations soon started to pose another problem of drug resistance in the treatment of malaria [61, 62]. As described earlier, the SP combination targets DHPS and DHFR and point mutations in their genes decrease the susceptibility of *P. falciparum*, which also relates to the number of mutations. In the early twentieth century, it was shown how cross-resistance between drugs, drug pharmacokinetics, overusage of drugs, and inadequate treatment led to the SP drug resistance [63–66]. So far, six-point mutations (A16V, C50R, N51I, C59R, S108N, I164L) have been linked to Pyr resistance, which occur as single, double, triple, and quadruple. Other six mutations, which have been structurally determined in *Pf*DHFR, are present as single (P33L, F57L/I, S58R, T61M, S117N/T, I173F/L), double (S58R-S117N; S117N-I173L), triple (S58R-S117N-I173L [RNL]; S58R-T61M-S117N/T [RMN/T], F57L-S58R-S117T [LRT]), and quadruple (S58R-T61M-S117N-I173L [RMNL]; F57L/I-S58R-T61M-S117T [L/IRMT]) mutations (Figure 5.4b). Sdx resistance corresponds to mutations in *Pf*DHPS, which are generally called SAKAA (Pf) and SAKAV (Pv) (SAKAA [S436A/F, A437G, K540E, A581G, A613S/T] SAKAV [S382A, A383G, K512E, A553G, V585A]) [67, 68]. The combinations of these mutations as double, triple, and quadruple have been reported in *Pf*DHPS and *Pv*DHPS [67]. The mutations leading to resistance of Sdx and Pyr show the specific order of occurrence when observed on the three-dimensional structures of DHPS and DHFR (Figure 5.4c). The problem has intensified with the emergence of full or super-resistant strains of Pf/Pv [69]. The isolates carrying combination of the triple mutations from DHFR and DHPS leading to fully resistant quintuple such as *Pf*DHFR (IRN) triple mutation in association with two mutations in *Pf*DHPS (GE) lead to fully resistant quintuple (N51I-C59R-S108N-A437G-K540E/IRN-GE). Similarly, a super-resistant sextuple is also reported in Pf, which occurs when the fully resistant quintuple also has another mutation A581G and results in a sextuple mutant. Such combinations have also been reported in Pv isolates and thus reduce the prophylactic period of Sdx and Pyr combination. The reduction results in clinical and parasitological treatment failure of SP.

5.4.3 Distribution of DHPS and DHFR Mutation Across Globe

5.4.3.1 *dhfr*

1. **South America:** Six countries in South America: Suriname, Brazil, Colombia, Ecuador, Haiti, and Panama dominating with ~33% strains with triple resistance among mutated Pf isolates. The documented mutations were reported to show varied prevalence. The observations were similar in the percent distribution of triple mutants of *Pv*DHFR.
2. **Africa:** The dominance of *Pf*DHFR triple mutants IRN has been reported in African continent. The double mutants of *Pf*DHFR (N51I-S108N) were reported to be prevalent in eastern and central regions of Sudan. Overall, IRN triple mutants dominate in African countries, which is suggested to be the result of evolution of the double mutants (C50R-N51I; N51I-S108N; 255 C59R-S108N) by sequential addition of mutations.
3. **Asia and Middle East:** In Asia, the double mutants are more prevalent such as (C59R-S108N) has been reported in Papua New Guinea (PNG), Hainan (China), Indonesia, Pakistan, and Solomon and Vanuatu (S&V) in Pf isolates. Similarly, the double mutants of *Pf*DHFR dominate the Middle Eastern countries, namely Yemen, Iran, and Afghanistan. In addition to these, triple mutants of *Pf*DHFR are reported from Myanmar and Malaysia as the dominating strains.
4. **India:** Here as well the double mutant prevails followed by triple, quadruple, and single mutations in *Pf*DHFR. The double mutations (C59R-S108N) are reported as the dominant mutation in West Bengal, Uttar Pradesh, Jharkhand, North-eastern states of India, and Odisha. The triple mutations have been observed in isolates from Meghalaya, Jharkhand, and North-East and quadruple mutation combination IRNL reported in samples from Andaman and Nicobar region of India.

5.4.3.2 *dhps*

1. **South America:** The countries, namely Peru, Brazil, and Suriname, dominate in *Pf*DHPS triple mutations, and single point mutations are found prevalent in Panama, Brazil, and Colombia. In *Pv*DHPS, only single (A383G) and double mutations (S382C-A383G) have been reported from Brazil/Colombia/Peru, and French Guiana, respectively.
2. **Asia and Middle East:** Similar to dominance of triple *Pf*DHPS mutations in South America, Asia and Middle-East countries show prevalence of triple mutations such as (AGEAA, SGEGA, and SGNGA). In Asia, these mutations have been shown to dominate in Yunnan (China), Thailand, Chin-Myanmar, Cambodia, Vietnam, Bangladesh, and Myanmar. The wild-type *Pf*DHPS sensitive to Sdx has shown prevalence only in certain regions of Asia, which includes Afghanistan, PNG, S&V, and Hainan (China). In *Pv*DHPS, single point mutations are more common and have been reported in isolates from Iran, Laos, Pakistan, Malaysia, Myanmar, and the Philippines.

3. **Africa:** The single point mutation of *Pf*DHPS dominates in Africa, for instance, single point mutations SAKAA have been reported from many countries in Africa. SGKAA is among the most common *Pf*DHPS mutations. Burkina Faso, Gabon, and Liberia isolates have shown single point mutations, which confer partial resistance. On the contrary, *Pv*DHPS exhibits mutations at very low frequency in Africa overall.
4. **India:** *Pf*DHPS triple mutations such as AGEAA and SGNGA dominate in North-eastern regions in India. The wild-type Sdx-sensitive *P. falciparum* has only been reported in Aligarh and Ghaziabad (UP), Baikunthpur (Chhattisgarh), Madhya Pradesh, and Odisha. *Pv*DHPS isolates have shown predominance of single and double mutants in various states of India. For example, SGKAV, SAKGV, and SGKGV have been reported in Rajasthan, Delhi, Tamil Nadu, West Bengal, and Karnataka. The single mutation A383G (SGKAV) is reported to be the most common among *Pv*DHPS isolates (Figure 5.4d).

5.4.4 WHO Guidelines to Use SP

As per WHO guidelines, the current treatment for *CQ*-resistant *P. falciparum* is SP given along with Artesunate in some countries. The guidelines for intermittent preventive treatment (IPT) suggest use of SP in pregnant women (IPTp) and infants (below 12 months of age) (IPTi) in the sub-Saharan African areas showing moderate to high transmission of malaria.

5.4.4.1 IPTp Guidelines

Some of the adverse outcomes of the malaria infection to pregnant women are maternal anemia, low birth weight, and preterm delivery and in severe cases can lead to death of mother and infant [70, 71]. As per WHOs guidelines, the interventions to control malaria, in malaria-endemic areas in Africa, should include case management, use of insecticidal nets and SP-based IPTp from the second trimester onward. The success of IPTp depends upon the number of doses administered depending upon visits to antenatal clinics. In addition to that, SP resistance is increasing and posing concerns related to SP-based IPTp policies [70].

5.4.4.2 IPTi Guidelines

In moderate-to-high transmission areas in Africa, the SP is provided as the IPTi considering it is still effective in the areas. The dosage is given at the time of the vaccination against diphtheria, tetanus, pertussis, and measles. The IPTi protects against clinical malaria, anemia, malaria parasitemia associated with hospital admissions and other causes of hospital admission in the first year of life. The treatment is decided on the basis of severity of malaria in the region concerned [72].

5.5 ACT Resistance

ART and its derivatives were first identified in the early 1970s as a collaborative effort by Chinese researchers. It was extracted from the plant Qinghao commonly known as sweet wormwood (*Artemisia annua*). ART made a remarkable contribution in the treatment of malaria and its drug-resistant forms, which were resistant to CQ, SP, and/or MQ [73–78]. ART (also known as Qinghaosu) is a sesquiterpene lactone compound of the traditional Chinese medicine (Figure 5.2). The compound was the result of Project 523 started by Chinese government to combat antimalarial CQ resistance in the parasite in South-East Asia and Sub-Saharan Africa [79]. The emergence of dichloro-diphenyl-trichloro-ethane (DDT) resistance in the vectors demanded further attention to develop potent drugs against malaria. Due to poor solubility of ART parent drug in water or oil, soluble derivatives were generated by reduction of the carbonyl group (Figure 5.2). Out of all the derivatives that were studied for the malaria treatment, DHA is pharmacologically most relevant. ART and its derivatives are among the most effective and rapid antimalarial drugs, however with the short elimination half-life from the plasma of approximately one hour. Subsequent studies were conducted in rodent and non-human primate models to understand the toxicity and dosage of the drug. The safety profile of ART was developed after the voluntary contribution of Professor Youyou Tu (the lead scientist of the project) and her colleagues. Eventually the clinical trials were carried out and ART and its derivatives came in use in China at the national level to treat malaria. The efficacy of ART and resurgence of drug resistance led to development of clinical studies in Africa.

As it was crucial to avoid ART monotherapy-associated potential breakout of malaria, combination therapies were suggested and developed. Also, short half-life of ART and its derivatives make them poor candidates for malaria prophylaxis, resulting in low cure rate and high chances of recrudescence. In the light of the aforementioned reasons, drugs showing synergistic effects with ART were selected and provided as combination therapy (Table 5.1). The novel combination therapy including lumefantrine and artemether was among the first ACTs. Another ACT, which was in development around the same time, was ART and PPQ. The group later proposed the two new drugs, artesunate and PPQ phosphate, to be used as ACT. The clinical trials in Vietnam led to the development of another novel regime after series of optimization. It was tested that DHA and PPQ phosphate had better efficacy than the others.

Currently, the treatment for malaria is prescribed on the basis of its complicated nature. As per the recommendations made by WHO, the *P. falciparum* uncomplicated malaria is treated by five ACTs from which the choice is made on the basis of local strains of *P. falciparum*. The *P. vivax* malaria is treated by ACT or CQ, provided the area does not have CQ-resistant strains of *P. vivax*. On the other hand, severe malaria can only be treated with ART derivative, artesunate, which is recommended to be followed by ACT. The monotherapy of ART is discouraged by the WHO to prevent development of ART-resistant strains. Despite all the efforts, the susceptibility to ACTs has been reduced and thus alarmed researchers to study ACT-resistant strains.

The first ART-resistant strain was generated by prolonged repeated exposure of ART for over five years to F32-Tanzania (African strain). The generated strain was named as F32-ART and was studied for mutations by sequencing the exome in

Table 5.1 Treatment of uncomplicated and severe malaria.

***Plasmodium* spp.**	**Drug treatment for uncomplicated malaria**	**Intensive care unit**
Plasmodium vivax or CQ-sensitive *Plasmodium falciparum*	CQ – 10 mg base/kg stat. 5 mg/kg (12, 24, and 36 h) **or** 10 mg/kg – 24 h and 5 mg/kg – 48 h; **or** Amodiaquine – 10 mg base/kg/day for 3 d	CQ 10 mg base/kg infused intravenously at constant rate over 8 h followed by 15 mg base/kg over 24 h
CQ-resistant *P. falciparum* sensitive to SP	Pyr 1.25 mg/kg + Sdx 25 mg/kg (single dose; three tablets in an adult) **or** Amodiaquine 10 mg base/kg/day for 3 d	Quinine dihydrochloride 7 mg salt/kg infused over 30 min followed by immediately 10 mg/kg over 4 h; or 20 mg salt/kg infused over 4 h. Maintenance dose: 10 mg salt/kg infused over 2–8 h at 8-h intervals Artemisinin derivatives 1. Artemether 3.2 mg/kg stat. by i.m. injection followed by 1.6 mg/kg daily 2. Artesunate 2.4 mg/kg stat. by i.v. injection followed by 1.2 mg/kg daily
CQ-resistant *P. vivax* and multidrug resistant *P. falciparum*	Oral artesunate 4 mg/kg daily for 3 d + mefloquine 25 mg base/kg (15 mg/kg on day 2, 10 mg/kg on day 3) **or** Artemether–lumefantrine 1.5/9 mg/kg twice daily for 3 d with food **or** Quinine 10 mg salt/kg three times daily plus tetracycline 4 mg/kg four times daily or doxycycline 3 mg/kg once daily or clindamycin 10 mg/kg twice daily for 7 d	

comparison to its clone grown in the absence of drug [80]. The study presented the evidence of eight single nucleotide polymorphisms (SNPs) in seven genes, which were further identified specifically on the basis of chronology in their appearance. Among these genes, the region, which was also previously identified in the genome wide association studies, conducted, independently, reported to belong to Kelch gene located on chromosome 13 [81, 82]. It was interesting to note that the K13 mutants were spatially and temporally located to western Cambodia, the region that reported resistance to ART. On the basis of the studies conducted on patients having delayed parasite clearance (DPC) and also presence of mutations in the K13 gene in the parasites isolated from patients, K13 gene mutations were identified as a molecular marker of resistance to ART and its derivatives [83]. The importance of K13 was further validated in studies where complementing the wild-type K13 knockout parasites with K13 mutant alleles, which were prevalent in resistant zones in Cambodia, led to an increase in survival rate of the parasite in the presence of ART [84]. Moreover, when the mutations were corrected using CRISPR-Cas9 in the mutated strains observed in Cambodia, the survival rate of the parasite decreased in response to ART [85].

5.5.1 Mechanism of Action of ART

The polymorphism in the gene coding Kelch-like superfamily protein, Kelch-13 (K13), has been reported in ACT-resistant strains. These mutations have been studied extensively to determine their association with decreased susceptibility to ACTs. Although the consensus on ART targets has not been reached yet, several studies highlighted the association of protein targets involved in the ART mechanism of action to the mutations observed in *P. falciparum* Kelch 13 (*Pf*K13) [86]. The mutation *Pf*K13 C580Y has been observed as the primary marker for the ART resistance [83]. ART gets activated upon cleavage of Endoperoxide Bridge and thereby produces free radicals to alkylate the drug targets so as to kill malarial parasites. Other studies have suggested multiple targets of ART, which might lead to interference with the proteome of the parasite [87, 88]. The gene that encodes *Pf*K13 is located on the chromosome 13 and as mentioned above, belongs to the superfamily of about 60 members. The protein expression is observed in all the stages of intraerythrocytic asexual cycle and gametocytes. The protein localization suggests partial presence in endoplasmic reticulum. The protein has been predicted to have a role in quality assurance of the proteins and also exhibits resistance to cancer drugs, which leads to proteopathy [89]. It has also been reported to be essential for the survival of *P. falciparum* [90] by knockout studies where the phenotype is linked to the essentiality in the survival of ring stage or transition of ring stage to trophozoite [91]. In another study, mutated *Pf*K13 carrying parasites, which are resistant to ART, have been shown to reprogram the developmental cycle and exhibit a prolonged ring stage in the infected erythrocytes [92].

The crystal structure of K13 was first reported from *P. falciparum* in the year 2015. It is a 726 amino acid residue long protein and has been studied as a dimer protein in the crystallographic studies. The structure of K13 reveals an *N*-terminus BTB/POZ (zinc-finger domain [ZFD]) domain with six Kelch domains. The dimerization occurs due to the ZFD and the Kelch domains have been reported to have a role in ubiquitylation and proteasomal degradation of the substrates. The mutations associated with ART were mapped to the K13 dimeric structure in the previous studies and the dimeric interface was further analyzed. The K13 mutations were sparsely scattered on the surface as well as inter-monomeric surface, and thus these analyses were not able to draw any conclusion to link K13 mutations that may lead to ART failure.

Several mechanisms have been reported behind ART resistance, which may work together to decrease the susceptibility to the ACTs. Mutations in the *Pf*K13 have been linked to decreased expression of genes required in DNA replication in addition to other responses during stress such as upregulation of unfolded protein response pathways and proteasome pathways. It has also shown to have role in phosphorylation of eukaryotic initiation factor 2, subunit-α (eIF2-α). On the other hand, the mutation of *Pf*K13 reduces the binding of polyubiquitination of *Pf*PI3K and its binding to *Pf*K13. This leads to limited proteolysis of *Pf*PI3K and thereby increases the level of kinase and its product phosphatidylinositol-3-phosphate.

5.5.2 ART Resistance and ACT Failure

According to WHO, ACT resistance is understood as the DPC rate in response to treatment by artesunate monotherapy or with an ACT. In treatment-sensitive strains, the parasite clearance half-life is ~2 hours, which is >5 hours in the ACT-resistant parasites. Generally, the patients infected with ART-resistant parasites show parasite presence even after the three days of the treatment. Recently, in addition to gene manipulation studies, extensive genome-wide association studies (GWAS) have been conducted in order to understand the reason behind reduced susceptibility to the ACTs. However, until today, any conclusive hypothesis, which can link K13 mutations to ART resistance, is absent. In a recent study, researchers have suggested to use structural modeling in order to map the effect of K13 mutations and their role reduction of ART susceptibility. So far, over 200 mutations have been reported in K13 from various *P. falciparum* strains. Out of these, 50 of these have been assessed for ART/ACT resistance using delayed parasite clearance at day 3 (DPC3), parasite clearance half-life (PCHL), *in-vitro* and *ex-vivo* ring stage survival assays (RSAs). Mutations F446I, N458Y/I, M476I/V, Y493H, R539T, I543T, P553L, R561H, C580Y have been assessed and validated for lower susceptibility to ART *ex vivo* and further 11 candidate mutations need validation (P441L, G449A, C469Y, A481V, N537I, G538V, V568G, P574L, N672S, F673I, A675V) for ART resistance.

PfK13 C580Y is the predominant marker of ART/ACT resistance and prevalent in parasites found in South East Asia particularly in Thailand–Cambodia border areas, Vietnam, and south of Laos. On the other hand, among other mutations reported to be associated with ART resistance, F446I is quite common in northern Myanmar and the China–Myanmar border area, whereas Y493H, R539T, and I543T are prevalent in strains found in Myanmar–Thailand–Cambodia border area. Some mutations such as F495L from the China–Myanmar border [93] have shown high RSA values, whereas same mutation reported from sub-Saharan Africa had no role in ART resistance.

5.5.3 WHO Guidelines

As per the latest guidelines set by WHO, ACTs should be used for the treatment of uncomplicated malaria by *P. falciparum* [7]. The recommended ACTs include artemether plus lumefantrine, artesunate plus amodiaquine/MFQ, DHA plus PPQ, and artesunate plus SP with regime time of three days. In low transmission areas, it is suggested to give a single dose of 0.25 mg/kg primaquine with ACT in order to control transmission. For the uncomplicated non-*falciparum* malaria in the areas with CQ-resistant/susceptible infections, ACTs can be used to treat adults and children. The former treatment should exclude pregnant women in their first trimester. To treat severe malaria in adults and children, WHO suggests artesunate to be given intramuscular or intravenous for at least 24 hours until the patient is able to tolerate oral medication. If intramuscular injections are unavailable, children of age <6 years should be given a single rectal dose of artesunate (10 mg/kg) followed by proper care (Figure 5.5).

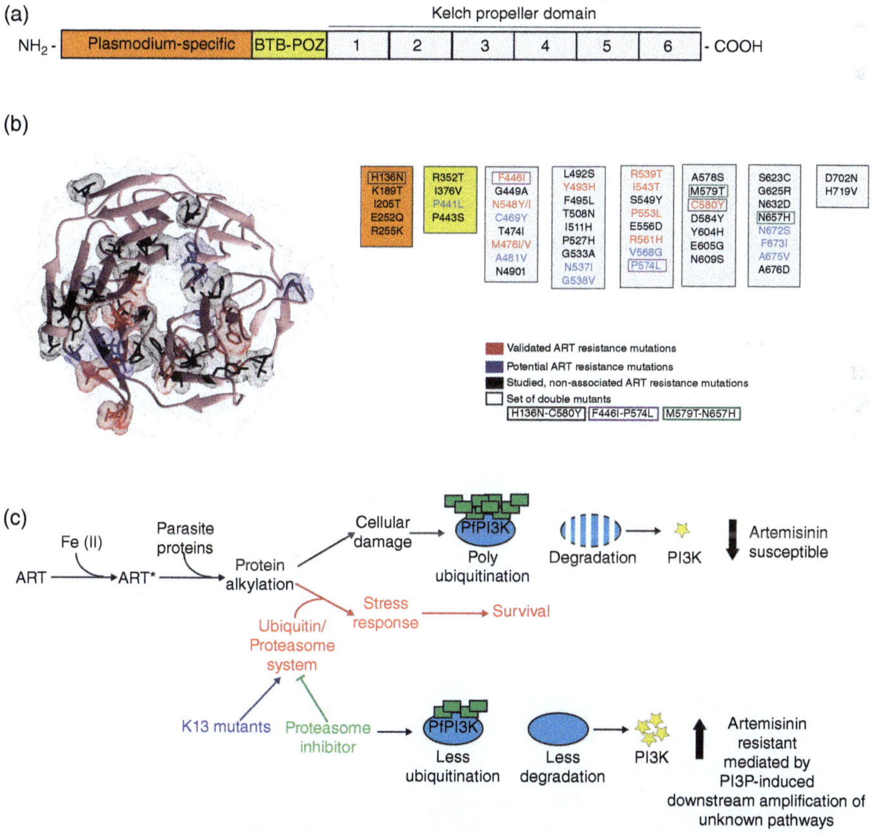

Figure 5.5 Structural distribution of ART-resistant mutations on Kelch 13 protein. (a) The domain diagram of the Kelch-13 protein from *Plasmodium* spp. highlighting the *Plasmodium*-specific domain, BTB-POZ domain, and the six-Kelch propeller domains. (b) The spatial distribution of the ART-resistant Kelch 13 mutations. (c) The proposed mechanism of the ART resistance and ART susceptibility owed to the Kelch 13 mutants are shown.

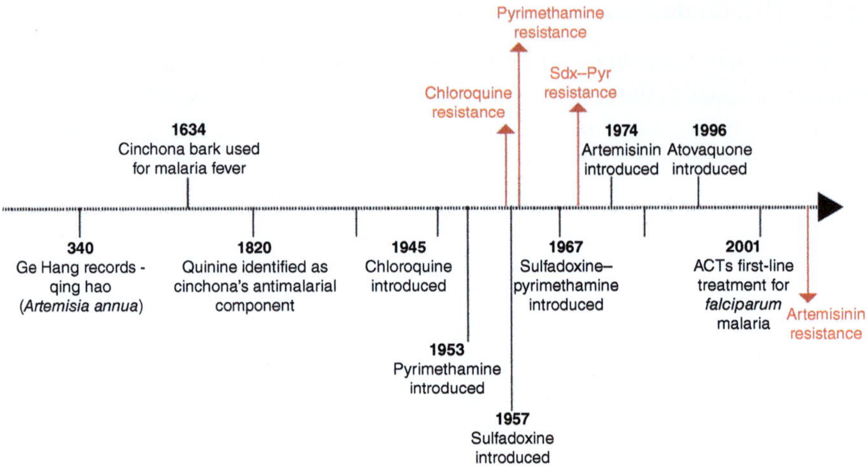

Figure 5.6 Timeline of key antimalarial resistance events.

5.6 Conclusion: The Road Ahead

The emergence of antimalarial drug-resistant *Plasmodium* spp. threatens the efforts to control and eradicate malaria globally. Figure 5.6 summarizes the timeline for the introduction of key antimalarial drugs and the first report on the incidence of drug resistance for *Plasmodium* spp. In this chapter, we provided an overview of the mechanism of action, the emergence of drug-resistant mutations, and the WHO guidelines for the use of three key antimalarial drugs, i.e. CQ, SP, and ACT. It is important to emphasize that the efforts to identify drug resistance and prevent its spread are as crucial as the need to develop novel antimalarial drugs. There is immediate need for new medicines and strategies to use the current medications before malaria wins the battle against humanity that has continued for thousands of years.

References

1 Delves, M., Plouffe, D., Scheurer, C. et al. (2012). The activities of current anti-malarial drugs on the life cycle stages of *Plasmodium*: a comparative study with human and rodent parasites. *PLoS Medicine* 9: e1001169. https://doi.org/10.1371/journal.pmed.1001169.

2 Phillips, M.A., Burrows, J.N., Manyando, C. et al. (2017). Malaria. *Nature Reviews. Disease Primers* 3: 17050. https://doi.org/10.1038/nrdp.2017.50.

3 Verhave, J.P. (2013). Experimental, therapeutic and natural transmission of *Plasmodium vivax* tertian malaria: scientific and anecdotal data on the history of Dutch malaria studies. *Parasites & Vectors* 6: 19. https://doi.org/10.1186/1756-3305-6-19.

4 White, N.J. (2011). Determinants of relapse periodicity in *Plasmodium vivax* malaria. *Malaria Journal* 10: 297. https://doi.org/10.1186/1475-2875-10-297.

5 Imwong, M., Stepniewska, K., Tripura, R. et al. (2016). Numerical distributions of parasite densities during asymptomatic malaria. *The Journal of Infectious Diseases* 213: 1322–1329. https://doi.org/10.1093/infdis/jiv596.

6 Basch, P.F. (1999). *Textbook of International Health*. USA: Oxford University Press.

7 WHO (2019). *World Malaria Report 2019*. Geneva: World Health Organization.

8 Bustos, M.D., Wongsrichanalai, C., Delacollette, C. et al. (2013). Monitoring antimalarial drug efficacy in the Greater Mekong Subregion: an overview of in vivo results from 2008 to 2010. *The Southeast Asian Journal of Tropical Medicine and Public Health* 44 (Suppl 1): 201–230; discussion 306–7.

9 Cowell, A.N. and Winzeler, E.A. (2019). The genomic architecture of antimalarial drug resistance. *Briefings in Functional Genomics* 18: 314–328. https://doi.org/10.1093/bfgp/elz008.

10 Imwong, M., Dhorda, M., Myo Tun, K., et al. (2020). Molecular epidemiology of resistance to antimalarial drugs in the Greater Mekong subregion: an observational study. *The Lancet Infectious Diseases*, https://doi.org/10.1016/S1473-3099(20)30228-0.

11 Noedl, H., Se, Y., Schaecher, K. et al. (2008). Evidence of artemisinin-resistant malaria in western Cambodia. *The New England Journal of Medicine* 359: 2619–2620. https://doi.org/10.1056/NEJMc0805011.

12 National Research Council (2003). *Malaria Control During Mass Population Movements and Natural Disasters*. Washington, DC: The National Academies Press https://doi.org/10.17226/10539.

13 Tse, E.G., Korsik, M., and Todd, M.H. (2019). The past, present and future of anti-malarial medicines. *Malaria Journal* 18: 93. https://doi.org/10.1186/s12936-019-2724-z.

14 Lee, M.R. (2002). Plants against malaria. Part 1: Cinchona or the Peruvian bark. *The Journal of the Royal College of Physicians of Edinburgh* 32: 189–196.

15 Croft, S. (2001). Antimalarial chemotherapy: mechanisms of action, resistance and new directions in drug discovery. *Drug Discovery Today* 6: 1151. https://doi.org/10.1016/s1359-6446(01)02035-9.

16 Woodward, R.B. and Doering, W.E. (1944). The total synthesis of quinine. *Journal of the American Chemical Society* 66: 849. https://doi.org/10.1021/ja01233a516.

17 Woodward, R.B. and Doering, W.E. (1945). The total synthesis of quinine. *Journal of the American Chemical Society* 67: 860–874. https://doi.org/10.1021/ja01221a051.

18 Jensen, M. and Mehlhorn, H. (2009). Seventy-five years of Resochin in the fight against malaria. *Parasitology Research* 105: 609–627. https://doi.org/10.1007/s00436-009-1524-8.

19 Rodriguez-Caruncho, C. and Bielsa Marsol, I. (2014). Antimalarials in dermatology: mechanism of action, indications, and side effects. *Actas Dermo-Sifiliográficas* 105: 243–252. https://doi.org/10.1016/j.adengl.2012.10.021.

20 CDC (2019). Malaria information and prophylaxis by country [Online]. Centers for Disease Control and Prevention, Global Health. Available: https://www.cdc.gov/malaria/travelers/country_table/a.html (accessed 22 October 2021).

21 Price, R.N., Von Seidlein, L., Valecha, N. et al. (2014). Global extent of chloroquine-resistant *Plasmodium vivax*: a systematic review and meta-analysis. *The Lancet Infectious Diseases* 14: 982–991. https://doi.org/10.1016/S1473-3099(14)70855-2.

22 Francis, S.E., Sullivan, D.J., and Goldberg, D.E. (1997). Hemoglobin metabolism in the malaria parasite *Plasmodium falciparum*. *Annual Review of Microbiology* 51: 97–123. https://doi.org/10.1146/annurev.micro.51.1.97.

23 Heller, L.E. and Roepe, P.D. (2018). Quantification of free ferriprotoporphyrin IX heme and hemozoin for artemisinin sensitive versus delayed clearance phenotype *Plasmodium falciparum* malarial parasites. *Biochemistry* 57: 6927–6934. https://doi.org/10.1021/acs.biochem.8b00959.

24 Pagola, S., Stephens, P.W., Bohle, D.S. et al. (2000). The structure of malaria pigment β-haematin. *Nature* 404: 307–310. https://doi.org/10.1038/35005132.

25 Dzekunov, S.M., Ursos, L.M., and Roepe, P.D. (2000). Digestive vacuolar pH of intact intraerythrocytic *P. falciparum* either sensitive or resistant to chloroquine. *Molecular and Biochemical Parasitology* 110: 107–124. https://doi.org/10.1016/s0166-6851(00)00261-9.

26 Bennett, T.N., Kosar, A.D., Ursos, L.M. et al. (2004). Drug resistance-associated pfCRT mutations confer decreased *Plasmodium falciparum* digestive vacuolar pH. *Molecular and Biochemical Parasitology* 133: 99–114. https://doi.org/10.1016/j.molbiopara.2003.09.008.

27 Coronado, L.M., Nadovich, C.T., and Spadafora, C. (2014). Malarial hemozoin: from target to tool. *Biochimica et Biophysica Acta* 1840: 2032–2041. https://doi.org/10.1016/j.bbagen.2014.02.009.

28 Saliba, K.J., Folb, P.I., and Smith, P.J. (1998). Role for the *Plasmodium falciparum* digestive vacuole in chloroquine resistance. *Biochemical Pharmacology* 56: 313–320. https://doi.org/10.1016/s0006-2952(98)00140-3.

29 Yayon, A. (1985). The antimalarial mode of action of chloroquine. *Reviews in Clinical & Basic Pharmacology* 5: 99–139.

30 Su, X., Kirkman, L.A., Fujioka, H. et al. (1997). Complex polymorphisms in an approximately 330 kDa protein are linked to chloroquine-resistant *P. falciparum* in Southeast Asia and Africa. *Cell* 91: 593–603. https://doi.org/10.1016/s0092-8674(00)80447-x.

31 Wellems, T.E., Walker-Jonah, A., and Panton, L.J. (1991). Genetic mapping of the chloroquine-resistance locus on *Plasmodium falciparum* chromosome 7. *Proceedings of the National Academy of Sciences of the United States of America* 88: 3382–3386. https://doi.org/10.1073/pnas.88.8.3382.

32 Fidock, D.A., Nomura, T., Talley, A.K. et al. (2000). Mutations in the *P. falciparum* digestive vacuole transmembrane protein PfCRT and evidence for their role in chloroquine resistance. *Molecular Cell* 6: 861–871. https://doi.org/10.1016/s1097-2765(05)00077-8.

33 Cooper, R.A., Ferdig, M.T., Su, X.Z. et al. (2002). Alternative mutations at position 76 of the vacuolar transmembrane protein PfCRT are associated with chloroquine resistance and unique stereospecific quinine and quinidine responses in *Plasmodium falciparum. Molecular Pharmacology* 61: 35–42. https://doi.org/10.1124/mol.61.1.35.

34 Martin, R.E. and Kirk, K. (2004). The malaria parasite's chloroquine resistance transporter is a member of the drug/metabolite transporter superfamily. *Molecular Biology and Evolution* 21: 1938–1949. https://doi.org/10.1093/molbev/msh205.

35 Juliano, R.L. and Ling, V. (1976). A surface glycoprotein modulating drug permeability in Chinese hamster ovary cell mutants. *Biochimica et Biophysica Acta* 455: 152–162. https://doi.org/10.1016/0005-2736(76)90160-7.

36 Gerlach, J.H., Endicott, J.A., Juranka, P.F. et al. (1986). Homology between P-glycoprotein and a bacterial haemolysin transport protein suggests a model for multidrug resistance. *Nature* 324: 485–489. https://doi.org/10.1038/324485a0.

37 Cowman, A.F., Karcz, S., Galatis, D. et al. (1991). A P-glycoprotein homologue of *Plasmodium falciparum* is localized on the digestive vacuole. *The Journal of Cell Biology* 113: 1033–1042. https://doi.org/10.1083/jcb.113.5.1033.

38 Lim, A.S. and Cowman, A.F. (1993). Phosphorylation of a P-glycoprotein homologue in *Plasmodium falciparum. Molecular and Biochemical Parasitology* 62: 293–302. https://doi.org/10.1016/0166-6851(93)90118-h.

39 Foote, S.J., Kyle, D.E., Martin, R.K. et al. (1990). Several alleles of the multidrug-resistance gene are closely linked to chloroquine resistance in *Plasmodium falciparum. Nature* 345: 255–258. https://doi.org/10.1038/345255a0.

40 Babiker, H.A., Pringle, S.J., Abdel-Muhsin, A. et al. (2001). High-level chloroquine resistance in Sudanese isolates of *Plasmodium falciparum* is associated with mutations in the chloroquine resistance transporter gene *pfcrt* and the multidrug resistance gene *pfmdr1. The Journal of Infectious Diseases* 183: 1535–1538. https://doi.org/10.1086/320195.

41 Harinasuta, T., Suntharasamai, P., and Viravan, C. (1965). Chloroquine-resistant falciparum malaria in Thailand. *Lancet* 2: 657–660. https://doi.org/10.1016/s0140-6736(65)90395-8.

42 Moore, D.V. and Lanier, J.E. (1961). Observations on two *Plasmodium falciparum* infections with an abnormal response to chloroquine. *The American Journal of Tropical Medicine and Hygiene* 10: 5–9. https://doi.org/10.4269/ajtmh.1961.10.5.

43 Grimmond, T.R., Donovan, K.O., and Riley, I.D. (1976). Chloroquine resistant malaria in Papua New Guinea. *Papua and New Guinea Medical Journal* 19: 184–185.

44 Lobel, H.O., Campbell, C.C., Schwartz, I.K. et al. (1985). Recent trends in the importation of malaria caused by *Plasmodium falciparum* into the United States from Africa. *The Journal of Infectious Diseases* 152: 613–617. https://doi.org/10.1093/infdis/152.3.613.

45 Talisuna, A.O., Bloland, P., and D'alessandro, U. (2004). History, dynamics, and public health importance of malaria parasite resistance. *Clinical Microbiology Reviews* 17: 235–254. https://doi.org/10.1128/cmr.17.1.235-254.2004.

46 Trape, J.F. (2001). The public health impact of chloroquine resistance in Africa. *The American Journal of Tropical Medicine and Hygiene* 64: 12–17. https://doi.org/10.4269/ajtmh.2001.64.12.

47 Balikagala, B., Sakurai-Yatsushiro, M., Tachibana, S.I. et al. (2020). Recovery and stable persistence of chloroquine sensitivity in *Plasmodium falciparum* parasites after its discontinued use in Northern Uganda. *Malaria Journal* 19: 76. https://doi.org/10.1186/s12936-020-03157-0.

48 Laufer, M.K., Thesing, P.C., Eddington, N.D. et al. (2006). Return of chloroquine antimalarial efficacy in Malawi. *The New England Journal of Medicine* 355: 1959–1966. https://doi.org/10.1056/NEJMoa062032.

49 Ocan, M., Akena, D., Nsobya, S. et al. (2019). Persistence of chloroquine resistance alleles in malaria endemic countries: a systematic review of burden and risk factors. *Malaria Journal* 18: 76. https://doi.org/10.1186/s12936-019-2716-z.

50 Das, S., Tripathy, S., Chattopadhayay, S. et al. (2017). Progressive increase in point mutations associates chloroquine resistance: even after withdrawal of chloroquine use in India. *International Journal for Parasitology: Drugs and Drug Resistance* 7: 251–261. https://doi.org/10.1016/j.ijpddr.2017.06.002.

51 WHO (2018). *World Malaria Report 2018*. Geneva: World Health Organization.

52 Curd, F.H.S., Davey, D.G., and Rose, F.L. (1945). Studies on synthetic antimalarial drugs. *Annals of Tropical Medicine and Parasitology* 39: 208–216. https://doi.org/10.1080/00034983.1945.11685237.

53 Falco, E.A., Goodwin, L.G., Hitchings, G.H. et al. (1951). 2:4-Diaminopyrimidines – a new series of antimalarials. *British Journal of Pharmacology and Chemotherapy* 6: 185–200. https://doi.org/10.1111/j.1476-5381.1951.tb00634.x.

54 Miller, K.D., Lobel, H.O., Pappaioanou, M. et al. (1986). Failures of combined chloroquine and Fansidar prophylaxis in American travelers to East Africa. *The Journal of Infectious Diseases* 154: 689–691. https://doi.org/10.1093/infdis/154.4.689.

55 Bzik, D.J., Li, W.B., Horii, T. et al. (1987). Molecular cloning and sequence analysis of the *Plasmodium falciparum* dihydrofolate reductase-thymidylate synthase gene. *Proceedings of the National Academy of Sciences of the United States of America* 84: 8360–8364. https://doi.org/10.1073/pnas.84.23.8360.

56 Hyde, J.E. (2005). Exploring the folate pathway in *Plasmodium falciparum*. *Acta Tropica* 94: 191–206. https://doi.org/10.1016/j.actatropica.2005.04.002.

57 Peters, W. (1970). *Chemotherapy and Drug Resistance in Malaria*. Academic Press.

58 Triglia, T. and Cowman, A.F. (1994). Primary structure and expression of the dihydropteroate synthetase gene of *Plasmodium falciparum*. *Proceedings of the National Academy of Sciences of the United States of America* 91: 7149–7153. https://doi.org/10.1073/pnas.91.15.7149.

59 Chulay, J.D., Watkins, W.M., and Sixsmith, D.G. (1984). Synergistic antimalarial activity of pyrimethamine and sulfadoxine against *Plasmodium falciparum* in vitro. *The American Journal of Tropical Medicine and Hygiene* 33: 325–330. https://doi.org/10.4269/ajtmh.1984.33.325.

60 Bloland, P., Kazembe, P., Oloo, A. et al. (1998). Chloroquine in Africa: critical assessment and recommendations for monitoring and evaluating chloroquine therapy efficacy in sub-Saharan Africa. *Tropical Medicine & International Health* 3: 543–552.

61 Wernsdorfer, W.H. (1994). Epidemiology of drug resistance in malaria. *Acta Tropica* 56: 143–156. https://doi.org/10.1016/0001-706x(94)90060-4.

62 White, N.J. (1992). Antimalarial drug resistance: the pace quickens. *The Journal of Antimicrobial Chemotherapy* 30: 571–585. https://doi.org/10.1093/jac/30.5.571.

63 Hastings, I.M., Watkins, W.M., and White, N.J. (2002). The evolution of drug-resistant malaria: the role of drug elimination half-life. *Philosophical Transactions of the Royal Society of London. Series B, Biological Sciences* 357: 505–519. https://doi.org/10.1098/rstb.2001.1036.

64 Iyer, J.K., Milhous, W.K., Cortese, J.F. et al. (2001). *Plasmodium falciparum* cross-resistance between trimethoprim and pyrimethamine. *Lancet* 358: 1066–1067. https://doi.org/10.1016/S0140-6736(01)06201-8.

65 Simpson, J.A., Watkins, E.R., Price, R.N. et al. (2000). Mefloquine pharmacokinetic–pharmacodynamic models: implications for dosing and resistance. *Antimicrobial Agents and Chemotherapy* 44: 3414–3424. https://doi.org/10.1128/aac.44.12.3414-3424.2000.

66 White, N. (1999). Antimalarial drug resistance and combination chemotherapy. *Philosophical Transactions of the Royal Society of London. Series B, Biological Sciences* 354: 739–749. https://doi.org/10.1098/rstb.1999.0426.

67 Korsinczky, M., Fischer, K., Chen, N. et al. (2004). Sulfadoxine resistance in *Plasmodium vivax* is associated with a specific amino acid in dihydropteroate synthase at the putative sulfadoxine-binding site. *Antimicrobial Agents and Chemotherapy* 48: 2214–2222. https://doi.org/10.1128/AAC.48.6.2214-2222.2004.

68 Wang, P., Lee, C.S., Bayoumi, R. et al. (1997). Resistance to antifolates in *Plasmodium falciparum* monitored by sequence analysis of dihydropteroate synthetase and dihydrofolate reductase alleles in a large number of field samples of diverse origins. *Molecular and Biochemical Parasitology* 89: 161–177. https://doi.org/10.1016/s0166-6851(97)00114-x.

69 Naidoo, I. and Roper, C. (2013). Mapping 'partially resistant', 'fully resistant', and 'super resistant' malaria. *Trends in Parasitology* 29: 505–515. https://doi.org/10.1016/j.pt.2013.08.002.

70 Harrington, W.E., Mutabingwa, T.K., Kabyemela, E. et al. (2011). Intermittent treatment to prevent pregnancy malaria does not confer benefit in an area of widespread drug resistance. *Clinical Infectious Diseases* 53: 224–230. https://doi.org/10.1093/cid/cir376.

71 Rogerson, S.J., Desai, M., Mayor, A. et al. (2018). Burden, pathology, and costs of malaria in pregnancy: new developments for an old problem. *The Lancet Infectious Diseases* 18: e107–e118. https://doi.org/10.1016/S1473-3099(18)30066-5.

72 Hartman, T.K., Rogerson, S.J., and Fischer, P.R. (2010). The impact of maternal malaria on newborns. *Annals of Tropical Paediatrics* 30: 271–282. https://doi.org/10.1179/146532810X12858955921032.

73 Gesase, S., Gosling, R.D., Hashim, R. et al. (2009). High resistance of *Plasmodium falciparum* to sulphadoxine/pyrimethamine in northern Tanzania and the emergence of dhps resistance mutation at Codon 581. *PLoS One* 4: e4569. https://doi.org/10.1371/journal.pone.0004569.

74 Mixson-Hayden, T., Jain, V., Mccollum, A.M. et al. (2010). Evidence of selective sweeps in genes conferring resistance to chloroquine and pyrimethamine in *Plasmodium falciparum* isolates in India. *Antimicrobial Agents and Chemotherapy* 54: 997–1006. https://doi.org/10.1128/AAC.00846-09.

75 Payne, D. (1987). Spread of chloroquine resistance in *Plasmodium falciparum*. *Parasitology Today* 3: 241–246. https://doi.org/10.1016/0169-4758(87)90147-5.

76 Shah, N.K., Dhillon, G.P., Dash, A.P. et al. (2011). Antimalarial drug resistance of *Plasmodium falciparum* in India: changes over time and space. *The Lancet Infectious Diseases* 11: 57–64. https://doi.org/10.1016/S1473-3099(10)70214-0.

77 Verdrager, J. (1986). Epidemiology of the emergence and spread of drug-resistant falciparum malaria in South-East Asia and Australasia. *The Journal of Tropical Medicine and Hygiene* 89: 277–289.

78 Verdrager, J. (1995). Localized permanent epidemics: the genesis of chloroquine resistance in *Plasmodium falciparum*. *The Southeast Asian Journal of Tropical Medicine and Public Health* 26: 23–28.

79 Tu, Y. (2011). The discovery of artemisinin (qinghaosu) and gifts from Chinese medicine. *Nature Medicine* 17: 1217–1220. https://doi.org/10.1038/nm.2471.

80 Witkowski, B., Lelièvre, J., Barragán, M.J. et al. (2010). Increased tolerance to artemisinin in *Plasmodium falciparum* is mediated by a quiescence mechanism. *Antimicrobial Agents and Chemotherapy* 54: 1872–1877. https://doi.org/10.1128/AAC.01636-09.

81 Cheeseman, I.H., Miller, B.A., Nair, S. et al. (2012). A major genome region underlying artemisinin resistance in malaria. *Science* 336: 79–82. https://doi.org/10.1126/science.1215966.

82 Miotto, O., Almagro-Garcia, J., Manske, M. et al. (2013). Multiple populations of artemisinin-resistant *Plasmodium falciparum* in Cambodia. *Nature Genetics* 45: 648–655. https://doi.org/10.1038/ng.2624.

83 Ariey, F., Witkowski, B., Amaratunga, C. et al. (2014). A molecular marker of artemisinin-resistant *Plasmodium falciparum* malaria. *Nature* 505: 50–55. https://doi.org/10.1038/nature12876.

84 Straimer, J., Gnädig, N.F., Witkowski, B. et al. (2015). Drug resistance. K13-propeller mutations confer artemisinin resistance in *Plasmodium falciparum* clinical isolates. *Science* 347: 428–431. https://doi.org/10.1126/science.1260867.

85 Ghorbal, M., Gorman, M., Macpherson, C.R. et al. (2014). Genome editing in the human malaria parasite *Plasmodium falciparum* using the CRISPR-Cas9 system. *Nature Biotechnology* 32: 819–821. https://doi.org/10.1038/nbt.2925.

86 Mbengue, A., Bhattacharjee, S., Pandharkar, T. et al. (2015). A molecular mechanism of artemisinin resistance in *Plasmodium falciparum* malaria. *Nature* 520: 683–687. https://doi.org/10.1038/nature14412.

87 Ismail, H.M., Barton, V., Phanchana, M. et al. (2016). Artemisinin activity-based probes identify multiple molecular targets within the asexual stage of the malaria parasites *Plasmodium falciparum* 3D7. *Proceedings of the National Academy of Sciences of the United States of America* 113: 2080–2085. https://doi.org/10.1073/pnas.1600459113.

88 Wang, J., Zhang, C.J., Chia, W.N. et al. (2015). Haem-activated promiscuous targeting of artemisinin in *Plasmodium falciparum*. *Nature Communications* 6: 10111. https://doi.org/10.1038/ncomms10111.

89 Nikesitch, N., Tao, C., Lai, K. et al. (2016). Predicting the response of multiple myeloma to the proteasome inhibitor Bortezomib by evaluation of the unfolded protein response. *Blood Cancer Journal* 6: e432. https://doi.org/10.1038/bcj.2016.40.

90 Zhang, M., Wang, C., Otto, T.D. et al. (2018). Uncovering the essential genes of the human malaria parasite by saturation mutagenesis. *Science* 360: https://doi.org/10.1126/science.aap7847.

91 Birnbaum, J., Flemming, S., Reichard, N. et al. (2017). A genetic system to study *Plasmodium falciparum* protein function. *Nature Methods* 14: 450–456. https://doi.org/10.1038/nmeth.4223.

92 Hott, A., Casandra, D., Sparks, K.N. et al. (2015). Artemisinin-resistant *Plasmodium falciparum* parasites exhibit altered patterns of development in infected erythrocytes. *Antimicrobial Agents and Chemotherapy* 59: 3156–3167. https://doi.org/10.1128/AAC.00197-15.

93 Wang, Z., Wang, Y., Cabrera, M. et al. (2015). Artemisinin resistance at the China–Myanmar border and association with mutations in the K13 propeller gene. *Antimicrobial Agents and Chemotherapy* 59: 6952–6959. https://doi.org/10.1128/AAC.01255-15.

6

Current Therapies and New Drug Targets for the Future Drug Development of Drug Resistant Malaria

Pooja Mittal[1] and Rupesh K. Gautam[2]

[1] *RIMT University, School of Pharmaceutical Sciences, Mandi Gobindgarh, Punjab, India*
[2] *Maharishi Markandeshwar University, MM School of Pharmacy, Sadopur, Ambala, Haryana 134007, India*

6.1 Introduction

The term *malaria* is an Italian term, which means bad air. This term was coined by Dr. Francisco Torti when he found that the people infected with this disease are from marshy lands with foul air. Later on in 1880, the French army physician discovered that this disease is caused by the protozoan. Malaria is caused by the parasite of *Plasmodium* genus. It is transmitted via the bites of infected female mosquito of *Anopheles* species. Two species of *Plasmodium* exist, i.e. *P. falciparum and P. vivax*, but the infection caused by the former one is deadliest. Children and pregnant women are at high risk of morbidity if they develop malaria [1].

In 2017, the statistics supplied by World Health Organization says that, there were 219 million cases of malaria worldwide where 2 million cases of malaria were increased from the past year, which also resulted in 435 000 deaths. Per day data includes approximately 1190 deaths, which include mostly young children. However, from 2000, the figures of malaria cases had been decreased by 37% worldwide, but the continuous data has shown that this decrease phase is now plateauing slowly. Five strains of malaria parasite are present, among which *Plasmodium falciparum* is the most dangerous one. Almost half of the world population is at risk of developing malaria where Africa has the maximum share of approximately 90% in both, i.e. cases development and deaths [2–5].

The rise in cases of malaria-related morbidity and the development of drug-resistant malaria have motivated the researchers to find the molecular pathway and pathogenesis of the disease so that new molecular targets can be evaluated to combat this deadliest disease completely. The knowledge of sanitation and healthy living style has led to the eradication of malaria up to some extent, but still a lot of work has to be done. The multifaceted life cycle with various stages needs to be studied at the molecular level so that numerous potential targets can be generated for the development of some vaccine or some treatment formulation for the complete eradication of this deadly disease [1, 6].

Drug Development for Malaria: Novel Approaches for Prevention and Treatment, First Edition.
Edited by Pravin Kendrekar.

6.2 Life Cycle of *Plasmodium falciparum*

Plasmodium species work with the help of two hosts, i.e. vertebrates and mosquito. The sporozoites infect the *Anopheles* mosquitoes and get transferred to human host with the bite of infected mosquito, then get loaded into the parenchymal cells of the liver where they get multiplied and form the tissue schizonts, which forms the pre-erythrocytic phase of the malarial infection and lasts upto 5–16 days depending upon the species. After this, the merozoite enters into the erythrocytic phase and starts invading the erythrocytes. Hypnozoites are formed in the exoerythrocytic phase, which is the dormant phase of malarial infection. Some hypnozoites remain dormant for six to eight months in case of *Plasmodium vivax* and *Plasmodium ovale* infections, but not in case of *P. falciparum* and *Plasmodium malariae* infections. The schizonts containing erythrocytes rupture and release up to 6–32 merozoites. Here comes the stage of feeling chills and fever. This stage of identification requires the management via drugs. The released merozoite starts the new cycle, and the process continues till the death of the host or the management by the drug therapy [7].

Some merozoites are differentiated into male as well as female gametocytes, which are taken up by the female *Anopheles* mosquito during the blood meal and there they undergo the sexual cycle, which is known as sporogony generating zygotes. These zygotes invade the middle gut wall of the mosquito and here they develop the oocysts. The oocysts grow and rupture to release the sporozoites, which infect the salivary glands of the mosquitos. Infection to a new human host via infected *Anopheles* mosquitoes starts a new cycle [5, 8, 9] (Figure 6.1).

6.3 Current Antimalarial Therapy and Their Shortcomings

Currently used marketed antimalarial drugs can be divided into three broad categories depending upon their chemical structures and their metabolism [10–12]. The drugs along with their categories are mentioned in Table 6.1.

Quinine was isolated in 1820 and was effectively used in the management of malaria. Further, more compounds were synthesized by using this plant material, but with the time course, the new strains of plasmodium started originating, and they were least responsive to the quinine therapy. This phenomenon is called as development of resistance [13, 14].

Quinine: It was isolated from the Cinchona bark and had become the most effective treatment of malaria. In 1980, the resistance to quinine was first reported, and from 2006, it was stopped to be used as first-line treatment, but still it is present in WHO list of essential medicines. It is used in the treatment of severe cases where artemisinins are no longer available [15–17].

Mepacrine: This drug was used throughout the Second World War under the brand name of Atabrine. This is a derivative of methylene blue; however, this drug was refused by the companies from past decade, but the derivatives of methylene blue are the area of interest of today's research. Mepacrine has been withdrawn from the market as it was causing serious toxic and psychosis effects [18, 19].

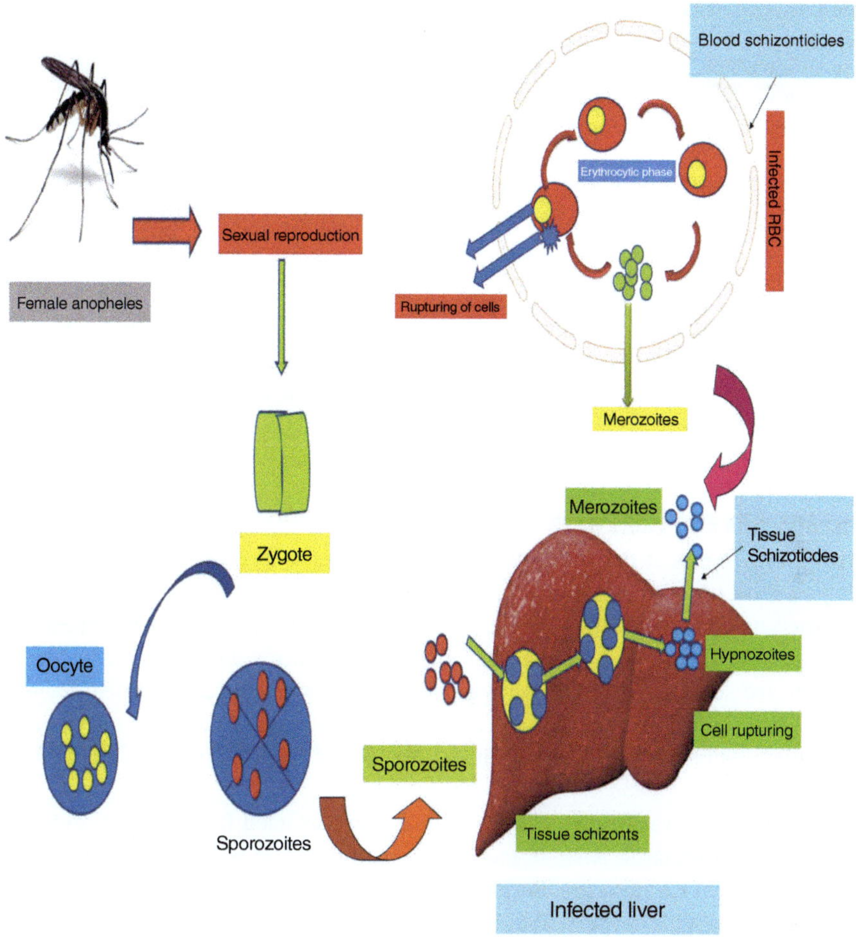

Figure 6.1 Life cycle and various stages of malarial parasite *Plasmodium falciparum*.

Chloroquine: From 1940, chloroquine (CQ) was used as an effective antimalarial drug, which has least side effects, but the cases to CQ were reported in 1950, when the multiple strains of *Plasmodium* species were reported. The new strains of parasite are now utilized in potency analyzing studies. Still CQ is in the list of WHO essential medicines and is utilized in the areas where the resistance has not developed till date [20, 21].

Mefloquine: In 1970, mefloquine (MQ) was developed in Indian army, and it is the effective medicine that is still being used for the management of malaria. No cases of resistance had been found so for with MQ. Initially it was used for the treatment of CQ-resistant malaria and is used for both curative and prophylactic purposes. It is structurally related to quinine drugs and works by disruption of RBCs at the blood stage of parasite. Nowadays, these drugs are used in combinations to prevent the resistance to the therapy. Lariam is a brand name of the racemic mixture of MQ; however, it is also not widely used nowadays with a precipitation that it will cause toxicity to the central nervous system [22].

Table 6.1 Classification of currently used antimalarial drugs.

Aryl aminoalcohol compounds	Antifolate compounds	Artemisinin compounds
Quinine, Quinidine, Halofantrine, Lumafantrine, Chloroquine, Mefloquine, Amodiaquine, Cycloquine etc.	Proguanil, Pyrimathamine, Trimethoprim, etc.	Artemisinin, Dihydroartemisinin, Artesunate, etc.

Halofantrine (HF): It was developed between 1960 and 1970. Initially it was used for the treatment of all forms of Plasmodium parasite while its use was diminished over the period of time as it was found to cause cardiotoxicity. Currently, it is being used only for curative purpose not for the prophylactic purpose under the brand name of Halfan, but the patient should not be suffering from any heart-related disease [23].

Artemisinins and their derivatives: It was firstly isolated in 1970 from the plant *Artimisia annua*. It comes under the list of Chinese herbal medicines list, and it possess a great positive impact on malaria. It had shown its great impact on all the multidrug-resistant forms of *P. falciparum*. Artemisinins, artemether, and artesunate are the most important forms of artemisinins. Prodrugs are also used, which are semisynthetic derivatives of artemisinins. Dihydroartemisinin is an active metabolite of the prodrug of artemisinin; however, slowly, the resistance to artemisinins had also developed, and it was firstly reported in 2008 in California [24, 25].

Amodiaquine: It was firstly isolated in 1948 and was used for uncomplicated and mild cases of malaria. Also, it was used in combination of artesunate under the brand name of Camoquine. Similar to CQ, amidaquine is also thought to cause complexation with heme, which will prevent the formation of hemazoin [26, 27].

Piperaquine: It was developed in 1960 in China and was initially used as a replacement to CQ as the developed resistance to CQ had diminished its use alone. Although its mechanism is not clearly understood, but it is believed to interfere in vacuole formation where it will interfere in heme detoxification process. Now a days, it is being used in combination with dihydroartemisinin for the treatment of malaria [28, 29].

Lumefantrine: It was first isolated in 1976 in China and was sold under the brand name of Coartem. Exact mechanism of action of this drug is unknown; however, it was found to inhibit the nucleic acid and protein synthesis in the parasite. Currently, it is being utilized in combination with artemisinin [30–33].

6.4 Drug Targets for Current Antimalarial Therapy

Currently available antimalarial drugs target the asexual erythrocytic stages of the malarial parasite; hence they are named as schizonticidal drugs, whereas the tissue schizonticidal drugs attack the hypozoites present in the liver of host. Gametocidal antimalarial drugs are also available, which kill the asexual erythrocytic forms of the parasite present in the bloodstream. CQ, Quinine and mefloquinine are the typical examples of schizonticidal drugs while pyrimethamine, sulfonamine, and sulfones are the examples of schizonticidal drugs, whereas proguanil and primaquine are faster acting and potent schizonticidal drugs. The basis of classification of various drugs is the major metabolic pathway of all these drugs. The major pathways involved in the metabolism of these drugs are oxidative stress, nucleic acid metabolism, heme toxification, and fatty acid synthesis, which have been targeted for the treatment of malaria. The resistance to the available antimalarial drugs develops within the body of the host during the course of chemotherapy [34]. The emergence of resistance is the major obstacle in the management of this disease, which calls for the need to identify newer molecular targets for the better treatment of this deadly disease. According to the latest research data, no potent antimalarial drug is available, which is developed rationally to inhibit the new molecular targets of the disease or which can prevent the emergence of resistance by the disease [35]. However, the antimalarial activity was shown by all the available drugs during *in-vivo* studies, which results in uncertainty in their mechanisms of actions. Till date, no promising evidences are present, which can claim the reason of originating resistance with the current therapy; however, molecular, pharmacological, and genetic approaches have concluded that the reason of emergence of resistance is the mutation or the gene duplication on the genes of their key enzymes or transporters. Like resistance of CQ is due to the mutation in *Pfndr1* and *Pfcrt* genes. A point mutation of dihydrofolate reductase and dihydroprotease synthase is the reason of resistance development in antifolates. It has also been shown that the incomplete cure provided by the antimalarial drugs resulted in the production of drug-resistant mutants. This increasing spread of drug-resistant malaria has created an enormous pressure on the healthcare system to come up with a solution that can provide the effective treatment without causing the resistance to the medication [36, 37].

6.4.1 Drug-Resistant Malaria and Identification of New Targets

To cure the malaria, a consistent effort over this time period is going on. Development of drug resistance is the most difficult hurdle in the successful antimalarial therapy, and the whole of the antimalarial research is oriented toward the eradication of the spread of this resistance. The drug targets are being studied at their molecular level. In spite of the urgent requirement, pharmaceutical companies are looking for new treatment compounds with a newer mechanism of action. They are exploiting the metabolic and chemical pathways of the parasite in the hope to develop some new drug targets. These studies are underway to provide the new specific inhibitors, which can act as new drug targets [4, 38, 39]. An overview of the various new drug targets is shown in Figure 6.2 and Table 6.2.

6.4.1.1 Food Vacuole as Drug Targets

Food vacuoles are formulated by the fusion of food molecules during the developmental stages of malaria parasite in the host body. This formed organelle causes the degradation of 60–80% of the hemoglobin of the host and thus provides a pool of the

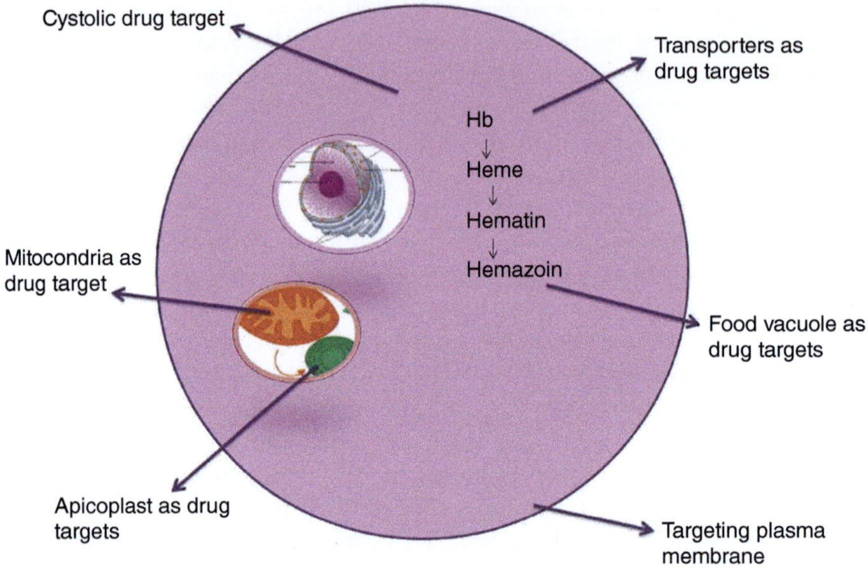

Figure 6.2 Illustration of various new drug targets for antimalarial therapy.

amino acids necessary for the growth of the malaria parasite inside the host body. Targeting this pathway can prove to be a promising approach for the treatment of malaria in this era.

Targeting protease enzyme: The initiation of this pathway occurs by the series of protease enzymes, which digest the hemoglobin into small fragments. During this process, heme is released as a toxic by-product, which gets converted into hemazoin containing 95% of free iron that was produced during the digestion of hemoglobin. Hemoglobin is the main product and serves as the main source of amino acids for malarial parasites. In the acidic environment of food vacuole, the hydrolysis of hemoglobin into small peptides and their transfer to the cells of the parasites are done by some aspartic enzymes. These peptides are essential for the growth of parasites as they provide essential amino acids to them. Four aspartic proteases, namely Plasmepsins I, II, and IV and metaloproteases, cysteine proteases, histoaspartic protease, and some dipeptidyl aminopeptidase 1 are involved in the process of proteolysis. These enzymes play an essential role in antimalarial therapy as they help in degradation of hemoglobin and help the parasites in their survival so they could be an important target for the treatment. The inhibitors of these proteases also play important role as they help in dissection of the molecular mechanisms, interrupt the merozoite release, and thereby prevent the parasite growth and hence can be developed into antimalarial therapy. Human immunodeficiency virus (HIV) protease inhibitors can also be used as potent antimalarial drugs as they affect the erythrocytic stage of the parasite. For example, when ritonavir and saquinavir combined with CQ, they provide the promising results, but their primary target and their exact mechanism of action are not yet investigated completely [49–51].

Table 6.2 Current drug targets and their related metabolic pathways to be targeted.

Main drug targets	Metabolic pathways that can be targeted	References
Food vacuole as drug targets	• Inhibition of protease • Interfere with hemazoin formation	[38]
Targeting plasma membrane	• Inhibiting membrane biosynthesis • New permeability pathways to stop the supply of nutrients	[40]
Transporters as drug targets	• Inhibiting phosphatidyl choline synthesis	[36, 41]
Cystolic drug targets	• Folate pathway • Glycolysis pathway • Purine biosynthesis • Nucleotide synthesis • Shikimic acid pathway • Thiol metabolism • Protein kinase	[4, 42, 43]
Apicoplast drug targets	• Fatty acid biosynthesis • Isopropenoid biosynthesis • Heme biosynthesis • Plastic DNA replication • Protein farnesylation	[44–46]
Mitochondria as drug targets	• Inhibit dihyroorotate dehydrogenase • Inhibit dihydrofolate reductase • Targeting NADPH reductase	[47, 48]

Inhibition of hemazoin crystal formation: Degradation of the hemoglobin inside the human host results in the release of a large amount of heme as a by-product, which is very much toxic to the parasites. Heme can damage the cell membrane of the parasite because of its peroxidative properties [52]. The conversion of heme to hemazoin is the most important pathway in *P. falciparum*, which involves two-step reaction. In the first step, heme gets converted into hematin, which is then converted into hemazoin with the help of histidine-rich protein 2 (HRP-2) so targeting of this pathway or targeting of HRP-2 protein could be the potential target for antimalarial therapy. Hemozin is a crystalline polymer, which is identical to beta hematin. Hematin is a known target for many schizonticidal drugs such as quinine, chloroquinine, mefloquinine, and HF, etc. These drugs prevent the detoxification of the hematin and also convert the same to a microcrystalline dimer complex known as hemazoin. Recent research on antimalarials has also revealed the fact that artemisinin binds to heme for its antimalarial activity, and hence, prevention of heme sequestering for its conversion to hemazoin can be the new molecular target for patent antimalarial action [36].

Targeting heme detoxification: For parasite survival, it is essential to remove the toxic heme. To assist in the toxic removal process, it is converted into hemazoin as well as heme is also degraded by hydrogen peroxide released during the conversion of oxyhemoglobin to methemoglobin. It has also been evaluated that,

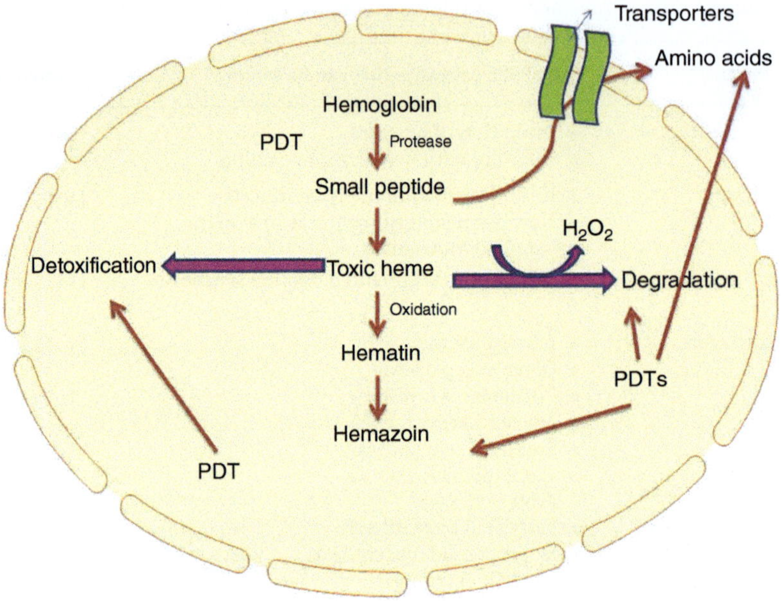

Figure 6.3 Potential drug targets in food vacuole.

on degradation of hemoglobin, peptides are released, which are transported to cytoplasm where they are further digested to produce the amino acids, which are taken up by the parasite for their survival. So, the transporters must be there, which helps in terminal degradation of peptides into amino acids. So, targeting of these transporters can be a vital target for the new antimalarials [2, 3, 15] (Figure 6.3).

Inhibiting proteasome: Proteasome is a protein complex, which degrades the proteins via breaking the peptide bonds. This is a part of the essential biological pathway by which the cells regulate the concentration of proteins inside the cells. Therefore, targeting of proteasome could also provide a potential target for the antimalarial activity. Development of protease inhibitors was also investigated for the treatment of tuberculosis. Inhibition of protease enzyme can induce apoptosis in cancer cells also, so they can be the potential targets for anticancer therapy as well [6, 18, 22, 40].

Apicoplasts as drug targets: Apicoplast is a type of plastid present inside the parasite. This is a non-photosynthetic plastid, which is responsible for various biochemical pathways. Among the various pathways, fatty acid biosynthesis, isoprenoid precursors, and heme synthesis are the vital pathways that are essential for the survival of the parasite. However, these pathways are absent in the human hosts, so these are parasite-specific, which can be targeted.

Synthesis of fatty acids as target: Biosynthesis of the fatty acids is essential for the growth of parasite within the host cell as huge amount of fatty acids are needed for the biosynthesis of cell membranes, and they also protect the parasites from the defense mechanism of the host. Fatty acids are also essential for cell

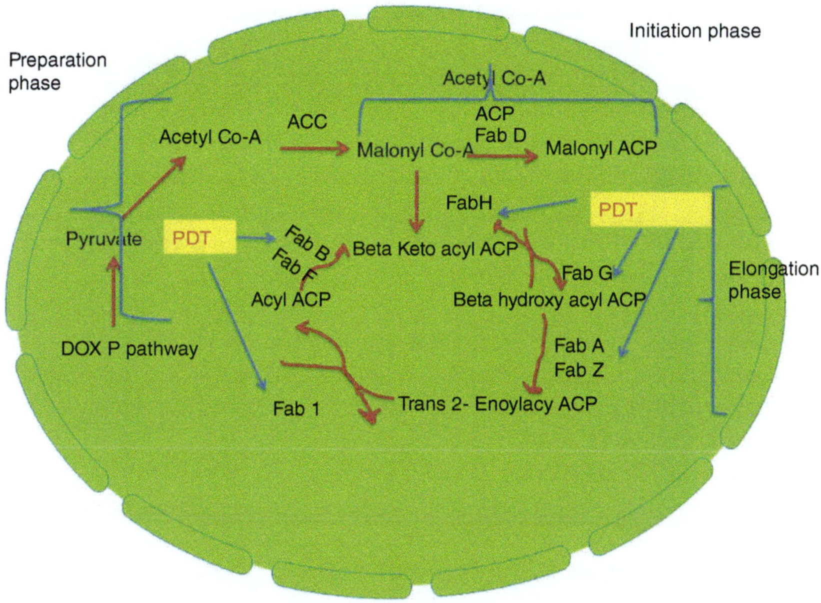

Figure 6.4 Various phases of fatty acid synthesis in apicoplasts as potential drug targets (PDTs).

growth, differentiation, and are the huge source of energy. Biosynthetic pathways of human host (FAS I) and parasite (FAS II) are different from each other, thereby can act as potential targets for the antimalarial treatment [23, 26, 38].

Various phases are involved in the fatty acid synthesis such as preparation phase, initiation phase, and elongation phase. Each phase involves a number of enzymes or proteins, which can be targeted for the antimalarial action. The various phases and enzymes involved are depicted in Figure 6.4.

Targeting heme biosynthesis: Malarial parasites synthesize heme by de novo pathway. Synthesis of the same needs aminoleulinic acid (ALA), which is the main precursor of heme synthesis. ALA is synthesized by glycine and succinyl CoA inside the host cell by using ALA dehydratase enzymes. The parasite imports the required enzymes and other precursor materials from the host red blood cells, and inhibition of this transporter can act as a valid target for antimalarial therapy. CQ, artemisinin, and other schizonticidal drugs act by interfering the heme metabolism.

DNA translation: It had been observed that the DNA of apicoplast has their own coding potential, i.e. they underwent some processes such as replication, transcription, and translation, etc. to produce the new DNA material. These processes are similar to that of prokaryotic replication process. Many antibacterial compounds are known, which inhibit the prokaryotic machinery to replicate; macrolids, clindamycin, tetracycline, etc. inhibit the various stages of protein synthesis; quinolones inhibit DNA gyrase enzyme while rifampicin inhibits RNA polymerase enzyme. All these mentioned compounds can result in delayed death. Moreover, at the protein synthesis level, it had been observed that peptide deformylase, which has the ability to deformylate the *N*-formylmethionine into a newly synthesized protein, could also act as a potential target [13, 16, 24, 47, 52].

Lipoic acid biosynthetic pathway: This pathway had been extensively investigated in case of *Plasmodium* species as this pathway provides the major part of lipoate cofactor required for the functioning of pyruvate dehydrogenase, which is involved in FAS II pathway. Lipoate is a sulfur containing octanoic acid derivative, which is essentially required for the growth of pathogens. Targeting of lipoate could act as a potential target for the antimalarial therapy [40].

Also, the apicoplast has its own genome, which encodes for about 30 proteins and most of the proteins present in apicoplasts are nuclear encoded. The genome of *P. falciparum* is 5–10 times more studied than any other species. Therefore, the protein trafficking becomes an important target for antimalarial therapy in case of *P. falciparum* species [3, 6, 23].

Cytoplasmic metabolic processes as drug targets: A number of metabolic processes occur inside the parasite's cystole, which involve a number of enzymes. Hence, these enzymes can act as potential drug targets for the advanced antimalarial therapy [13, 26, 46–48].

6.4.1.2 Shikimic Acid Pathway Targeting

Shikimic acid pathway is a metabolic route pathway, which is followed in all fungi, bacteria, algae, parasites, and plant species for the generation of aromatic amino acids. All the *Plasmodium* species also require amino acids for their survival. The Shikimic acid pathway is a multistep reaction, which requires the involvement of various enzymes or the catalysts at all the stages. Targeting of these enzymes can be the potential drug target for antimalarial therapy. Moreover, the shikimate pathway is absent in mammals, so it can be excellent drug target for the chemotherapy also [6, 38]. The various stages and the enzymes involved in all the stages are shown in Figure 6.5.

This pathway consists of seven stages , which generate chorismate as an important molecule of the carbohydrate metabolism. Chorismate is further utilized for the synthesis of various important molecules such as tryptophan, ubiquinone, tyrosine, vitamin K, and *para*-amino benzoic acid, which are utilized in folate synthesis. Moreover, the various enzymes are being utilized at various stages of shikimate pathway; chorismate synthase and 5-enol-pyruvylshikimate-3-phosphate are the potential drug targets. Chorismate synthase is identified as the promising drug target as it is essential for the normal growth of the parasite cells.

6.4.1.3 Targeting Folate Pathway and Methionine Synthesis Pathway

Folate pathway is an essential pathway for the growth of cells as this provides a folate cofactor, which is needed for the DNA synthesis. Hence, the inhibition of this pathway could lead to the sequential death of the cells as new DNAs will not be able to get synthesized, which ultimately leads to the death of the parasite. Dihydrofolate synthesis requires the involvement of seven enzymes at various stages; however, out of these seven enzymes, only two enzymes have been extensively studied for antimalarial therapy, which are dihydrofolate reductase (DHFR) and

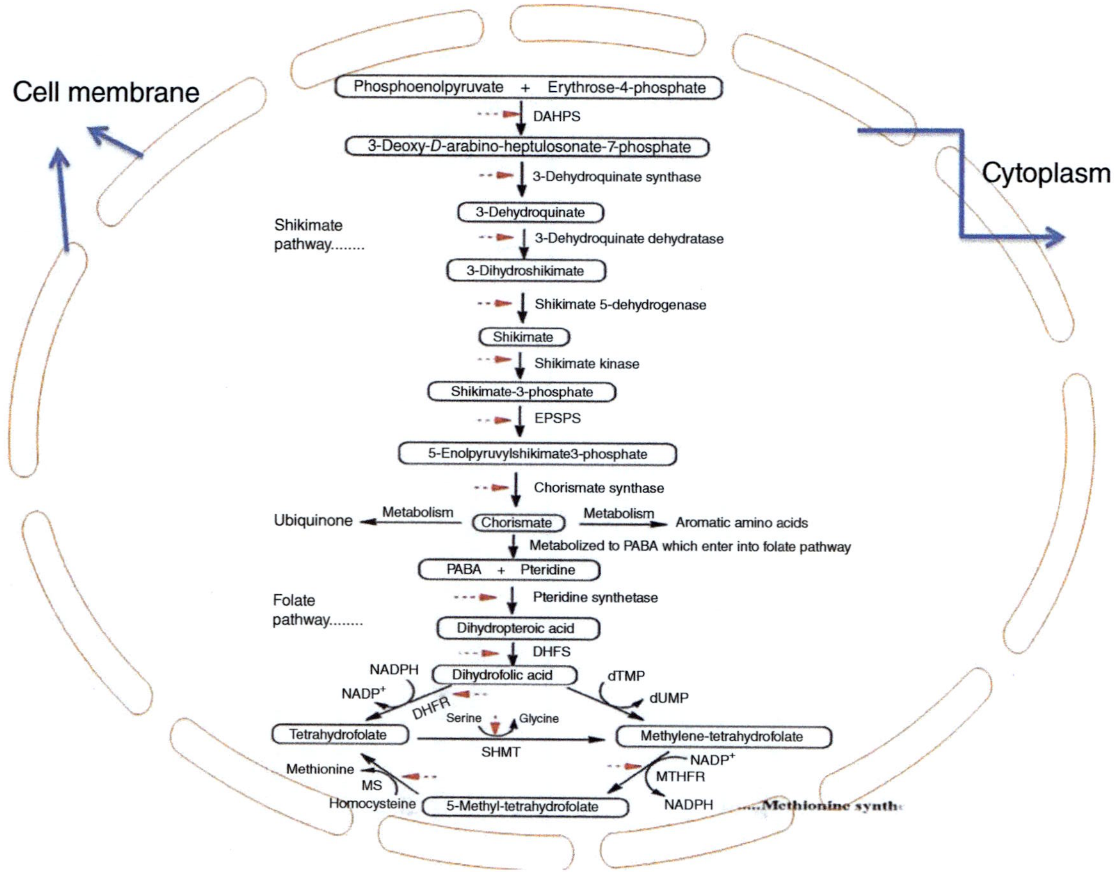

Figure 6.5 Shikimate acid pathway showing the various stages and potential drug targets at all the stages.

dihydropteroate synthase (DHPS). These enzymes are absent in the mammals, so these targets can be evaluated for further investigations also [13, 16, 27, 49, 50].

6.4.1.4 Glycolytic Pathway Inhibition

Plasmodium parasite depends on glucose as it is the primary source of energy that is required for all the metabolic processes. The main enzyme of this pathway is lactate dehydrogenase (LDH), which codes for some unique amino acids and that amino acids can serve as the potential drug targets.

A much attention is given to LDH enzyme and LDH inhibitors such as gossypol derivatives and napthoic acid derivatives have been developed. Oxamate is a competitive inhibitor, which also has the high affinity for LDH [24, 46, 49, 50]. All the key steps, required enzymes, and the potential drug targets have been mentioned in Figure 6.6.

6.4.2 Mitochondria as Drug Targets

Mitochondria is an essential part of *Plasmodium* parasites as it serves the two basic functions, i.e. electron transport and synthesis of proteins. Both the functions are essential for the physiological functions of the body. However, there is a significant difference between the molecular mechanism of parasite's mitochondria and host mitochondria so it can be served as a potential drug target for antimalarial chemotherapy [1, 30, 52].

6.4.2.1 Targeting Electron Transport Chain

The electron transport chain of parasite contains five dehydrogenases, e.g. NADH:ubiquinone oxidoreductase, glycerol-3 phosphate dehydrogenase, succinate:ubiquonone oxidoreductase, and malate quinine oxidoreductase. The activity of dehydrogenase serves the electrons to downstream. This can serve as a potential drug target for antimalarial activity.

There is structural difference between the cytoplasm of host and parasite, and the mitochondrial differences between two serve as another potential target for antimalarial therapy [4, 7, 11, 19, 43].

6.4.2.2 Inhibition of Dihydroorate Dehydrogenase

Malarial parasite is dependent on the de novo synthesis as it cannot synthesize the pyrimidine of its own. Pyrimidines are the essential macromolecules, which are essential for the synthesis of DNA, RNA, phospholipids, and glycoproteins. Dihyroorate dehydrogenase enzyme is a flavin-based mononucleotide-dependent enzyme, which catalyzes the one of the rate-limiting steps of de novo pathway of pyrimidine synthesis. The electrons synthesized in the above step will be directly fed into electron transport chain. Inhibition of dihyroorate dehydrogenase enzyme can serve as a potential drug target for antimalarial therapy [8, 17, 34, 45].

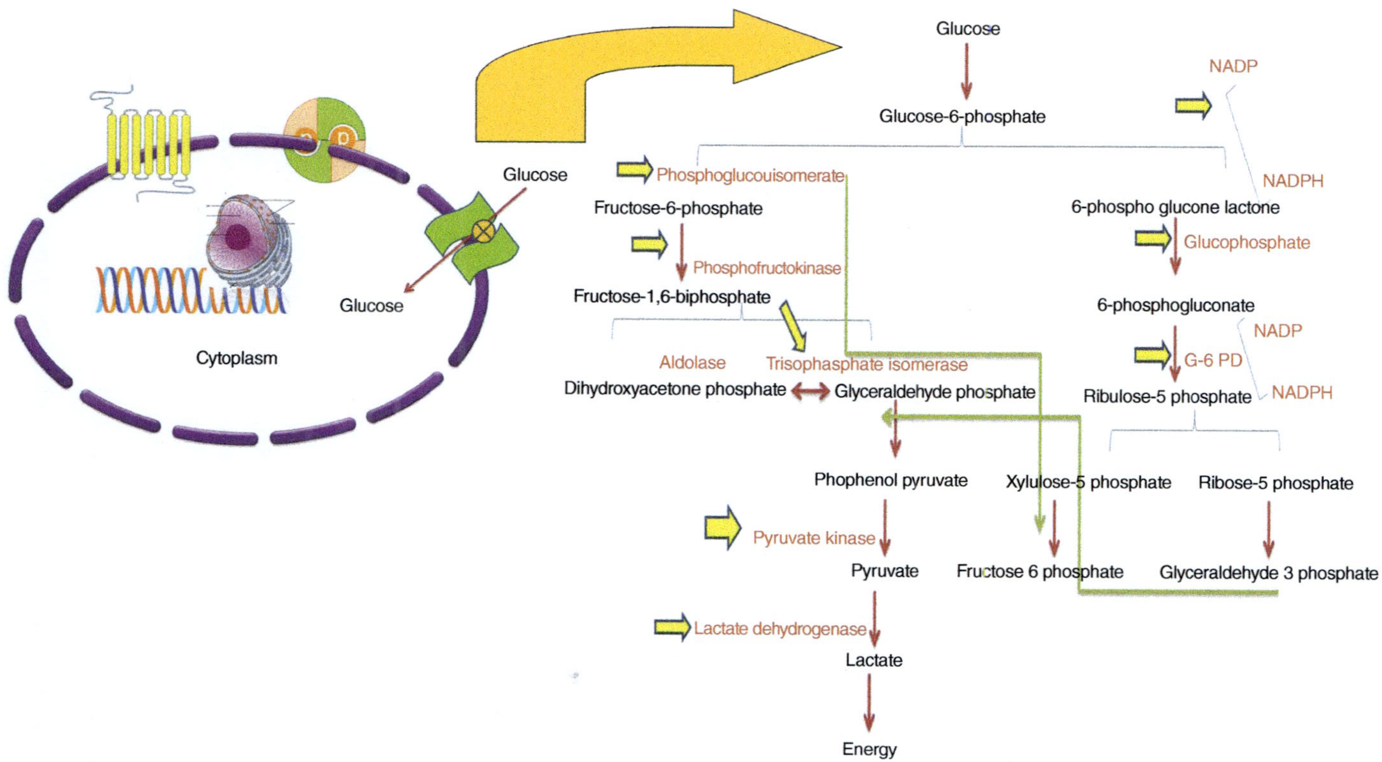

Figure 6.6 Various steps of glycolysis pathway. Yellow arrow shows the potential drug targets.

6.5 Future Drug Development for the Treatment of Malaria

Malaria drug discovery is now facing some challenging attributes in the new era of technology due to resistance to existing methods of treatment. These saturations lead to the development of new emerging methods in the field of treatment such as nanotechnology, which have high therapeutic values, minimal toxicity, and targeted drug delivery. In this, nanocarriers are used, which help in protection of drugs and vaccines from extracellular degradation and help in achieving specific drug delivery with enhanced efficacy [9, 21, 29].

6.5.1 Benefits of Nanocarriers

1. Help in improving the pharmacokinetic profile of the drugs.
2. Increased target site and help in minimizing the side effects.
3. Could combat drug resistance.
4. Dosing frequency reduced, which helps in rise of time of action.
5. Particle aggregations reduced and blockage is minimized.

To achieve all these tremendous benefits, a large number of nanocarriers have been used such as lipid-based drug delivery, liposomes, nanostructured lipid carrier, solid lipid nanoparticles, polymer-based nanocarriers, and micro-emulsifying drug delivery carriers [5].

6.5.2 Lipid-Based Drug Delivery

Among the various polymeric molecules only those compounds are sued that are physiologically compatible with the prime drug moiety. The lipid-based drug carriers such as solid lipid nanoparticles and nanostructure lipid carriers enhance the bioavailability of hydrophobic drugs, provide the sustained release thereby provide the cost-effectiveness and they are biocompatible and biodegradable as well.

6.5.3 Liposomes (as Nanocarriers)

They consist of spindle-shaped vesicles made of phospholipids present in the bilayers. This bilayer is composed by two parts such as aqueous and lipid part. The hydrophobic drugs get entrapped in the lipid part, whereas hydrophilic drugs can be included in the aqueous part. Some of the well-known examples of this are plain liposomes and PEGylated liposomes. These liposomes are widely used in the treatment of malaria as they enhance the circulation time and decrease the intrinsic toxicity and immunogenicity [5, 42, 43].

6.5.4 Nanostructured Lipid Carriers

They are well known as the second generation lipid carriers, which are extensively used to combat the drawbacks of solid lipid nanoparticles.

They are mainly used to incorporate the hydrophobic drugs in a mixture of lipids as liquid and solid phases, which result in the formation of liquid lipid matrix; in this liquid lipid matrix, the drug gets accumulated and leads to various changes in release rate and stability.

6.5.5 Solid Lipid Nanocarriers

This method is alternative to abovementioned methods. The biocompatible lipids, which are used in the formation of solid lipid nanocarriers, are precirol, cetyl alcohol, compritol, glycerylmonostearate, cetylpalmitate, stearic acid, tristearin, and trimyristin. These carriers were used in the optimum drug delivery for both lipophilic and hydrophilic drugs.

Self-micro-emulsifying drug delivery carriers are composed of a mixture of active medicament such as surfactant, co-surfactant, and oil. In this, the fine oil molecules are suspended in water results in formation of o/w. These types of carriers were mainly used in the release of hydrophobic drugs [4, 13, 42, 47].

6.6 Conclusion

In summary, current antimalarial therapy as well as the future drug targets has been reviewed. Complex life cycle of malarial parasite is hindering the efficient working of present antimalarial drugs, which is causing the resistance, but the complex life cycle was studied and the tedious biochemical pathways of the parasite resulted in discovery of new molecular promising drug targets, which can serve as efficient antimalarial therapy. In this chapter, we tried to explain the well-validated promising drug targets and the advancement in drug discovery of the same. The application of docking studies, genomic-based identification of drug targets, rational drug design will fasten the process of drug development for antimalarial therapy.

References

1 Edwin, G.T., Korsik, M., and Todd, M.H. (2019). The past, present and future of anti-malarial medicines. *Malaria Journal* 18: 93.

2 Aregawi, M., Cibulskis, R.E., Otten, M., and Williams, R. (2009). *World Malaria Report 2009*. World Health Organization.

3 Barber, B.E., Rajahram, G.S., Grigg, M.J. et al. (2017). World malaria report: time to acknowledge *Plasmodium knowlesi* malaria. *Malaria Journal* 16: 1–3.

4 Kumar, S., Bhardwaj, T., Prasad, D., and Singh, R.K. (2018). Drug targets for resistant malaria: historic to future perspectives. *Biomedicine & Pharmacotherapy* 104: 8–27.

5 Raphemot, R., Posfai, D., and Derbyshire, E.R. (2016). Current therapies and future possibilities for drug development against liver-stage malaria. *The Journal of Clinical Investigation* 126: 2013–2020.

6 Cibulskis, R.E., Alonso, P., Aponte, J. et al. (2016). Malaria: global progress 2000–2015 and future challenges. *Infectious Diseases of Poverty* 5: 1–8.

7 Lalloo, D.G., Olukoya, P., and Olliaro, P. (2006). Malaria in adolescence: burden of disease, consequences, and opportunities for intervention. *The Lancet Infectious Diseases* 6: 780–793.

8 Mueller, E.A., Van Vugt, M., Kirch, W. et al. (2006). Efficacy and safety of the six-dose regimen of artemether–lumefantrine for treatment of uncomplicated *Plasmodium falciparum* malaria in adolescents and adults: a pooled analysis of individual patient data from randomized clinical trials. *Acta Tropica* 100: 41–53.

9 Uddenfeldt Wort, U., Warsame, M., and Brabin, B.J. (2006). Birth outcomes in adolescent pregnancy in an area with intense malaria transmission in Tanzania. *Acta Obstetricia et Gynecologica Scandinavica* 85: 949–954.

10 Kitchen, A. and Chiodini, P. (2006). Malaria and blood transfusion. *Vox Sanguinis* 90: 77–84.

11 Martinelli, A., Moreira, R., and Cravo, P. (2008). Malaria combination therapies: advantages and shortcomings. *Mini Reviews in Medicinal Chemistry* 8: 201–212.

12 Nájera, J.A. (2001). Malaria control: achievements, problems and strategies. *Parassitologia* 43: 1–89.

13 Dhingra, V., Rao, K.V., and Narasu, M.L. (1999). Current status of artemisinin and its derivatives as antimalarial drugs. *Life Sciences* 66: 279–300.

14 Kain, K.C., Harrington, M.A., Tennyson, S., and Keystone, J.S. (1998). Imported malaria: prospective analysis of problems in diagnosis and management. *Clinical Infectious Diseases* 27: 142–149.

15 Anvikar, A.R., Arora, U., Sonal, G. et al. (2014). Antimalarial drug policy in India: past, present & future. *The Indian Journal of Medical Research* 139: 205.

16 Delves, M., Angrisano, F., and Blagborough, A. (2018). Antimalarial transmission-blocking interventions: past, present, and future. *Trends in Parasitology* 34: 735–746.

17 Petri, M. (1998). *Hydroxychloroquine: Past, Present, Future*. Thousand Oaks, CA: Sage Publications Sage CA.

18 Biagini, G.A., O'Neill, P.M., Nzila, A. et al. (2003). Antimalarial chemotherapy: young guns or back to the future? *Trends in Parasitology* 19: 479–487.

19 Muhammad, I. and Samoylenko, V. (2007). Antimalarial quassinoids: past, present and future. *Expert Opinion on Drug Discovery* 2: 1065–1084.

20 O'Neill, P.M., Bray, P.G., Hawley, S.R. et al. (1998). 4-Aminoquinolines—past, present, and future; a chemical perspective. *Pharmacology & Therapeutics* 77: 29–58.

21 Wallace, D. (2001). Antimalarials—the 'real' advance in lupus. *Lupus* 10: 385–387.

22 Basco, L., Gillotin, C., Gimenez, F. et al. (1992). In vitro activity of the enantiomers of mefloquine, halofantrine and enpiroline against *Plasmodium falciparum*. *British Journal of Clinical Pharmacology* 33: 517–520.

23 Cowman, A.F., Galatis, D., and Thompson, J.K. (1994). Selection for mefloquine resistance in *Plasmodium falciparum* is linked to amplification of the *pfmdr1* gene and cross-resistance to halofantrine and quinine. *Proceedings of the National Academy of Sciences of the United States of America* 91: 1143–1147.

24 Duraisingh, M.T., Roper, C., Walliker, D., and Warhurst, D.C. (2000). Increased sensitivity to the antimalarials mefloquine and artemisinin is conferred by mutations in the *pfmdr1* gene of *Plasmodium falciparum*. *Molecular Microbiology* 36: 955–961.

25 Rojas-Rivero, L., Gay, F., Bustos, M. et al. (1992). Mefloquine-halofantrine cross-resistance in *Plasmodium falciparum* induced by intermittent mefloquine pressure. *The American Journal of Tropical Medicine and Hygiene* 47: 372–377.

26 de Sousa, A.C.C., Diaz, N.C., de Souza, A.M.T. et al. (2015). Molecular modeling study of a series of amodiaquine analogues with antimalarial activity. *Medicinal Chemistry Research* 24: 3529–3536.

27 Guglielmo, S., Bertinaria, M., Rolando, B. et al. (2009). A new series of amodiaquine analogues modified in the basic side chain with in vitro antileishmanial and antiplasmodial activity. *European Journal of Medicinal Chemistry* 44: 5071–5079.

28 Go, M., Ngiam, T., and Wan, A.S. (1981). Synthesis of some novel amodiaquine analogs as potential antimalarial and antifilarial compounds. *Journal of Medicinal Chemistry* 24: 1471–1475.

29 Vennerstrom, J.L., Ellis, W.Y., Ager, A.L. et al. (1992). Bisquinolines. 1. *N,N*-bis(7-chloroquinolin-4-yl) alkanediamines with potential against chloroquine-resistant malaria. *Journal of Medicinal Chemistry* 35: 2129–2134.

30 Ezzet, F., Van Vugt, M., Nosten, F. et al. (2000). Pharmacokinetics and pharmacodynamics of lumefantrine (benflumetol) in acute falciparum malaria. *Antimicrobial Agents and Chemotherapy* 44: 697–704.

31 Van Vugt, M., Looareesuwan, S., Wilairatana, P. et al. (2000). Artemether–lumefantrine for the treatment of multidrug-resistant falciparum malaria. *Transactions of the Royal Society of Tropical Medicine and Hygiene* 94: 545–548.

32 White, N.J., Van Vugt, M., and Ezzet, F.D. (1999). Clinical pharmacokinetics and pharmacodynamics of artemether–lumefantrine. *Clinical Pharmacokinetics* 37: 105–125.

33 WorldWide Antimalarial Resistance Network (WWARN) Lumefantrine PK/PD Study Group (2015). Artemether–lumefantrine treatment of uncomplicated *Plasmodium falciparum* malaria: a systematic review and meta-analysis of day 7 lumefantrine concentrations and therapeutic response using individual patient data. *BMC Medicine* 13: 227.

34 Sun, W., Tanaka, T.Q., Magle, C.T. et al. (2014). Chemical signatures and new drug targets for gametocytocidal drug development. *Scientific Reports* 4: 3743.

35 Krauth-Siegel, R.L., Bauer, H., and Schirmer, R.H. (2005). Dithiol proteins as guardians of the intracellular redox milieu in parasites: old and new drug targets in trypanosomes and malaria-causing plasmodia. *Angewandte Chemie International Edition* 44: 690–715.

36 Alam, A., Goyal, M., Iqbal, M.S. et al. (2009). Novel antimalarial drug targets: hope for new antimalarial drugs. *Expert Review of Clinical Pharmacology* 2: 469–489.

37 Waters, N.C. and Geyer, J.A. (2003). Cyclin-dependent protein kinases as therapeutic drug targets for antimalarial drug development. *Expert Opinion on Therapeutic Targets* 7: 7–17.

38 Coombs, G.H., Goldberg, D.E., Klemba, M. et al. (2001). Aspartic proteases of *Plasmodium falciparum* and other parasitic protozoa as drug targets. *Trends in Parasitology* 17: 532–537.

39 Teixeira, C., Gomes, J.R.B., and Gomes, P. (2011). Falcipains, *Plasmodium falciparum* cysteine proteases as key drug targets against malaria. *Current Medicinal Chemistry* 18: 1555–1572.

40 Ben Mamoun, C., Prigge, S.T., and Vial, H. (2010). Targeting the lipid metabolic pathways for the treatment of malaria. *Drug Development Research* 71: 44–55.

41 Slavic, K., Krishna, S., Derbyshire, E.T., and Staines, H.M. (2011). Plasmodial sugar transporters as anti-malarial drug targets and comparisons with other protozoa. *Malaria Journal* 10: 1–10.

42 Padmanaban, G., Nagaraj, V.A., and Rangarajan, P.N. (2007). Drugs and drug targets against malaria. *Current Science* 92 (11): 38–91.

43 McFadden, G.I. and Roos, D.S. (1999). Apicomplexan plastids as drug targets. *Trends in Microbiology* 7: 328–333.

44 Wiesner, J. and Jomaa, H. (2007). Isoprenoid biosynthesis of the apicoplast as drug target. *Current Drug Targets* 8: 3–13.

45 Ralph, S.A., D'Ombrain, M.C., and McFadden, G.I. (2001). The apicoplast as an antimalarial drug target. *Drug Resistance Updates* 4: 145–151.

46 Goodman, C.D. and McFadden, G.I. (2013). Targeting apicoplasts in malaria parasites. *Expert Opinion on Therapeutic Targets* 17: 167–177.

47 Doggett, J.S., Nilsen, A., Forquer, I. et al. (2012). Endochin-like quinolones are highly efficacious against acute and latent experimental toxoplasmosis. *Proceedings of the National Academy of Sciences of the United States of America* 109: 15936–15941.

48 Gobert, G.N. and Jones, M.K. (2008). Discovering new schistosome drug targets: the role of transcriptomics. *Current Drug Targets* 9: 922–930.

49 Hans, R.H. (2009). *Novel Antimalarial and Antitubercular Agents Based on Natural Products*. University of Cape Town.

50 Hrckova, G. and Velebny, S. (2012). *Pharmacological Potential of Selected Natural Compounds in the Control of Parasitic Diseases*. Springer Science & Business Media.

51 Khanye, S.D. (2010). *Synthesis and Antimalarial Evaluation of Gold Thiosemicarbazone Complexes and Polyamine-Thiosemicarbazone Dendrimers*. University of Cape Town.

52 e Silva, L.R., Montoia, A., Amorim, R.C. et al. (2012). Comparative in vitro and in vivo antimalarial activity of the indole alkaloids ellipticine, olivacine, cryptolepine and a synthetic cryptolepine analog. *Phytomedicine* 20: 71–76.

Part III

Drug Development

7

Assays for Antimalarial Drug Discovery

Varun Gorki, Neha S. Walter, and Sukhbir Kaur

Panjab University, Parasitology Laboratory, Department of Zoology, Sector-14, Chandigarh 160014, India

7.1 Introduction

The slow and unnoticed progression of resistant strains of *Plasmodium* spp. has necessitated the need to look for new alternatives to contain malaria. The goal is indeed crystal-clear that any processed chemical which is pronounced as a drug must be safe, affordable, and should combat the resistant strain of human parasite. Toxicity and drug efficacy are basic parameters in the selection of compounds which is a long-streamlined process. Assessment of the activity of any test compound or drug involves two basic approaches, i.e. screening and analysis in the *in vitro* system and further evaluation in the *in vivo* system. Efficacy testing using both approaches is essential to establish any candidate drug or compound as lead molecule which can further be evaluated in clinical trials.

The *in vitro* approach comprises isolation of parasites from their natural environment and maintaining them in controlled laboratory conditions. The parasites are then exposed to various concentrations of the drug molecules to assess their antimalarial efficacy. Testing of the test compounds or drugs can be carried out on different life cycle stages of the parasite, i.e. the pre-erythrocytic stage, erythrocytic stages, and the gametocytic stage. While most assays target the erythrocytic stages which are responsible for the clinical symptoms of diseases, there are assays targeting the pre-erythrocytic and gametocytic stage of the parasite.

On the other hand, the *in vivo* approach involves the testing of the drug candidates on animal models. In this approach, ethical issues need to be given proper considerations prior to performing these studies. The major advantage of this approach is that it involves the metabolism of the host which is lacking in the *in vitro* system. There are certain drugs which become active only after metabolization and hence do not show interesting activity in the *in vitro* system [1]. Thus, efficacy testing in both systems is crucial to establish any compound or drug as an antimalarial.

In this chapter, the authors outlines the various assays utilized to assess the *in vitro* and *in vivo* antimalarial efficacy of the drug molecules (Figure 7.1). It also provides

Varun Gorki and Neha S. Walter contributed equally to the work.

Drug Development for Malaria: Novel Approaches for Prevention and Treatment, First Edition.
Edited by Pravin Kendrekar.

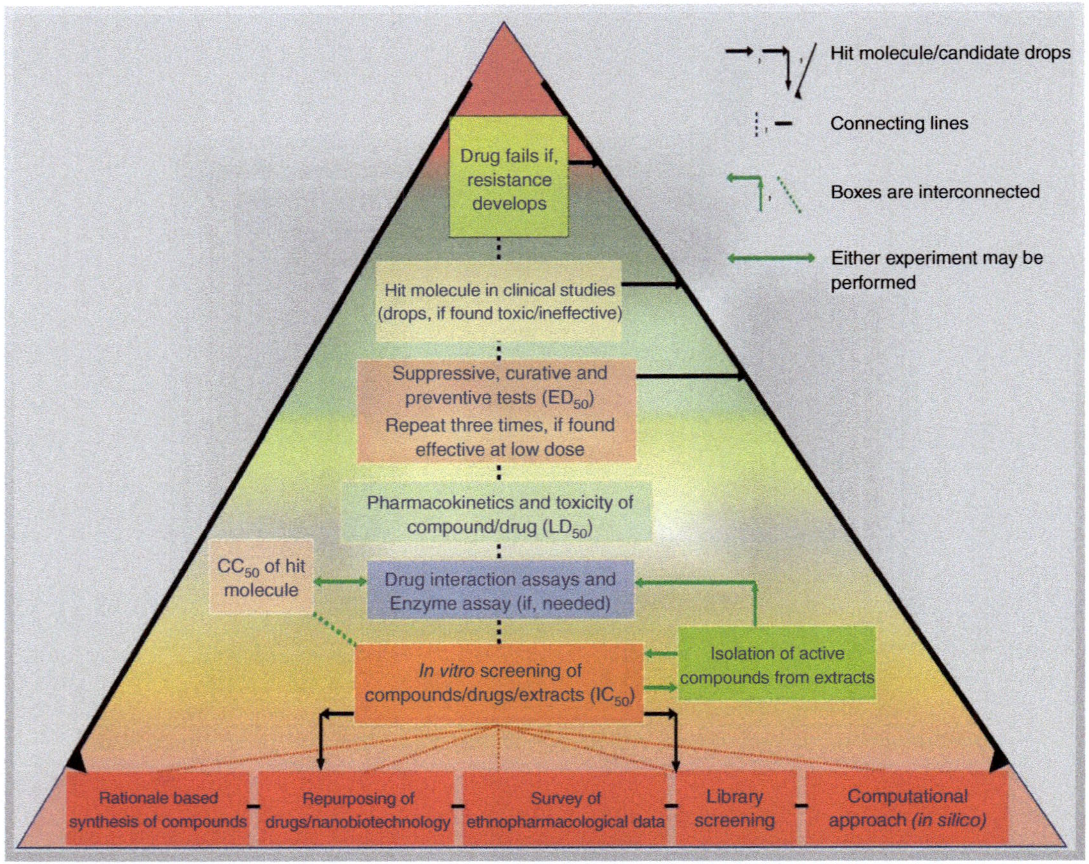

Figure 7.1 Schematic rendition of assays employed in anti-plasmodial drug discovery. The color scheme in the background reflects the intensity of candid efforts required at the particular stage of the drug discovery process.

description of the toxicity assays routinely used in the laboratory to establish the safety and selectivity of these candidate drugs toward the parasite, which is very crucial before establishing their antiplasmodial efficacy. There are several assays to test the *in vitro* and *in vivo* toxicity of any compound or drug under consideration. However, the prime focus of this chapter is on the *in vitro* and *in vivo* oral toxicity protocols relevant only to the antimalarial testing of compounds.

7.2 *In Vitro* Assays for Antimalarial Drug Discovery

Most of the currently available antimalarial drugs have been derived from traditionally used medicinal plants, by the development of their synthetic analogues, by modification of the natural product or repurposing drugs used for treatment of other pathogenic diseases. *In vitro* assays are the linchpin for assessment of antiplasmodial efficacy of any compound or drug. The screening of the antimalarial activity of any compound or drug *in vitro* depends on the ability to maintain the *in vitro* culture of *Plasmodium*. Since the early twentieth century, short-term *Plasmodium falciparum* culture was described. But a major breakthrough in this regard was made when method to maintain continuous cultures of *P. falciparum* erythrocytic stages in human erythrocytes (Figure 7.2) was described and delineated by Trager and Jenson in 1976 [2]. The parasite is maintained in RPMI (Roswell Park Memorial Institute)-1640 culture medium supplemented with 10% human serum or Albumax and WBC-free erythrocytes at 2–5% hematocrit with *N*-(2-hydroxyethyl) piperazine-*N*′-(2-ethanesulfonic acid) (HEPES), and sodium bicarbonate. The culture is kept at 37 °C under reduced oxygen atmosphere (3–5% oxygen, 5% carbon

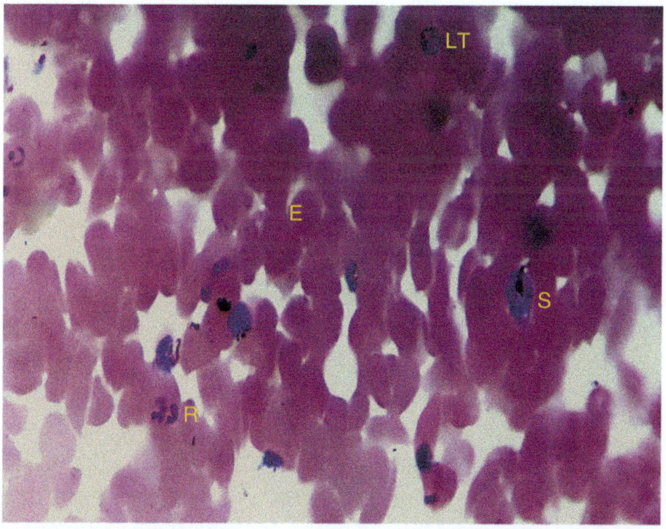

Figure 7.2 Asexual blood stages of *P. falciparum* (1000×). (R-ring, E-erythrocyte, LT-late trophozoite, S-schizont).

dioxide, 90–92% nitrogen). *Plasmodium* strains resistant as well as sensitive can be cultured, and the efficacy of different drugs/compounds can easily be assessed.

Different methods are employed to test the antimalarial activity of various candidate drugs.

7.2.1 Schizont Maturation Inhibition Assay (Microscopic Test)

The simplest method to test the antimalarial activity of any compound involves incubation of the parasite synchronized to ring stages in 96-well plates with different concentrations of the test sample for 48–72 hours [3]. Two types of controls are used in this assay, i.e. negative control (parasite culture without drugs) and positive control (parasite culture with chloroquine or any standard antimalarial drug). The percent parasitemia in treated wells in comparison to control well is then calculated by the preparation of Giemsa-stained thin blood smears microscopically (1000×). The schizont maturation inhibition assay involves counting of the number of schizonts in the treated well in comparison to the control to determine the percent inhibition and the half maximal inhibitory concentration (IC_{50}). IC_{50} value corresponds to the 50% inhibition of the parasite in culture at the specific concentration of test compound/drug by impeding the biological activity. This method is very accurate, easy to perform, and permits direct visualization of the effect of drug treatment on the growth of the parasite inside the red blood cells (RBCs) [4]. Nevertheless, the technique is laborious and requires an expert microscopist to limit the variability in the results.

7.2.2 *In Vitro* Micro Test Technique

It is a commonly used method based on the maturation of parasite into schizonts and counting the number of parasites microscopically [5]. The test was developed by Rieckmann et al. [6] This test provides information about the quantitative drug response of *P. falciparum* irrespective of patient's immune system. The Micro test kit is pre-dosed with several drugs and patient's blood sample is added to each well and incubated with suitable medium. This is followed by preparation of thick blood smears from each well. The number of schizonts in control well is compared to drug treated well out of total 200 asexual parasites to determine the response of the drug as percentage. The major advantage of this method is its simplicity and requirement of only a small quantity of capillary blood. However, the interpretation of the results is arduous and time-consuming.

7.2.3 Radioisotope Assay

Another method to determine the level of parasite inhibition is based on the uptake of ^{3}H-hypoxanthine by the parasite for DNA synthesis and purine salvage. It is the most common method for large-scale testing of the antimalarial activity of any compound *in vitro*. Different concentrations of test sample are added to parasite culture containing reduced concentrations of hypoxanthine. After this the culture is incubated with ^{3}H-hypoxanthine followed by cell harvesting. The radioactive cell counts are measured with liquid scintillation counter. The incorporation of ^{3}H hypoxanthine is directly proportional to the number of *P. falciparum*-infected erythrocytes. Linear regression analysis on linear segments of dose response curves is carried out to determine the IC_{50} value [7]. The technique is rapid and not subject to human error as compared with microscopy. However, the major drawbacks of this method are high cost of the equipment, complexity, high-throughput screening, and use of radioactive substances [8].

7.2.4 Colorimetric Assay (Plasmodium Lactate Dehydrogenase Assay [pLDH])

Colorimetric detection of lactate dehydrogenase (LDH) enzyme of *P. falciparum* is another assay for the assessment of *in vitro* antimalarial efficacy of any drug. This drug sensitivity assay was developed in 1993 by Makler et al. [9]. Plasmodium Lactate Dehydrogenase (pLDH) enzyme catalyzes the conversion of lactate to pyruvate (the last step of glycolysis) in the presence of 3-acetyl pyridine adenine dinucleotide (APAD) as coenzyme. The enzyme of the parasite is different from the human LDH at structural as well as immunological level. The detection of pLDH is specific in the presence of APAD instead of nicotinamide adenine dinucleotide (NAD) by the human enzyme. This assay can be performed using both laboratory adapted and clinical isolates of the parasite. pLDH assay is performed in 24- or 96-well culture plates which are frozen and thawed after the incubation period. The haemolysed cell suspension is transferred to fresh 96-well plates followed by addition of various reagents (MalstatR solution, nitro blue tetrazolium [NBT], phenazine ethosulfate). The NBT gets reduced to a blue formazan derivative by APAD and is detected spectrophotometrically at 650 nm [10]. The optical density is plotted against the drug concentrations to calculate the IC_{50} value. Parasitemia level of 0.02% from *in vitro* culture can be detected using this method.

7.2.5 ELISA-Based Methods

7.2.5.1 DELI Assay

Two Enzyme-Linked Immuno-Sorbent Assay (ELISA)-based methods (pLDH and Histidine-Rich Protein II [HRP II]) are also used for the assessment of antiplasmodial efficacy of drugs. Druilhe et al. described the "double-site enzyme-linked lactate dehydrogenase immune-detection" (DELI) assay in 2001 based on the principle of detection of pLDH by specific monoclonal antibodies immobilized on a dipstick (routinely used for diagnosis of malaria in epidemiological surveys) [11]. The DELI assay is a highly sensitive method. It is accomplished in microtiter plates wherein the parasitized blood is incubated with various concentrations of the drugs. Thereafter, the test plates are frozen and thawed three times to ensure hemolysis and liberation of the pLDH enzyme. The lysate is diluted with PBS (phosphate buffered saline) and transferred to fresh 96-well plates pre-coated with pLDH-specific monoclonal antibodies. The ensuing steps are similar to conventional ELISA. The color development is measured spectrophotometrically at 450 nm.

7.2.5.2 Assay Based on Histidine-Rich Protein II (HRP II) of *P. falciparum*

The second ELISA-based method is similar to the DELI assay but is based on the measurement of the HRP II of *P. falciparum* [12–14]. This protein is produced by the parasite during its growth and development. The levels of HRP II are proportional to the parasite density. The only difference between the HRP II assay and DELI assay is the longer incubation period (72 hours) in the former, which provides an additional advantage of testing the activity of slow-acting drugs. The HRP II assay is very sensitive, simple, does not require radioisotopes, and can be performed using commercially available ELISA kits using both laboratory-adapted or clinical isolates of the parasite.

7.2.6 Flow Cytometry

It is also used to assess the antimalarial activity of test samples based on the fact that DNA is absent in erythrocytes [15]. The parasite is fixed with glutaraldehyde after incubation with various concentrations of test compounds, and the infected cells are stained by fluorescent DNA dyes such as hydroethidine, thiazole orange, acridine orange, ethidium bromide, or the parasite nucleus is stained with DAPI (4′,6-diamidino-2-phenylindole). After staining the cells are excited with laser or ultraviolet light, depending on the dye used. The treated and control cultures are then counted by flow cytometry. The fluorescence intensity is directly proportional to the parasitemia. Different parasite stages can also be distinguished using appropriate gating. The advantage of flow cytometry is that it provides high throughput and is rapid, sensitive, and automated; however, the technique is expensive, requires well-equipped laboratory, sophisticated equipment, and skilled technicians [16].

The green fluorescent protein (PfGFP) obtained from the bioluminescent jellyfish (*Aequorea victoria*) is genetically incorporated into *Plasmodium falciparum* strain as a marker to study gene expression and protein localization in vitro [17]. This approach can also be employed in chemotherapy studies, which can be quantified by flow cytometry [18]. The assay can be used to study the growth-inhibitory activity of antibodies and antimalarial drugs [19]. The PfGFP-transformed parasites could be maintained in continuous culture for over a year without any modification in their fluorescence profile, which further validates its use for chemotherapy studies. The technique is highly sensitive, simple, rapid, reproducible, and suitable for high-throughput applications. The results obtained using PfGFP are comparable to those employing radioisotopic methods and have greater reproducibility than light microscopy [4].

7.2.7 Fluorometric Assay

It is based on measurement of infected RBCs by DNA labelling with fluorochromes which can be used for *in vitro* drug susceptibility assay without using flow cytometry

[20]. After incubation, the RBCs are lysed using distilled water or saponin. The pellet obtained by centrifugation is dissolved in guanidinium or sodium dodecyl sulfate solution followed by staining with DNA-binding fluorochromes. SYBR Green I can also be used to stain the DNA [21]. Additionally, DNA extraction can also be carried out to remove the malarial pigment hemozoin which can cause quenching. The fluorescence intensity of each well is measured using a fluorescence spectrophotometer or fluorescence-activated microplate reader to determine the parasite DNA in treated and control wells [22, 23].

DNA-based fluorimetric methods using the fluorochrome PicoGreen are also used to check the susceptibility of parasite to test sample. PicoGreen intercalates into the dsDNA (double-stranded DNA) resulting in increase in fluorescence emission [24]. The amount of fluorescence is positively co-related with percent parasitemia between 0.1% and 15%. The method can be used to determine the parasite inhibition (IC_{50}) of potential antimalarial drugs. This method is sensitive, rapid, and results are similar to [^{3}H]-hypoxanthine assay [25].

7.2.8 β-Hematin Formation (Haemozoin Test)

Plasmodium parasites are known to ingest the hemoglobin and convert it into the malaria pigment haemozoin by a process known as Ferriprotoporphyrin IX (FP) biomineralization. The inhibition of this process is utilized to screen compounds for their antiplasmodial activity [26]. The method involves incubation of test compounds/drugs (50 μl) with 50 μl hemin chloride which is freshly dissolved in dimethyl sulfoxide (DMSO) and 0.5 M sodium acetate buffer (100 μl) in 96-well plates for 18–24 hours at 37 °C and 5.5 pH. The components of the mixture should be added in the following sequence, i.e. hemin chloride solution, the buffer, and finally the solvent or the solution of drug. After incubation, the samples are transferred into a 96-well Multi-Screen plate size (Millipore MAR4 N04 10) individually fitted with glass fiber filters. The solvent is aspirated through the filter by applying vacuum, followed by washing the wells with DMSO (200 μl per well). The β-haematin adhering to the filters is then dissolved in 200 μl of 0.1 N NaOH per well. Finally, 150 μl from each well is transferred into a parallel well in a 96-well plate and the absorbance read at 405 nm. Results are expressed as percent inhibition of β-haematin formation using the following formula (% inhibition = 100[O.D. control – O.D. drug]/[O.D. control]).

7.2.9 Drug Interaction Assay and Isobologram Analysis

Isobologram analysis is performed to ascertain the effect of drug combinations. It is an important tool to assess whether the chosen combinations are additive, synergistic, or antagonistic to each other [27, 28]. Dose–response assays over a range of individual concentrations using fixed ratio method [27] or checkerboard technique [29] are used to conduct this analysis. The combination of atovaquone–proguanil was identified using this analysis.

Fivelman et al. [30] and Bhattacharya et al. [31] described the method to assay the effect of drugs combinations (along with their sevenfold serial dilution) on parasite maturation in flat-bottom 96-well plates. The experimental well consists of medium (100 μl) with or without drugs and 1% parasitized erythrocytes with 1% hematocrit. After seeding of wells, the plates are incubated in a candle-jar at 37 °C for the 48 hours asexual cycle followed by preparing of Giemsa-stained thin blood films and counting the number of parasites to determine the parasitemia.

The fractional inhibitory concentration (FIC) is then calculated by the formula (FIC = Concentration of synthetic compound/drugs in combination to produce IC_{50}/Concentration of synthetic compound/drugs alone required to produce IC_{50}). Isobologram is plotted with mean FIC to determine the interactions between the drugs. The sum FIC value for each combination is determined to classify the drug interactions (additive, synergistic, or antagonistic).

7.2.10 PCR-Based Methods

Molecular methods based on polymerase chain reaction (PCR) detection are also becoming popular in endemic areas, which are used to detect mutations in the parasite genome responsible for development of resistance [32]. These methods are useful for determining the level and spread of resistance. Molecular methods are very suitable in endemic areas for studying a large number of samples and are advantageous over other *in vitro* tests in which parasite culture is required, which is a time-consuming process. PCR is also used to detect point mutations in the parasite genome which are responsible for development of resistance [16].

7.2.11 *In Vitro* Assays Targeting Exo-erythrocytic and Sexual Stages of the Parasite

7.2.11.1 Exo-erythrocytic Schizontocidal Assay

In addition to the aforementioned assays targeting the erythrocytic stages of the parasite, assays have been described to test the efficacy of the antimalarial drugs against the exo-erythrocytic and sexual stages of *Plasmodium*. The most commonly used method to evaluate the antiplasmodial efficacy of the drugs against the liver stage is the antimalarial exo-erythrocytic schizontocidal assay. The assay involves the *in vitro* cultivation of the exo-erythrocytic stages of *Plasmodium berghei* ANKA or *Plasmodium yoelii* by infecting HepG2 cell line by sporozoites produced in the salivary glands of the *Anopheles* mosquitoes [33, 34]. The drug activity is assessed by counting the number of hepatic cells containing the schizonts in the sporozoites infected cultures [35]. Alternatively, it has been proposed to count the infected cells using qRT (quantitative Real Time)-PCR [35]. The screening of drugs targeting liver stages *in vitro* as well as *in vivo* can be effectively performed using luminescence-based analysis [36].

7.2.11.2 Ex-flagellation Assay

The efficacy screening of the compounds as transmission blocking drugs involves gametocytocidal activity (targeting the sexual of the parasite). The ex-flagellation assay is used to assess the effect on micro-gametogenesis (formation of flagellar microgametes from microgametocytes). The assay is based on the formation of multicellular ex-flagellation centers by microgametes which adhere to the neighboring erythrocytes [37]. Gametogenesis is triggered artificially *in vitro* by increasing the pH from 7 to 8 [38] and simultaneously decreasing the temperature by 5 °C [39]. The formation of ex-flagellation centers can be observed microscopically to assess successful gametogenesis. However, the method is laborious and cannot be automated. Alternatively, the DNA staining dyes can be used to analyze the cells by flow cytometry [40] or by fluorescent microscopy. Assays have been developed based on incorporation of ^{3}H-hypoxanthine into newly synthesized DNA of microgametes in 96-cell plates to monitor gametocyte activation [41].

Additionally, to test the transmission blocking ability of any drug, test compounds are added to *P. falciparum* gametocytes produced *in vitro* [42]. Also, assays employing feeding of starved mosquitoes with a blood meal containing infectious gametocytes via artificial membrane feeding apparatus are useful. After a week, the mosquito midguts are dissected and the number of oocysts in treated and control groups can be compared by light microscopy [43].

Thus, different assays are used for *in vitro* screening of efficacy of compounds/drugs. Of all the assays used, inhibition of schizont maturation is the most widely used assay for *in vitro* testing of any drug/compound. The results of *in vitro* antiplasmodial activity of extracts/drugs are mostly classified according to the criteria given by Lekana-Douki et al. based on WHO recommendations and other studies, which classifies compounds as highly active ($IC_{50} < 5\,\mu g/ml$), promising activity ($IC_{50} = 5$–$15\,\mu g/ml$), moderate activity ($IC_{50} = 15$–$50\,\mu g/ml$), and inactive ($IC_{50} > 50\,\mu g/ml$) [44]. Some authors express IC_{50} value in μM, where $IC_{50} < 1\,\mu M$ is considered to be excellent antiplasmodial activity. The major advantage of *in vitro* screening methods is that they are simple, rapid, and allow evaluation of a large number of compounds simultaneously along with assessment of intrinsic activity of any drug. In addition, isobologram analysis is useful to study the synergistic, additive, or antagonistic interactions between the drug combinations. However, there are certain limitations such as drugs acting through an active metabolite cannot be identified, toxic compounds can be selected, and skilled personnel and laboratory infrastructure are needed [16]. Experiment design and selection of *Plasmodium* strain must be done prior to *in vitro* study despite knowing and getting the running culture from other authentic sources. Taking all the aspects in mind while performing such experiments, all the necessary measures must be considered. Drawing the inferences and reaching to the conclusion is another consequential step where computation of data must be performed with earnestness.

7.3 *In Vivo* Assays for Antimalarial Drug Discovery

After the *in vitro* analysis, most of the lead molecules fail to be promising novel entity *in vivo*. Species of *Plasmodium* infecting humans cannot cause infection in non-primate animal models. Therefore, murine parasite is best known experimental

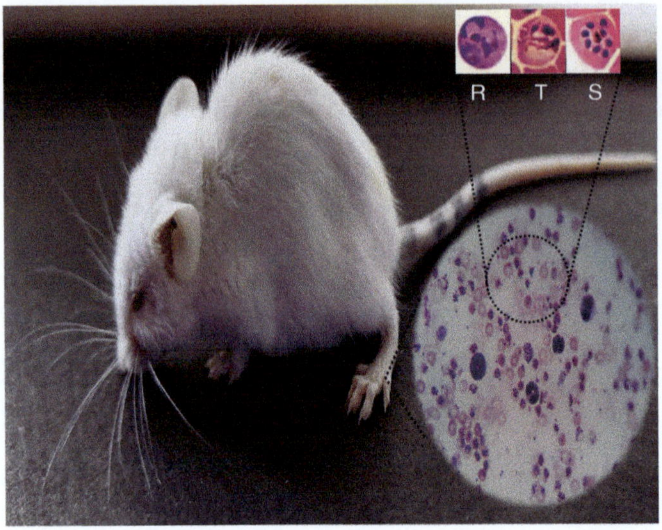

Figure 7.3 Balb/C mouse infected with *Plasmodium berghei* (NK-65) and thin blood smear (1000×) exhibiting asynchronous (Ring, Trophozoites, Schizonts) infection.

model in this field. Except in the immune-compromised mice model in which *P. falciparum*-infected RBCs can sustain, other human *Plasmodium* species are unable to infect other animal models [45]. For any drug/novel/lead compound discovery, *in vivo* determination of efficacy of such entity is the prerequisite process [46]. Thanks to Vincke and Lips, who discovered murine parasite in 1948 in Central Africa, the *in vivo* assessment of antiplasmodial efficacy of any drug/compounds is performed using rodent malaria parasites, and hence, halofantrine, mefloquine, and artemisinin derivatives were discovered [47–50]. Murine strains are well characterized, extensively studied, and their correlation with human parasite is well documented [51].

There are four species of the *Plasmodium* infecting rodents, namely *P. berghei, P. yoelii, P. chabaudi*, and *P. vinckei*. Out of these, *P. berghei*-infected mouse [52, 53] is most widely used for initial drug evaluation (Figure 7.3). The choice of rodent malaria parasite species and mouse model is also crucial before designing an experiment. For example, *P. vinckei* and *P. chabaudi* generate high synchronous infection and can be used to study parasite stage specificity, and chronic infection produced by *P. chabaudi* is useful in studies on immunomodulators [8].

Various assays used to evaluate the *in vivo* activity of the antimalarial drugs are described below:

7.3.1 Peters' 4-Day Test

The 4-day suppressive test [54, 55] is used to see the effects of four daily doses of test sample on blood parasitemia (on day 4 post inoculation) and mean survival time in treated and untreated groups. The rodent infection is initiated by intraperitoneal or intravenous injection of 10^6–10^7 infected erythrocytes from an infected to a naïve rodent. The test sample can be administered via oral, intraperitoneal, intravenous, or subcutaneous routes. Chloroquine is often used as the reference drug (ED_{50} 1.5–1.8 mg against ANKA strain) which is mandatory to make comparison with other experimental groups. On day 5, the percent parasitemia is assessed using Toluidine blue/Leishman/Giemsa-stained thin blood smears to calculate the percent chemosuppression in each experimental group in comparison to the infected/untreated control group. The effective dose (ED_{50}), defined as the concentration of the drug that produces a biological response in 50% of the subjects/test population, is also calculated.

The percent parasitemia is also checked weekly (day 7, day 14, day 21, and day 28) during the follow-up period [56, 57]. Mean survival time (MST) in days is also calculated during this period. Additionally, biochemical (liver and kidney function) [58], immunological (cytokine analysis), and histopathological (liver, kidney, spleen) parameters can be checked during different days in the treated mice (Figure 7.4) to assess the effect of compound/drug treatment on these vital functions of the rodent host. This provides a detailed study of the impact of compound/drug in controlling the infection, its safety to the vital organs of the host, and immunological response (if any) generated during the course of treatment. A slight variation in the overall treatment regimen is followed in case of ANKA strain of *P. berghei* (Figure 7.5). The protocol involves assessment for experimental cerebral malaria (ECM), characteristic of ANKA strain. Hence, efficacy screening of compounds/drug can be performed against ECM in mice using this model.

The classification of *in vivo* antimalarial activity is done based on the classification given by Muñoz et al. [59], according to which the results of *in vivo* antimalarial activity can be categorized as moderate, good, and very good if the extract/drug displays a percent growth inhibition equal to or greater than 50% at a dose of 500, 250, and 100 mg/kg, respectively.

Compound found to be active in the 4-day test can further be tested in secondary tests [8], which are discussed as follows:

7.3.2 Dose Ranging Full 4-Day Test

In this test, four doses of the compound are tested by different routes of administration followed by assessment of percent parasitemia using Giemsa-stained thin blood smears. The therapeutically effective dose (ED_{50}) is determined by plotting the log dose against probit activity. The dose ranging test also provides an insight into the relative potency and bioavailability [16].

7.3.3 Onset/Recrudescence Test

In this assay, the test population is first inoculated with the parasite. On day 3 post-infection, mice are subcutaneously or orally treated with single dose of the lead compound/drug, while the infected control mice are given the vehicle alone. Giemsa-stained blood smears are prepared at 12 and 24 hours interval and then everyday till day 33 post-infection. The percent parasitemia is assessed. The results

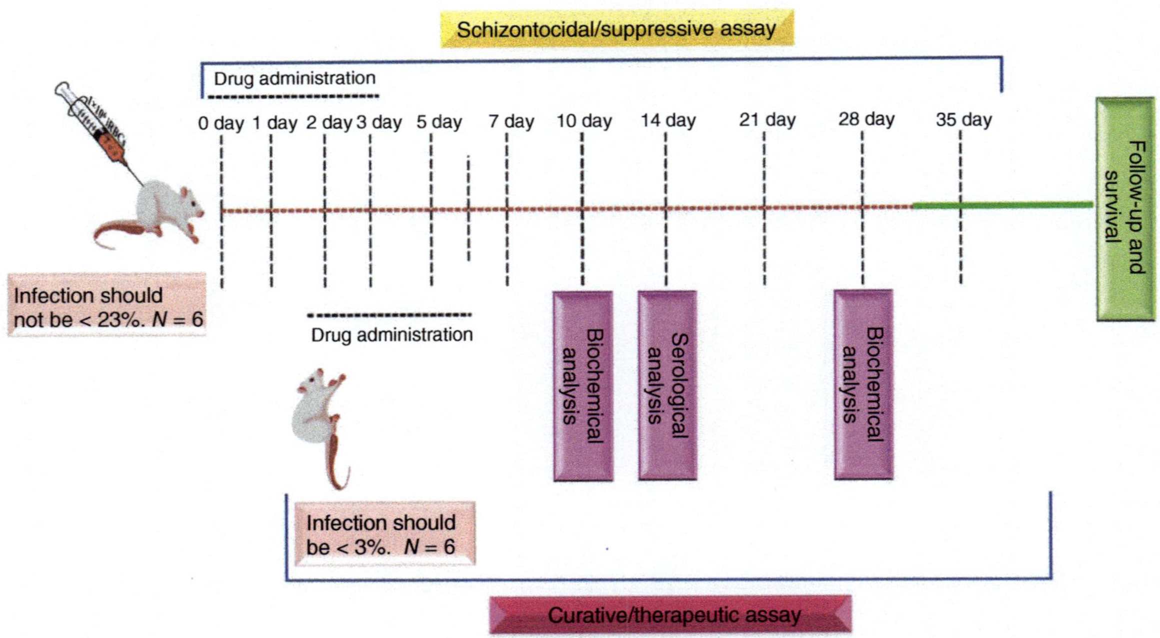

Figure 7.4 Schematic rendition of suppressive (schizontocidal) and curative test for the assessment of *in vivo* activity of test compound/drug.

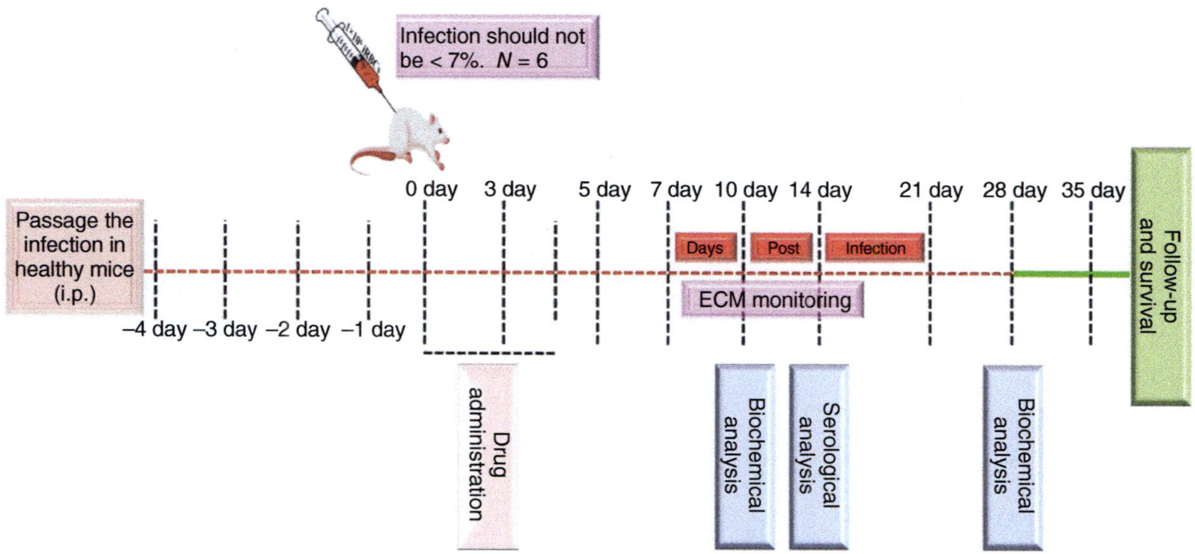

Figure 7.5 Schematic rendition of suppressive (schizontocidal) test for the assessment of *in vivo* activity of test compound/drug against *Plasmodium berghei* ANKA.

obtained are expressed in terms of rapidity of onset of activity, i.e. parasite clearance, time taken for onset of recrudescence, rise in parasitemia, and duration of survival in days [16, 60].

7.3.4 Preventive Test

Test compounds can also be evaluated for their preventive/repository activity against malaria [61]. In this test, the experimental mice are administered with the compounds for four days (D0–D3) prior to infection. On the fifth day (D4), they are inoculated with the parasite. Seventy-two hours post-treatment on D7, thin blood smears are prepared to assess the percent parasitemia and chemosuppression in each experimental group. This is followed by weekly (D14, D21, and D28) monitoring of the percent parasitemia during the one-month follow-up period. The MST (in days) of the experimental animals is also determined.

7.3.5 Curative Test

The therapeutic efficacy of the compound is tested using the curative test [62]. In this test, the experimental animals are first inoculated with the parasite and the infection is allowed to be established in the host providing a more clinical aspect of the infection. On day 3 post infection, the treatment is initiated and continued for five days. The infection is monitored weekly using Giemsa-stained thin blood smears to assess the percent parasitemia and chemosuppression in each experimental group. The biochemical, immunological, and histopathological studies are performed during the follow-up period, and the MST (in days) is also calculated (Figure 7.3).

7.3.6 Hill's Test for Causal Prophylaxis and Residual Activity

This test involves infection of the Charles River strain of mice with N67 strain of *P. yoelii* sporozoites from *Anopheles stephensi* [16, 60]. The sporozoites are obtained 8–11 days after the infected blood meal, and 10^4–10^5sub sporozoites are intravenously injected into the mice. The test compound is assessed for its causal prophylactic and residual effects upon blood stage parasites in four different phases.

Phase 1: In this phase, the compound is tested for its causal prophylactic activity. Treatment with the compound is initiated three hours post-inoculation of the sporozoites. Parasitemia is assessed using blood films for next 14 days until 2% parasitemia is evident. The compound is considered to be 100% protective (causal prophylactic) if parasitemia is not detected during the 14-day study.

Phase 2: After phase 1, the compound is assessed for residual activity against blood stage infection. In this phase, single dose of the compound is administered 48 hours before intravenous inoculation of 10^4 trophozoites. The time interval to obtain 2% parasitemia is compared with the infected control. No residual activity is observed if time taken to obtain 2% parasitemia is similar in both the groups.

Phase 3: In this phase, the compounds are assessed for prolonged residual activity. The mice are first inoculated with the sporozoites, and after three hours they are treated with the test compounds. After 48 hours, 0.2 ml blood is withdrawn from each mouse and intraperitoneally injected into a naïve mouse. The parasitemia is assessed in the recipient mice for 14 days or until development of patency. If <50% of the recipients develop parasitemia, then compound is considered to exhibit some residual activity. However, if >75% recipient mice exhibit patent infection, the compound is categorized as having no residual activity.

Phase 4: This phase provides an additional test to ascertain whether or not a compound has residual activity. Experimental mice are first treated with the compound followed by intravenous injection with 10^4 trophozoites 48 hours post-treatment. After three to four hours, 0.2 ml of blood is taken from the treated mice and injected to naive recipient mice. Parasitemia is assessed using blood films, and the time taken to obtain 2% parasitemia is then compared with the infected control. Similar time interval in both groups is indicative of no effect of the compound on the parasite, hence, no residual activity.

7.3.7 Assays with *P. berghei* Green Fluorescent Protein (PbGFP)

The strain of *P. berghei* transformed using the green fluorescent protein (GFP) can be employed to assess the *in vivo* efficacy of the compounds [63]. The assay using PbGFP is similar to the Peters' 4-day test. Parasite inhibition in the control and treated groups is rapidly quantified using flow cytometry. The infected RBCs can be identified on the basis of their specific light-scattering properties. The results obtained using this technique are comparable to light microscopy. The major advantage of using PbGFP is that the parasitemia can be quantified rapidly in a single drop of blood allowing screening of a large number of compounds rapidly [4].

7.3.8 Assays Employing Immunocompromised Mice

A novel method to test the antimalarial efficacy is based on the use of immunocompromised mice [45], which can sustain *P. falciparum* infection due to lack of T and LAK (lymphokine activated killer) cells. The *P. falciparum*-infected RBCs (huRBC) are grafted into these immunodeficient BXN laboratory mice. The neutrophils are controlled by NIMP-R 14 monoclonal antibody, and dichloromethylene diphosphate is administered to reduce tissue macrophages. *P. falciparum* (sensitive [NF54] and multi-drug-resistant [T24] strain) infected human red blood cells (PfhuRBC) are grafted into the mice. The strains retain their usual drug susceptibility in the mice. The drug administration is done when the infection becomes stable for six days and ring forms are evident in the blood smears. This is the first murine model in which *P. falciparum* can be maintained *in vivo* [16].

However, there are several limitations of using immunocompromised mice such as limited reproducibility and variable kinetics of infection, requirement of intraperitoneal route of infection, and use of chemicals which may interact with the antimalarial compounds. In order to overcome these drawbacks, a non-myelodepleted mice ($NOD^{scid/\beta 2m-/-}$ mice) defective in natural killer (NK) cell activity, serum complement, and macrophage activation was established as a new murine model of *P. falciparum* malaria [64]. These mice were engrafted with *P. falciparum*-infected human RBCs through serial passages intravenously to obtain persistent parasitemia. When treated with the standard antimalarials, these mice exhibited dose-dependent inhibitory activity, which validated this model for *in vivo* studies.

7.3.9 Primate Models for *In Vivo* Studies

Primate models are also very useful in preclinical drug development [65]. These provide a final confirmation of rodent efficacy results and clear prediction of the effect of drug candidate on humans. *Aotus* and *Saimiri* monkeys are susceptible to *P. falciparum* infection [66]. *Aotus* monkeys are recommended models by the WHO for studying malaria infection as this is the only model that can sustain both *P. vivax* and *P. falciparum* infection [16].

Infection of *Plasmodium cynomolgi* in *Rhesus* monkeys can also be used to assess schizontocidal, hypnozoitocidal, and prophylactic activity of test samples in a single model [67]. This model bears a close similarity with human infection caused by *P. vivax*. In this model, young, tuberculin-negative *Rhesus* monkeys (3.5–6 kg) are intravenously inoculated with *P. cynomolgi* sporozoites. Drug treatment is initiated one day before infection and is continued once daily till day 8 through a stomach tube. Blood smears are prepared daily for four to six weeks. However, if no infection is seen in animals after six weeks, the monkeys are re-infected (re-challenged) with a same inoculum. Animals which become infected during the course of time and also infected animals from re-challenged group are given further treatment when 0.1–0.5% infection is evident.

The experimental animals are given seven doses of the drug orally once daily and observed for 30 days. If no infection is evident, they are assessed twice weekly until they relapse. However, if infection is not cleared during the primary infection, they are treated with seven doses of chloroquine (5 mg/kg) once a day. No relapse after treatment with chloroquine indicates that the hypnozoites have been destroyed by the test drug [16]. Furthermore, after 8–12 weeks if no relapse is observed, the animals are splenectomized. The animals are again observed for four weeks, and if no infection is evident, the results are indicative of radical cure, though, in most cases relapses are observed within three weeks of splenectomy.

Recently, the Japanese macaque (*Macaca fuscata*) has been reported to be useful as an alternative model for studying the hypnozoite-induced relapsing *P. cynomolgi* infection. *M. fuscata* model is comparable to the *Rhesus* monkey model and can be employed for assessment of anti-hypnozoite activity of drugs [68].

Thus, these primate models provide better prediction of activity and pharmacokinetics of these candidate drugs in humans than the rodent models leading to a logical transition toward clinical studies [69]. *Aotus* and *Saimiri* monkeys are also excellent models for testing vaccines.

7.3.10 Sporontocidal Assays

Assays evaluating the sporontocidal activity (targeting the development of the parasite in the mosquito) of the antimalarials have also been developed. The experimental mice are intraperitoneally inoculated with the parasite, and the presence of mature gametocytes in the blood is confirmed by observing ex-flagellation centers microscopically. These mice are treated with the compounds/drugs and placed over cages containing the mosquitoes. After 10 days, the mosquitoes are dissected and their midguts are examined to assess the presence of oocysts under the microscope [70, 71]. The oocysts can be easily and rapidly detected using GFP transformed rodent malaria parasites wherein the fluorescence generated can be detected using a fluorescent microscope.

After day 21 post-infection, the transmission-blocking activity is examined by detecting the presence of sporozoites in the mosquito salivary glands using phase-contrast microscopy [72–74]. Alternatively, these mosquitoes are allowed to feed on uninfected mice and the parasitemia is subsequently assessed in the mice.

7.3.11 Anti-sporozoite Assay

This assay involves treating the experimental mice with the compound/extract orally for six consecutive days. Thereafter, each animal is individually exposed to 2–12 infected mosquitoes. The treatment is further continued for seven more days. From day 5, post sporozoite inoculation, Giemsa-stained thin blood smears are prepared daily to determine the malaria pre-patent period (PPP) and the course of the parasitemia. The survival/mortality of the treated animals is also monitored for 30 days post sporozoite inoculation. The standard antimalarial primaquine is utilized as the positive control (reference drug) in this assay.

Thus, various assays are used to evaluate the *in vivo* antiplasmodial efficacy of any compound or drug under consideration. The Peters' 4-day suppressive test remains the fundamental test to evaluate the efficacy of any compound. Besides, the *Plasmodium* species (*Plasmodium gallinaceum*) infecting chickens (avian model) were also used to assess the antimalarial activity of the drugs [75]. However, the avian models became unpopular for malaria research mainly because of the introduction of rodent models which are convenient to handle, and being mammalian models, they are more pertinent to human malaria infection [16].

7.4 *Ex Vivo* Assays for Antimalarial Drug Discovery

Ex vivo assays provide a powerful tool to study human malaria parasite biology and to assess the antimalarial activity of the drugs. The *ex vivo* studies involve the manipulation of clinical samples of *Plasmodium* spp. in an artificial environment for no longer than 48 hours. Russell et al. [76] developed field-based flow cytometry for *ex vivo* characterization of freshly isolated clinical isolates of *P. vivax* and *P. falciparum* using SYBR green and dihydroethidium as an alternative to microscopy. Witkowski et al. [77] also assessed an *ex vivo* ring-stage survival assay (RSA) for surveillance of artemisinin-resistant *P. falciparum*. A flow cytometric approach for the detection of haemozoin (Hz) was developed by Rebelo et al. [78] for reagent-free assessment of parasite maturation and analysis of drug effects on *ex vivo* culture of parasites in malaria patient samples. Chang et al. [79] developed an optimized *ex vivo* antimalarial susceptibility assay for rodent malaria parasites. The assay utilizes a single-step 65% Percoll gradient that separates the ring stages from the trophozoites and schizonts. This results in the synchronization growth of the parasite, regardless of the species used. This method facilitates the monitoring of parasite maturation which can lead to the understanding of pathobiology of parasite. This *ex-vivo* maturation assay is also utilized to assess the antimalarial activity of the drugs by flow cytometry.

7.5 Assays for Assessment of *In Vitro* Toxicity

There is constant demand to look for new alternatives which are rapid, rational, and economical instead of evaluating toxicity in animal models. Hence, cell line cultures are a promising aspect. To discern any toxicity and biological activity of unknown chemical entity, it must go through a series of toxicity tests. Toxicity profiling comprises of both *in vitro* and *in vivo* testing. Human cells have two sorts of aspects, i.e. basal cell function and organ-specific function. The former deals with the common structure and function of cells while the latter concerns with the precise functioning and structural features of cells typical to organs. Therefore, basal cytotoxicity always leads to specific cytotoxicity [80]. As far as the structure–activity relationship and other specific signal targeting are concerned, such toxicity assays are reliable and provide valuable information of lethal range and its action via live imaging.

Many benchmarks are employed as end-products to compute toxicity which comprises of alteration in morphology, bursting of cells, plasmolysis, seeping of cytosolic enzymes in complete media, various staining/dyes, etc. Normally, cancerous cells are employed followed by specific basal primary cell culture. Further, cancer cell lines, for instance, HeLa cells, RAW-264.07 (Figure 7.6), and others illustrating constant rate of division, are easily vulnerable to test substance due to the presence of microtubules, microfilaments, enzymes, mRNA, DNA, and others as targets. Besides, primary culture (Fibroblast cell culture) provides greater cognizance by retaining intact morphology and cell division. Such assays also aid in providing insight into parasite uptake by immune cells and pathogenesis. Considering this aspect, designing and selection of cell-line is mandatory as per the nature of test substance and basal toxicity profile. Solvent in which test substance has to be dissolved and cells without treatment must be added in design study.

7.5.1 MTT Assay

MTT (3-[4,5-dimethylthiazol-2-yl]-2,5 diphenyl tetrazolium bromide) assay is a well-established, reliable, and high-throughput test to determine the viability

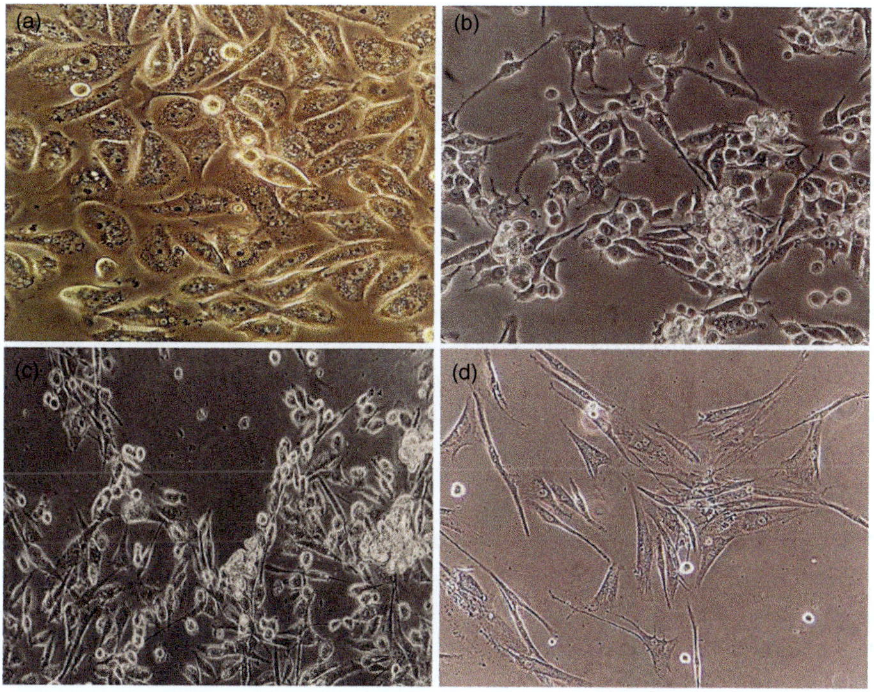

Figure 7.6 HeLa (a), RAW 264.7 macrophage (b), MCF-7 (c) cell lines and primary culture of dermal fibroblasts (d).

(IC_{50} and CC_{50}) and cell sensitivity against the chemicals/natural products' extracts/isolated components without the need for the counting of cells [81]. This assay covers a wide area of research such as to screen the various drugs on human samples/cell lines, evaluate cross-resistance between related and unrelated drugs, etc. The principle relies on the fact that the viability of cells is directly proportional to mitochondrial activity which turns MTT into formazan crystals. Hence, a decrease in the number of living cells affects the crystal formation, and these are easily solubilized by adding DMSO, methanol, and ethanol and concentration can be measured at 540 and 720 nm using ELISA plate reader [82].

While setting up toxicity assays in laboratory conditions, other aspects which must be omitted are as follows:

A. Contamination
B. Seeding of smaller number of cells
C. Addition of inadequate amount of media
D. Addition of excess of antibiotics
E. Insufficient supply of CO_2
F. Pipetting error
G. Concentrated form of DMSO used for dissolving the test substances.

Mostly round and flat-bottom plates are of choice. It is mandatory to have space for control (without drugs) and blank wells (without cells). Physical characteristics of test entity must be noticed as few chemical substances create influence on neighboring wells. Some test substances are colored and exhibit absorbance so in such instances, there must be wells that contain solemnly test substances. To avoid evaporation impact on experiment, outer layer of well plate must be filled with PBS (PBS + Antibiotics). To minimize the variability of the results more often, cells are seeded in triplicate and content/volume of cells is usually kept constant (10 000–15 000) and adjusted within minimum amount of suspended media which is further calibrated to final volume of the well. When it seems that cells are fully turgid and confluent under the inverted microscope, process of trypsinization is initiated [82]. It is performed by two means either manually by scraping or by enzymatic activity, i.e. addition of trypsin (33–37 °C) in culture vial for three to six minutes followed by mild centrifugation. Cells must be added in equal volume in each well without any jerk in pipetting. After adherence of cells to surface (incubation period may differ) test substance in various concentrations would be added. After the suitable incubation of plate MTT (10 μl) is added (5 mg/ml or 1 : 10 volume). The plate is shaken for three to five minutes and incubated for three to four hours. Hundred microliter of DMSO is added to solubilize the formazan crystals. Ten-minute incubation is provided before taking the reading at 450 nm in an ELISA reader. The percent cell viability is calculated in the drug-treated wells in comparison to the control wells, and the CC_{50} value is determined. CC_{50} (50% cytotoxic concentration) is defined as the concentration of the drug/compound required for reducing the cell viability by 50%.

7.5.2 XTT Assay

It is another colorimetric assay used to determine the *in vitro* cytotoxicity of any compound. The method is based on the tetrazolium salt XTT (2,3-bis(2-methoxy-4-nitro-5-sulphophenyl)-5-carboxanilide-2*H*-tetrazolium, monosodium salt). The principle of this assay is the reduction of XTT tetrazolium salt to an orange-colored formazan compound by metabolically active cells [83]. The assay is performed in 96-well plates and involves incubation of cells with XTT reagent for 2–24 hours resulting in the formation of orange color. The intensity of color is measured with a spectrophotometer, which has a linear relationship with the number of viable cells. The basic difference between MTT and XTT assay is that the former produces a water-insoluble formazan compound, which has to be dissolved before measuring the absorbance, while the formazan is water-soluble in the latter. XTT assay is simple, safe, and very useful for measuring the cell proliferation as well as for cytotoxicity [84].

7.5.3 LDH (Lactate Dehydrogenase) Assay

This assay is utilized to assess the *in vitro* cytotoxicity of any compound based on the estimation of LDH activity in the medium [85]. LDH assay is rapid, simple, and reliable. It is based on the principle of release of the LDH enzyme into the culture medium after damage to the cell membrane (indicative of cell death). The activity is assessed based on the diaphorase mediated conversion of iodonitrotetrazolium (INT), a tetrazolium salt into a red-color formazan. The initial step of the reaction involves conversion of lactate to pyruvate catalyzed by the LDH enzyme and reduction of NAD to NADH/H^+. The subsequent step involves the transfer of H/H^+ from NADH/H^+ to INT, which is reduced to red formazan and the absorbance is measured at 490 nm [86].

7.5.4 Protein Content Assay

It is used to measure the protein content of adherent and suspension cell cultures indirectly. The assay is based on the coloration with sulforhodamine B (SRB) which is a bright-pink aminoxanthene dye with two sulfonic groups. This dye binds to basic amino acid residues of protein under mildly acidic conditions in trichloroacetic acid (TCA) fixed cells. The absorbance is detected at 490 nm using a microplate reader. The assay is simple, rapid, sensitive, and reproducible and provides a sensitive index of cellular protein. SRB also produces strong fluorescence upon laser excitation at 488 nm which can be quantitatively measured by static fluorescence cytometry at a single-cell level [87].

7.5.5 Neutral Red Uptake Assay (NRU)

Neutral red uptake (NRU) is a commonly used test to evaluate the cell viability or cell toxicity. It utilizes the ability of viable cells to bind neutral red, a supravital dye in the lysosomes [88]. The dye is then extracted from the cells using acidified ethyl alcohol and quantified by measuring absorbance using a spectrophotometer. This assay is used to differentiate between damaged, viable, or dead cells [89] based on the capacity of the viable cells to maintain pH gradients through adenosine triphosphate (ATP) production and hence retain the dye. The assay is highly sensitive and can be used to determine cell viability or cytotoxic effects [90].

7.6 Assays for Assessment of *In Vivo* Toxicity

Animals are being employed either as sentinels to discern any possible perils in advance or as models to examine the physiological alteration, progression, and pathogenesis. In the last two to three decades, scientists have standardized the protocols for toxicity (minimum use of animal with least discomfort and pain) which generates assured data by reducing the bias, variance, and false-positive/negative results. Some of the crucial points ought to be noted before performing the toxicity test which comprises of cognizance of natural product isolate/drug/new chemical substance's stability, selection of route, frequency, time duration, intensity of test substance, and international rules and regulations.

Table 7.1 Categories depicted by EPA for acute toxicity.

Study	Category I	Category II	Category III	Category IV
Dermal LD_{50}	≤200 mg/kg	>200–2000 mg/kg	>2000–5000 mg/kg	>5000 mg/kg
Inhalation (4-h) LC_{50}	≤0.05 mg/l	>0.05–0.5 mg/l	>0.5–2 mg/l	>2 mg/l
Oral LD_{50}	≤50 mg/kg	>50–500 mg/kg	>500–5000 mg/kg	>5000 mg/kg

Source: EPA (1998) [92] and National Research Council (2006) [93].

Usually rodents (mice, rat, and rabbit) and dogs are used as models for toxicity assessment. Organisation for Economic Cooperation and Development (OECD) test guidance documents and guidelines must be considered [91]. EPA (U.S. Environmental Protection Agency) clearly illustrates that highest dose creates the toxicity and lowest dose does not (Table 7.1). The following definitions have been described in EPA document (Section 3 of TSCA [Toxic Substances Control Act] [92]).

- "**Acute oral toxicity** are the adverse effects occurring within a short time of oral administration of a single dose of a substance or multiple doses given within 24 hours."
- "**Delayed death** means that an animal does not die or appear moribund within 48 hours, but dies later during the 14-day observation period."
- "**Dose** is the amount of test substance administered. Dose is expressed as weight (g, mg [grams, milligrams]) or as weight of test substance per unit weight of test animal (e.g. mg/kg [milligrams/kilograms])."
- "**LD_{50}** (median lethal dose), oral, is a statistically derived single dose of a substance that can be expected to cause death in 50% of animals when administered by the oral route. The LD_{50} value is expressed in terms of weight of test substance per unit weight of test animal (mg/kg)."
- "**Limit dose** refers to a dose at an upper limitation on testing (2000–5000 mg/kg)."
- "**Moribund status** of an animal refers to being in a state of dying or inability to survive, even if treated."

7.6.1 Acute Toxicity

There are number of assays and every test/assay has its vicinity and is expanded by new protocols [94]. *In vitro* assessment fails due to organ-specific toxicity, lack of pharmacokinetic model in the *in vitro* culture, less understanding of the metabolism of a chemical compound, solubility issues (nano-formulation and few chemicals insoluble in DMSO); hence, the animal models are recruited for toxicity studies [95]. However, before the *in vivo* testing is done much of the information must be collected via cell culture. Any known and unknown substance/chemical/natural product imparts ramification up to a certain extent on organ/tissue, which is auto recovered by the body. However, the administration of test substances above their threshold level generates much impact, which leads to toxicity. So, chemical substances elicit chronic and acute toxicity that may be severe or mild.

The latter one appears in the body within 24 hours after the dose administration. EPA considers it as an "integral step in the assessment of [a chemical's] toxic potential under the regulatory framework of its pesticide and toxic substances programs" [92].

If a chemical entity is assessed to possess a low toxicity in the *in vitro* system, then limit test is a major parameter to measure the acute toxicity LD_{50} (lethal dose) *in vivo*, which is defined as a concentration of extract/drug/chemicals corresponding to 50% mortality in the test population. In addition to defining the upper limit in rodent, i.e. 5 g/body weight, it also illustrates other physiological impacts, time of onset, and degree of recovery in mice/rats [92].

7.6.1.1 Limit Test of Lorke

Among various tests, limit test of Lorke (LD_{50}) has a great impact to determine the *in vivo* toxicity [96]. Mice/rats must be kept according to the guidelines of OECD [97]. To perform an experiment three mice/rats of 25–30/250–270 g are taken and fasted for five hours. As per body weight test substance is dissolved in the desired solvent and administered to mice/rats. Animals are observed incessantly for two hours to look for clinical symptoms (abdominal cramps, fever, restlessness, vomiting, giddiness, and blur vision). The test population is monitored for 14 days after the administration to observe the adverse side effects in terms of mortality. If mice/rats die during this duration, lower dose 4 g/body weight is administered and the same process is repeated till the full survival obtained in the experiment. Further, biochemical analysis, serology, and histopathological examination of organs (liver and kidney) can be done at the end of the study to assess any alteration at the organ or tissue level.

7.6.1.2 Up and Down Procedure

All the chemical substances do not exhibit same toxicity pattern, and if it is more active physiologically or toxic than presumed, then basic test to assess toxicity is up-down procedure advocated by EPA [92]. Historically, during World War II, Dixan and Mood illustrated a method for testing the sensitivity of explosives [98] and later on in a few publications, Dixon and others explained this, but it was Bruce who nicely elaborated this aspect in biological research [99] and evaluated the uridine diphosphate (UDP) method but did not mention starting dose to be administered orally. In support of this, Ekwall justified with experimental prospective that CC_{50} presumably depicts the initial dose for acute toxicity [95]. This method utilizes a smaller number of rodents and preferably, females. It initiates with single dose and if animal survives, the dose is raised. In this case, it suffices to observe the test population for seven days as the animal would die early if chemical substance seemed toxic. The amount of dose is increased till the mortality is observed.

7.6.2 Chronic Toxicity

To set up the margin of safety and lessen the toxic manifestations of any chemical compound under consideration, chronic toxicity is of major concern. It determines the cumulative adverse impact of dose administered daily either through inhalation, dermal, or oral routes for at least more than 10 months. It is carried out with at least (preferably two) one non-rodent and one rodent species. Dog is preferred as non-rodent and rat as rodent species. Here, the test substance is administered and the animals are observed for more than 90 days to determine the LD_{50}. The test population is observed periodically. From this study various inferences can be obtained, for instance, effect of a test substance over the time on behavior, physiology, and at organ level [100]. It broadly comprises carcinogenicity and teratogenicity. EPA recommends separate norms and guidelines for carcinogenicity. The dose regimen is elected on the bases of previous toxicological data. There should be one group of control with three dose groups and include 40 rats (half of each sex)/8 dogs in each group. During the course of study, food intake, body weight should be monitored and clinical pathology should be evaluated at desired set of time. Gross anatomical analysis must be performed and all major organs must be preserved for histopathological examination [101].

Thus, both *in vitro* and *in vivo* toxicity studies need to be carried out for any compound exhibiting promising antimalarial activity before undergoing further evaluation in clinical trials. The candidate drug must not only be highly efficacious against the parasite, but it should also be non-toxic to the host. *In vitro* toxicity studies allow calculation of the selectivity index (SI), which is defined as ratio of the cytotoxic and antiparasitic activity of any compound/drug which can be used to define the criteria to proceed or not to the next steps [4]. Usually compounds exhibiting selectivity index (SI) >10 are classified as highly active antimalarial molecules with a potential for safe therapy [102]. Moreover, the selectivity index helps in ascertaining whether the compound exhibits specific antimalarial efficacy rather than general toxicity [103]. On the other hand, *in vivo* toxicity studies of any compound/drug provide initial information about its mode of toxic action and help in determining the dose for animal studies.

7.7 Conclusion

The drug susceptibility and toxicity assays form the basis of antimalarial drug research in the quest to look for newer antimalarial drugs. The identification of newer drugs to treat malaria is the need of the hour due to emergence of multi-drug-resistant strains of *Plasmodium*, particularly *P. falciparum*. All these assays have their own significance as well as limitations but are fundamental and indispensable tools in the antimalarial drug discovery studies. Also, more assays were targeting the asexual blood stages in the past; however, newer techniques are now being developed that can assess drug susceptibility of exo-erythrocytic stages of the parasite, thereby providing newer treatment options to target the parasite. Also, as the chances of development of resistance to these stages are quite low, therefore identification of the novel drug molecules against the exo-erythrocytic stages as well as the asexual blood stages can have a tremendous impact on the malaria control and eradication efforts.

References

1 Adebayo, J.O. and Krettli, A.U. (2011). Potential antimalarials from Nigerian plants: a review. *Journal of Ethnopharmacology* 133 (2): 289–302. https://doi:10.1016/j.jep.2010.11.024.

2 Trager, W., Jensen, J.B. (1976). Human malarial parasites in continuous culture. *Science* 193(4254): 673–675. doi:https://doi.org/10.1126/science.781840.

3 Lambros, C. and Vanderberg, J.P. (1979). Synchronization of *Plasmodium falciparum* erythrocytic stages in culture. *The Journal of Parasitology* 65 (3): 418–420.

4 Krettli, A.U., Adebayo, J.O., Krettli, L.G. (2009). Testing of natural products and synthetic molecules aiming at new antimalarials. *Current Drug Targets* 10(3): 261–270. doi:https://doi.org/10.2174/138945009787581203.

5 World Health Organization (2001). *In vitro* micro test (mark III) for the assessment of response of *Plasmodium falciparum* to chloroquine, mefloquine, quinine, amodiaquine, sulfadoxine, pyrimethamine and artemisinin. CTD/MAL/97, 20, World Health Organization, Geneva.

6 Rieckmann, K.H., Campbell, G.H., Sax, L.J. et al. (1978). Drug sensitivity of *Plasmodium falciparum*. An *in-vitro* microtechnique. *The Lancet* 1 (8054): 22–23. doi:https://doi.org/10.1016/s0140-6736(78)90365-3

7 Desjardins, R.E., Canfield, C.J., Haynes, J.D. et al. (1979). Quantitative assessment of antimalarial activity *in vitro* by a semiautomated microdilution technique. *Antimicrobial Agents and Chemotherapy* 16(6):710–718. doi:https://doi.org/10.1128/aac.16.6.710.

8 Fidock, D.A., Rosenthal, P.J., Croft, S.L. et al. (2004). Antimalarial drug discovery: efficacy models for compound screening. *Nature Reviews Drug Discovery* 3(6): 509–520. doi:https://doi.org/10.1038/nrd1416.

9 Makler, M.T., Ries, J.M., Williams, J.A. et al. (1993). Parasite lactate dehydrogenase as an assay for *Plasmodium falciparum* drug sensitivity. *American Journal of Tropical Medicine and Hygiene* 48(6):739–741. doi:https://doi.org/10.4269/ajtmh.1993.48.739.

10 Wright, C.W. (2005). Traditional antimalarial and the development of novel antimalarial drugs. *Journal of Ethnopharmacology* 100 (1, 2): 67–71. doi:https://doi.org/10.1016/j.jep.2005.05.012

11 Druilhe, P., Moreno, A., Blanc, C. et al. (2001). A colorimetric *in vitro* drug sensitivity assay for *Plasmodium falciparum* based on a highly sensitive double-site lactate dehydrogenase antigen-capture enzyme-linked immunosorbent assay. *American Journal of Tropical Medicine and Hygiene* 64(5, 6): 233–241. doi:https://doi.org/10.4269/ajtmh.2001.64.233.

12 Noedl, H., Wongsrichanalai, C., Miller, R.S. et al. (2002) *Plasmodium falciparum*: effect of anti-malarial drugs on the production and secretion characteristics of histidine-rich protein II. *Experimental Parasitology* 102(3, 4): 157–163. doi:https://doi.org/10.1016/s0014-4894(03)00051-1.

13 Noedl, H., Wernsdorfer, W.H., Miller, R.S. et al. (2002). Histidine-rich protein II: a novel approach to malaria drug sensitivity testing. *Antimicrobial Agents*

and Chemotherapy 46(6): 1658–1664. doi:https://doi.org/10.1128/aac.46.6.1658-1664.2002.

14 Noedl, H., Bronnert, J., Yingyuen, K. et al. (2005). Simple histidine-rich protein 2 double-site sandwich enzyme-linked immunosorbent assay for use in malaria drug sensitivity testing. *Antimicrobial Agents and Chemotherapy* 49(8): 3575–3577. doi:https://doi.org/10.1128/AAC.49.8.3575-3577.2005.

15 van Vianen, P. H., Thaithong, S., Reinders, P. P. et al. (1990). Automated flow cytometric analysis of drug susceptibility of malaria parasites. *The American Journal of Tropical Medicine and Hygiene* 43(6): 602–607. doi:https://doi.org/10.4269/ajtmh.1990.43.602.

16 Kalra, B.S., Chawla, S., Gupta, P. et al. 2006. Screening of antimalarial drugs: an overview. *Indian Journal of Pharmacology* 38: 5–12. doi:https://doi.org/10.4103/0253-7613.19846.

17 Sultan, A.A., Thathy, V., Nussenzweig, V. et al. (1999). Green fluorescent protein as a marker in *Plasmodium berghei* transformation. *Infection and Immunity* 67 (5): 2602–2606. https://doi.org/10.1128/IAI.67.5.2602-2606.1999.

18 Sanchez, B. A., Varotti, F. P., Rodrigues, F. G. et al. (2007). Validation of a *Plasmodium falciparum* parasite transformed with green fluorescent protein for antimalarial drug screening. *Journal of Microbiological Methods* 69(3): 518–522. doi:https://doi.org/10.1016/j.mimet.2007.03.001.

19 Wilson, D.W., Crabb, B.S., Beeson, J.G. (2010). Development of fluorescent *Plasmodium falciparum* for *in vitro* growth inhibition assays. *Malaria Journal* 9: 152. doi:https://doi.org/10.1186/1475-2875-9-152

20 Maji, A. K. (2018). Drug susceptibility testing methods of antimalarial agents. *Tropical Parasitology* 8(2): 70–76. doi:https://doi.org/10.4103/2229-5070.248695.

21 Bennett, T. N., Paguio, M., Gligorijevic, B. et al. (2004). Novel, rapid, and inexpensive cell-based quantification of antimalarial drug efficacy. *Antimicrobial Agents and Chemotherapy* 48(5):1807–1810. doi:https://doi.org/10.1128/aac.48.5.1807-1810.2004.

22 Smeijsters, L. J., Zijlstra, N. M., Franssen, F. F., et al. (1996). Simple, fast, and accurate fluorometric method to determine drug susceptibility of *Plasmodium falciparum* in 24-well suspension cultures. *Antimicrobial Agents and Chemotherapy* 40(4): 835–838. doi:https://doi.org/10.1128/AAC.40.4.835.

23 Smilkstein, M., Sriwilaijaroen, N., Kelly, J. X. et al. (2004). Simple and inexpensive fluorescence-based technique for high-throughput antimalarial drug screening. *Antimicrobial Agents and Chemotherapy* 48(5): 1803–1806. doi:https://doi.org/10.1128/aac.48.5.1803-1806.2004.

24 Corbett, Y., Herrera, L., Gonzalez, J. et al. (2004). A novel DNA-based microfluorimetric method to evaluate antimalarial drug activity. *The American Journal of Tropical Medicine and Hygiene* 70 (2): 119–124.

25 Quashie, N.B., de Koning, H.P., Ranford-Cartwright, L.C. (2006). An improved and highly sensitive microfluorimetric method for assessing susceptibility of *Plasmodium falciparum* to antimalarial drugs *in vitro*. *Malaria Journal* 5: 95. doi:https://doi.org/10.1186/1475-2875-5-95

26 Deharo, E., García, R. N., Oporto, P. et al. (2002). A non-radiolabelled ferriprotoporphyrin IX biomineralisation inhibition test for the high throughput screening of antimalarial compounds. *Experimental Parasitology* 100(4): 252–256. doi:https://doi.org/10.1016/s0014-4894(02)00027-9

27 Berenbaum, M. C. (1978). A method for testing for synergy with any number of agents. *The Journal of Infectious Diseases* 137(2): 122–130. doi:https://doi.org/10.1093/infdis/137.2.122.

28 Ohrt, C., Willingmyre, G.D., Lee, P. et al. (2002). Assessment of azithromycin in combination with other antimalarial drugs against *Plasmodium falciparum in vitro*. *Antimicrobial Agents and Chemotherapy* 46(8): 2518–2524. doi:https://doi.org/10.1128/aac.46.8.2518-2524.2002.

29 Canfield, C. J., Pudney, M., Gutteridge, W. E. (1995). Interactions of atovaquone with other antimalarial drugs against *Plasmodium falciparum in vitro*. *Experimental Parasitology* 80(3): 373–381. doi:https://doi.org/10.1006/expr.1995.1049.

30 Fivelman, Q. L., Adagu, I. S., Warhurst, D. C. (2004). Modified fixed-ratio isobologram method for studying *in vitro* interactions between atovaquone and proguanil or dihydroartemisinin against drug-resistant strains of *Plasmodium falciparum*. *Antimicrobial Agents and Chemotherapy* 48(11): 4097–4102. doi:https://doi.org/10.1128/AAC.48.11.4097-4102.2004.

31 Bhattacharya, A., Mishra, L.C., and Bhasin, V.K. (2008). *In vitro* activity of artemisinin in combination with clotrimazole or heat-treated amphotericin B against *Plasmodium falciparum*. *The American Journal of Tropical Medicine and Hygiene* 78 (5): 721–728.

32 Plowe, C. V., Djimde, A., Bouare, M. et al. (1995). Pyrimethamine and proguanil resistance-conferring mutations in *Plasmodium falciparum* dihydrofolate reductase: polymerase chain reaction methods for surveillance in Africa. *The American Journal of Tropical Medicine and Hygiene* 52(6): 565–568. doi:https://doi.org/10.4269/ajtmh.1995.52.565

33 Hollingdale, M. R., Leland, P., Schwartz, A. L. (1983). *In vitro* cultivation of the exoerythrocytic stage of *Plasmodium berghei* in a hepatoma cell line. *The American Journal of Tropical Medicine and Hygiene* 32(4), 682–684. doi:https://doi.org/10.4269/ajtmh.1983.32.682.

34 Gruner, A. C., Hez-Deroubaix, S., Snounou, G. et al. (2005). Insights into the *P. y. yoelii* hepatic stage transcriptome reveal complex transcriptional patterns. *Molecular and Biochemical Parasitology* 142(2): 184–192. doi:https://doi.org/10.1016/j.molbiopara.2005.03.019

35 Mahmoudi, N., Ciceron, L., Franetich, J. F. et al. (2003). *In vitro* activities of 25 quinolones and fluoroquinolones against liver and blood stage *Plasmodium* spp. *Antimicrobial Agents and Chemotherapy* 47(8): 2636–2639. doi:https://doi.org/10.1128/aac.47.8.2636-2639.2003

36 Bruña-Romero, O., Hafalla, J. C., González-Aseguinolaza, G. et al. (2001). Detection of malaria liver-stages in mice infected through the bite of a single *Anopheles* mosquito using a highly sensitive real-time PCR. *International Journal for Parasitology* 31(13): 1499–1502. doi:https://doi.org/10.1016/s0020-7519(01)00265-x.

37 Pradel, G. (2007). Proteins of the malaria parasite sexual stages: expression, function and potential for transmission blocking strategies. *Parasitology* 134(Pt. 14): 1911–1929. doi:https://doi.org/10.1017/S0031182007003381.

38 Nijhout, M. M., Carter, R. (1978). Gamete development in malaria parasites: bicarbonate-dependent stimulation by pH *in vitro*. *Parasitology* 76(1): 39–53. doi:https://doi.org/10.1017/s0031182000047375.

39 Sinden, R. E. (1983). The cell biology of sexual development in *Plasmodium*. *Parasitology* 86 (Pt 4): 7–28. doi:https://doi.org/10.1017/s0031182000050824.

40 Billker, O., Dechamps, S., Tewari, R. et al. (2004). Calcium and a calcium-dependent protein kinase regulate gamete formation and mosquito transmission in a malaria parasite. *Cell* 117(4), 503–514. doi:https://doi.org/10.1016/s0092-8674(04)00449-0

41 Raabe, A. C., Billker, O., Vial, H. J. et al. (2009). Quantitative assessment of DNA replication to monitor microgametogenesis in *Plasmodium berghei*. *Molecular and Biochemical Parasitology* 168(2): 172–176. doi:https://doi.org/10.1016/j.molbiopara.2009.08.004

42 Ponnudurai, T., Meuwissen, J. H., Leeuwenberg, A. D. et al. (1982). The production of mature gametocytes of *Plasmodium falciparum* in continuous cultures of different isolates infective to mosquitoes. *Transactions of the Royal Society of Tropical Medicine and Hygiene* 76(2): 242–250. doi:https://doi.org/10.1016/0035-9203(82)90289-9.

43 Templeton, T. J., Kaslow, D. C., Fidock, D. A. (2000). Developmental arrest of the human malaria parasite *Plasmodium falciparum* within the mosquito midgut via CTRP gene disruption. *Molecular Microbiology* 36(1): 1–9. doi:https://doi.org/10.1046/j.1365-2958.2000.01821.x.

44 Lekana-Douki, J. B., Bongui, J. B., Oyegue Liabagui, S. L. et al. (2011). *In vitro* antiplasmodial activity and cytotoxicity of nine plants traditionally used in Gabon. *Journal of Ethnopharmacology* 133(3): 1103–1108. doi:https://doi.org/10.1016/j.jep.2010.11.056.

45 Moreno, A., Badell, E., Van Rooijen, N. et al. (2001). Human malaria in immunocompromised mice: new *in vivo* model for chemotherapy studies. *Antimicrobial Agents and Chemotherapy* 45(6): 1847–1853. doi:https://doi.org/10.1128/AAC.45.6.1847-1853.2001

46 Childs, G. E., Lambros, C., Notsch, J. D. et al. (1984). Comparison of *in vitro* and *in vivo* antimalarial activities of 9-phenanthrenecarbinols. *Annals of Tropical Medicine and Parasitology* 78(1): 13–20. doi:https://doi.org/10.1080/00034983.1984.1181176.

47 Peters, W., Howells, R. E., Portus, J. et al. (1977). The chemotherapy of rodent malaria, XXVII. Studies on mefloquine (WR 142, 490). *Annals of Tropical Medicine and Parasitology* 71(4): 407–418. doi:https://doi.org/10.1080/00034983.1977.11687206.

48 Peters, W., Robinson, B. L., Ellis, D. S. (1987). The chemotherapy of rodent malaria. XLII. Halofantrine and halofantrine resistance. *Annals of Tropical Medicine and Parasitology* 81(5): 639–646. doi:https://doi.org/10.1080/00034983.1987.11812165.

49 Vennerstrom, J. L., Dong, Y., Andersen, S. L., et al. (2000). Synthesis and antimalarial activity of sixteen dispiro-1,2,4,5-tetraoxanes: alkyl-substituted 7,8,15,16-tetraoxadispiro[5.2.5. 2]hexadecanes. *Journal of Medicinal Chemistry* 43(14): 2753–2758. doi:https://doi.org/10.1021/jm0000766.

50 Posner, G. H., Paik, I. H., Sur, S. et al. (2003). Orally active, antimalarial, anticancer, artemisinin-derived trioxane dimers with high stability and efficacy. *Journal of Medicinal Chemistry* 46(6): 1060–1065. doi:https://doi.org/10.1021/jm020461q.

51 Sanni, L. A., Fonseca, L. F., Langhorne, J. (2002). Mouse models for erythrocytic-stage malaria. *Methods in Molecular Medicine* 72: 57–76. doi:https://doi.org/10.1385/1-59259-271-6:57.

52 Janse, C. (2020). Introduction to *Plasmodium berghei*. https://www.lumc.nl/org/parasitologie/research/malaria/berghei-model/introduction-berghei (accessed 22 October 2021).

53 Gorki, V., Singh, R., Walter, N. S. et al. (2018). Synthesis and evaluation of antiplasmodial efficacy of β-carboline derivatives against murine malaria. *ACS Omega* 3(10): 13200–13210. doi:https://doi.org/10.1021/acsomega.8b01833

54 Knight, D.J. and Peters, W. (1980). The antimalarial activity of *N*-benzyloxydihydrotriazines. I. The activity of clociguanil (BRL 50216) against rodent malaria, and studies on its mode of action. *Annals of Tropical Medicine and Parasitology* 74 (4): 393–404.

55 Peters, W. and Robinson, B.L. (1999). Malaria. In: *Handbook of Animal Models of Infection* (ed. O. Zak and M. Sande), 757–773. London: Academic Press.

56 Walter, N. S., Bagai, U., Kalia, S. (2013). Antimalarial activity of *Bergenia ciliata* (Haw.) Sternb. against *Plasmodium berghei*. *Parasitology Research* 112(9): 3123–3128. doi:https://doi.org/10.1007/s00436-013-3487-z

57 Walter, N., Bagai, U. (2016). Antimalarial efficacy of *Bergenia ciliata* (Saxifragaceae) leaf extract *in vitro* against *Plasmodium falciparum* and *in vivo* against *Plasmodium berghei*. *British Microbiology Research Journal* 17(6): 1–10. doi:https://doi.org/10.9734/BMRJ/2016/29262

58 Gorki, V., Walter, N. S., Singh, R. et al. (2020). β-Carboline derivatives tackling malaria: biological evaluation and docking analysis. *ACS Omega* 5(29): 17993–18006. doi:https://doi.org/10.1021/acsomega.0c01256

59 Muñoz, V., Sauvain, M., Bourdy, G. et al. (2000). The search for natural bioactive compounds through a multidisciplinary approach in Bolivia. Part II. Antimalarial activity of some plants used by Mosetene Indians. *Journal of Ethnopharmacology* 69(2): 139–155. doi:https://doi.org/10.1016/s0378-8741(99)00096-3.

60 Ager, A.L. Jr., (1984). Rodent malaria models. In: *Handbook of Experimental Pharmacology* (ed. W. Peters and W.H.G. Richards), 254–258. Berlin: Springer-Verlag.

61 Peters, W. (1965). Drug resistance in *Plasmodium berghei* Vincke and Lips, 1948. I. Chloroquine resistance. *Experimental Parasitology* 17(1): 80–89. doi:https://doi.org/10.1016/0014-4894(65)90012-3.

62 Ryley, J. F., Peters, W. (1970). The antimalarial activity of some quinolone esters. *Annals of Tropical Medicine and Parasitology* 64(2): 209–222. doi:https://doi.org/10.1080/00034983.1970.11686683.

63 Sanchez, B. A., Mota, M. M., Sultan, A. A. et al. (2004). *Plasmodium berghei* parasite transformed with green fluorescent protein for screening blood schizontocidal agents. *International Journal for Parasitology* 34(4): 485–490. doi:https://doi.org/10.1016/j.ijpara.2003.11.011

64 Angulo-Barturen, I., Jiménez-Díaz, M. B., Mulet, T. et al. (2008). A murine model of falciparum-malaria by *in vivo* selection of competent strains in non-myelodepleted mice engrafted with human erythrocytes. *PLoS One* 3(5): e2252. doi:https://doi.org/10.1371/journal.pone.0002252.

65 Carvalho, L.J.d.M., Alves, F.A., Oliveira, S.G.d. et al. (2003). Severe anaemia affects both splenectomized and non-splenectomized *P. falciparum* infected *Aotus infulatus* monkeys. *Memórias do Instituto Oswaldo Cruz* 98: 679–686. doi:https://doi.org/10.1590/S0074-02762003000500016.

66 Gysin, J. (1998). Animal models: Primates. In: *Malaria: Parasite Biology, Pathogenesis and Protection* (ed. I. Sherman), 419–441. Washington, DC: ASM Press.

67 Peters, W. (1987). Techniques of drug evaluation 1: primary screening. In: *Chemotherapy and Drug Resistance in Malaria*. Florida: Academic Press.

68 Kawai, S., Annoura, T., Araki, T., et al. (2020). Development of an effective alternative model for *in vivo* hypnozoite-induced relapse infection: a Japanese macaque (*Macaca fuscata*) model experimentally infected with *Plasmodium cynomolgi*. *Parasitology International* 76: 102096. doi:https://doi.org/10.1016/j.parint.2020.102096

69 Wengelnik, K., Vidal, V., Ancelin, M.L. et al. (2002). A class of potent antimalarials and their specific accumulation in infected erythrocytes. *Science* 295: 1311–1314.

70 Lucantoni, L., Yerbanga, R. S., Lupidi, G. et al. (2010). Transmission blocking activity of a standardized neem (*Azadirachta indica*) seed extract on the rodent malaria parasite *Plasmodium berghei* in its vector *Anopheles stephensi*. *Malaria Journal* 9: 66. doi:https://doi.org/10.1186/1475-2875-9-66.

71 Vale, N., Prudêncio, M., Marques, C. A. et al. (2009). Imidazoquines as antimalarial and antipneumocystis agents. *Journal of Medicinal Chemistry* 52(23): 7800–7807. doi:https://doi.org/10.1021/jm900738c.

72 Coleman, R. E. (1990). Sporontocidal activity of the antimalarial WR-238605 against *Plasmodium berghei* ANKA in *Anopheles stephensi*. *The American Journal of Tropical Medicine and Hygiene* 42(3): 196–205. doi:https://doi.org/10.4269/ajtmh.1990.42.196.

73 Coleman, R. E., Nath, A. K., Schneider, I. et al. (1994). Prevention of sporogony of *Plasmodium falciparum* and *P. berghei* in *Anopheles stephensi* mosquitoes by transmission-blocking antimalarials. *The American Journal of Tropical Medicine and Hygiene* 50(5): 646–653. doi:https://doi.org/10.4269/ajtmh.1994.50.646.

74 Coleman, R. E., Polsa, N., Eikarat, N. et al. (2001). Prevention of sporogony of *Plasmodium vivax* in *Anopheles dirus* mosquitoes by transmission-blocking antimalarials. *The American Journal of Tropical Medicine and Hygiene* 65(3): 214–218. doi:https://doi.org/10.4269/ajtmh.2001.65.214.

75 Krettli, A. U., Andrade-Neto, V. F., Brandão, M. G. et al. (2001). The search for new antimalarial drugs from plants used to treat fever and malaria or plants randomly selected: a review. *Memórias do Instituto Oswaldo Cruz* 96(8): 1033–1042. doi:https://doi.org/10.1590/s0074-02762001000800002

76 Russell, B., Malleret, B., Suwanarusk, R. et al. (2013). Field-based flow cytometry for *ex vivo* characterization of *Plasmodium vivax* and *P. falciparum* antimalarial sensitivity. *Antimicrobial Agents and Chemotherapy* 57(10): 5170–5174. doi:https://doi.org/10.1128/AAC.00682-13.

77 Witkowski, B., Amaratunga, C., Khim, N. et al. (2013). Novel phenotypic assays for the detection of artemisinin-resistant *Plasmodium falciparum* malaria in Cambodia: *in-vitro* and *ex-vivo* drug-response studies. *The Lancet Infectious Diseases* 13(12): 1043–1049. doi:https://doi.org/10.1016/S1473-3099(13)70252-4.

78 Rebelo, M., Tempera, C., Fernandes, J. F. et al. (2015). Assessing anti-malarial drug effects *ex vivo* using the haemozoin detection assay. *Malaria Journal* 14: 140. doi:https://doi.org/10.1186/s12936-015-0657-8.

79 Chang, Z. W., Malleret, B., Russell, B. et al. (2016). *Ex vivo* maturation assay for testing antimalarial sensitivity of rodent malaria parasites. *Antimicrobial Agents and Chemotherapy* 60(11): 6859–6866. doi:https://doi.org/10.1128/AAC.01292-16.

80 Ekwall, B. (1983). Screening of toxic compounds in mammalian cell cultures. *Annals of the New York Academy of Sciences* 407: 64–77. doi:https://doi.org/10.1111/j.1749-6632.1983.tb47814.x.

81 Mosmann T. (1983). Rapid colorimetric assay for cellular growth and survival: application to proliferation and cytotoxicity assays. *Journal of Immunological Methods* 65(1, 2): 55–63. doi:https://doi.org/10.1016/0022-1759(83)90303-4.

82 van Meerloo, J., Kaspers, G.J., Cloos, J. (2011). Cell sensitivity assays: the MTT assay. In: *Methods in Molecular Biology* (ed., N.J. Clifton), 731: 237–245. doi:https://doi.org/10.1007/978-1-61779-080-5_20.

83 Scudiero, D.A., Shoemaker, R.H., Paull, K.D. et al. (1988). Evaluation of a soluble tetrazolium/formazan assay for cell growth and drug sensitivity in culture using human and other tumor cell lines. *Cancer Research* 48 (17): 4827–4833.

84 Aslanturk OS. 2017. *In vitro* cytotoxicity and cell viability assays: principles, advantages, and disadvantages. In: *Genotoxicity – A Predictable Risk to Our Actual World*. (ed., M.L. Larramendy, S. Soloneski). IntechOpen. doi:https://doi.org/10.5772/intechopen.71923.

85 Decker, T., Lohmann-Matthes, M. L. (1988). A quick and simple method for the quantitation of lactate dehydrogenase release in measurements of cellular cytotoxicity and tumor necrosis factor (TNF) activity. *Journal of Immunological Methods* 115(1): 61–69. doi:https://doi.org/10.1016/0022-1759(88)90310-9.

86 Fotakis, G., Timbrell, J. A. (2006). *In vitro* cytotoxicity assays: comparison of LDH, neutral red, MTT and protein assay in hepatoma cell lines following exposure to cadmium chloride. *Toxicology Letters* 160(2): 171–177. doi:https://doi.org/10.1016/j.toxlet.2005.07.001.

87 Skehan, P., Storeng, R., Scudiero, D. et al. (1990). New colorimetric cytotoxicity assay for anticancer-drug screening. *Journal of the National Cancer Institute* 82(13): 1107–1112. doi:https://doi.org/10.1093/jnci/82.13.1107.

88 Zhang, S. Z., Lipsky, M. M., Trump, B. F. et al. (1990). Neutral red (NR) assay for cell viability and xenobiotic-induced cytotoxicity in primary cultures of human and rat hepatocytes. *Cell Biology and Toxicology* 6(2): 219–234. doi:https://doi.org/10.1007/BF00249595

89 Borenfreund, E., Puerner, J.A. (1985). A simple quantitative procedure using monolayer cultures for cytotoxicity assays (HTD/NR-90). *Journal of Tissue Culture Methods* 9: 7–9. doi:https://doi.org/10.1007/BF01666038.

90 Repetto, G., del Peso, A., Zurita, J. et al. (2008). Neutral red uptake assay for the estimation of cell viability/cytotoxicity. *Nature Protocols* 3(7): 1125–1131. doi:https://doi.org/10.1038/nprot.2008.75

91 OECD (Organisation for Economic Cooperation and Development) (2004). *OECD Guidelines for the Testing of Chemicals*, 15th Addendum. Paris: Organisation for Economic Cooperation and Development.

92 EPA (U.S. Environmental Protection Agency) (1998). Health effects test guidelines OPPTS 870.1100. Acute oral toxicity. EPA 712-C-98-190. Office of Prevention, Pesticides, and Toxic Substances, U.S. Environmental Protection Agency, Washington, DC. https://www.regulations.gov/document?D=EPA-HQ-OPPT-2009-0156-0003 (accessed 22 October 2021). https://www.epa.gov/test-guidelines-pesticides-and-toxic-substances/series-870-health-effects-test-guidelines (accessed 22 October 2021).

93 National Research Council (2006). *Toxicity Testing for Assessment of Environmental Agents: Interim Report*. Washington, DC: The National Academies Press https://doi.org/10.17226/11523.

94 Litchfield, J.T. Jr., and Wilcoxon, F. (1949). A simplified method of evaluating dose-effect experiments. *The Journal of Pharmacology and Experimental Therapeutics* 96 (2): 99–113.

95 Ekwall, B. (1983). Correlation between cytotoxicity *in vitro* and LD_{50}-values. *Acta Pharmacologica et Toxicologica* 52 Suppl 2: 80–99. doi:https://doi.org/10.1111/j.1600-0773.1983.tb02685.x

96 Lorke D. (1983). A new approach to practical acute toxicity testing. *Archives of Toxicology* 54(4): 275–287. doi:https://doi.org/10.1007/BF01234480.

97 OECD (1992). *OECD Guidelines for Testing of Chemicals*. No. 420: Acute oral toxicity-fixed dose method. Paris: Organisation for Economic Co-operation and Development.

98 Dixon, W.J. and Mood, A.M. (1948). A method for obtaining and analyzing sensitivity data. *Journal of the American Statistical Association* 43: 109–126.

99 Bruce, R.D. (1985). An up-and-down procedure for acute toxicity testing. *Toxicological Sciences* 5(1): 151–157. doi:https://doi.org/10.1093/toxsci/5.1.151.

100 Parasuraman, S. (2011). Toxicological screening. *Journal of Pharmacology and Pharmacotherapeutics* 2 (2): 74–79. https://doi:10.4103/0976-500X.81895.

101 EPA (U.S. Environmental Protection Agency) (1998). Health effects test guidelines OPPTS 870.4300. Combined chronic toxicity/carcinogenicity. EPA 712-C-98-212. Office of Prevention, Pesticides, and Toxic Substances, U.S. Environmental Protection Agency, Washington, DC.

102 Valdés, A. F., Martínez, J. M., Lizama, R. S. et al. (2010). *In vitro* antimalarial activity and cytotoxicity of some selected Cuban medicinal plants. *Revista do Instituto de Medicina Tropical de São Paulo* 52(4): 197–201. doi:https://doi.org/10.1590/s0036-46652010000400006.

103 Sarr, S. O., Perrotey, S., Fall, I. et al. (2011). *Icacina senegalensis* (Icacinaceae), traditionally used for the treatment of malaria, inhibits *in vitro Plasmodium falciparum* growth without host cell toxicity. *Malaria Journal* 10: 85. doi:https://doi.org/10.1186/1475-2875-10-85.

8

Aminoacyl-tRNA Synthetases as Malarial Drug Targets: A Structural Biology Perspective

Bharti Singal[1] and Jyoti Chhibber-Goel[2]

[1]Nanyang Technological University, School of Biological Sciences, 60 Nanyang Dr, 637551, Singapore
[2]International Centre for Genetic Engineering and Biotechnology, Molecular Medicine, Aruna Asaf Ali Marg, Vasant Kunj, New Delhi 110067, India

8.1 Introduction

Malaria is among the leading causes of mortality and morbidity worldwide and during 2018, around 228 million people succumbed to malaria. As per the same report, ~0.4 million deaths were reported in 2018 [1]. The ongoing regime for malaria treatment involves artemisinin-based combination (ACT) therapy and other drugs such as chloroquine (CQ) or Sulfadoxine-Pyrimethamine (SP). The ACTs (Artesunate [As] + Sulfadoxine [Sdx]) are administered once or twice a day for a 3-day duration. However, emerging drug resistance is alarming. In some countries, for CQ-resistant *Plasmodium falciparum* (*Pf*) malaria, As + SP combination therapy (ACT) is recommended [1]. The guidelines stated by the World Health Organization (WHO) suggests the use of Sulfadoxine + Pyrimethamine (SP) for intermittent preventive care (IPT) in pregnant women (IPTp) as well as in infants and children under five years of age (IPTi) in areas of moderate to high transmission [1]. Despite the availability of the antimalarial drugs, it is drug resistance resurgence that hampers the accelerated malaria control, elimination, and subsequent eradication. A look at the timeline of antimalarials highlights the proclivity of malaria parasites to develop drug resistance, thus emphasizing that malaria control requires constant discovery and development of antimalarial. For instance, CQ was first introduced in the year 1934 and recognized as a highly successful antimalarial. Eventually, about two decades later as early as 1957, resistance to CQ emerged in South East Asia (SEA) and Colombia [2]. In the 1970s, after the advent of CQ resistance, mefloquine and drug combinations of SP (Fansidar) were introduced, followed by the first report of SP resistance in the 1970s [3, 4]. Alarmingly, primaquine is currently the only approved therapy for treating the liver stages of *P. vivax* (*Pv*) hypnozoite. Similarly, ACT, which is the most commonly used malaria drug, is threatened by resistant strains of *Pf* recorded from SEA in 2009, followed by *Pv* in recent years

Bharti Singal and Jyoti Chhibber-Goel contributed equally.

Drug Development for Malaria: Novel Approaches for Prevention and Treatment, First Edition.
Edited by Pravin Kendrekar.

[5]. Due to the imminent return of drug resistant parasites against drug-based approaches, dependence on established potential drug candidates (PDCs) and novel drug scaffolds has become the key in recent years. In this chapter, we discuss the *Pf*/*Pv*-aminoacyl-tRNA synthetases (*Pf*/*Pv*-aaRSs) and the overwhelming wealth of the structural data. Such data offer an insight into the essence and efficacy of already established/validated drug targets and giving way to the growth of next-generation antimalarials.

8.2 *Pf*/*Pv*-aaRSs

8.2.1 *Pf*/*Pv* Genome

The *Plasmodium* spp. that infect humans are: *P. falciparum, P. vivax, P. malariae, P. ovale*, and *P. knowlesi*. *Pf*/*Pv* are the major cause of spreading malaria in the human population. The canonical *Pf* clone 3D7 was the first species to be sequenced within the genus *Plasmodium* [6]. The *Pf* genome is made up of about 5400 genes. This ~24 Mb genome has just ~19% GC material. The *Pf* genome forms part of 14 chromosomes with a size range of 0.6–3.3 Mb. The subtelomeric regions of the chromosomes have the greatest degree of variability in the sequence. The genome comprises 35 kb apicoplastic DNA that encodes 30 proteins and a 6 kb haploid mitochondrial DNA encoding cytochrome b and cytochrome c oxidase I and oxidase III [7]. The ~55% of the total genes are interrupted by introns. Similarly, the genome of other *Plasmodium* spp., which ranges from 23 to 27 Mb in size, also consists of three different genomes – nuclear, apicoplastic, and mitochondrial [8]. However, the GC content of these *Plasmodium* species varies from one another, for instance, *Pv* genome has GC content of ~42% [9]. The tRNA molecules required for the full collection of aaRSs genes are coded by the nuclear genome of *Pf* [10]. Most nuclear genome-encoded proteins target the apicoplast, an organelle involved in the metabolism of fatty acids and isoprenoids [11]. The antimalarial that can target multiple stages such as blood and liver stages of the parasite's life cycle are of utmost priority. Most existing medications, such as ART, lack the ability to affect the parasites in the liver stage. New eEF2 inhibitors have recently been identified as a potent drug and they target multiple stages of the parasite life [12]. The key principle for being a dual or multi-stage inhibitor is that the target should be relevant at all times [13].

The availability of the whole genome sequence of *Pf/Pv* has opened up potential novel targets with new structural scaffolds. Genome sequencing projects have provided the field of structural biology with new opportunities and challenges to broaden the understanding of molecular basis of life. The field of structural parasitology faces different challenges since proteins from *Plasmodium* genomes have proven to be more difficult than most, to express recombinantly in heterologous expression systems. The complicating factors include AT-richness of the *Pf*/*Pv* genome and prevalence of low complexity insertions. Structure genomics consortiums, along with other research groups, have overcome challenges for some parasitic proteins and have solved a number of 3D structures to date. Structural information on proteins from other human parasites is also scarce.

8.2.2 Aminoacyl-tRNA Synthetases (aaRSs)

Protein translation mechanisms are poorly understood in *Apicomplexa*, a phylum that includes deadly human pathogens such as malaria-causing *Plasmodium* spp. Bioinformatics showed that, as compared with bacteria and human counterparts, *Apicomplexans* possess a large fraction of aaRSs relative to their protein. This offers an opportunity to target this parasite's critical function as a path to killing the protozoan. Like all cells, malaria parasites possess aaRSs that are central for protein translation. These enzymes are crucial in sustaining the fidelity of translation by matching the tRNA to its corresponding amino acid and forming aa-tRNA adduct [14]. It is known that aaRSs also play roles in splicing, apoptosis, regulation of transcription, and translation. These are essential drivers for survival, growth, and proliferation. Detailed structure–function studies of crucial parasite proteins can provide new targets against malaria for drug discovery. Further, aaRSs, which are household enzymes, can also be targeted in multiple stages [14].

The aaRSs fall in to two classes – Class I comprises MRS, VRS, IRS, LRS, CRS, ERS, QRS, KRS, RRS, WRS, and YRS, while Class II comprises ARS, HRS, PRS, TRS, SRS, GRS, FRS, DRS, NRS, and KRS. Class I is characterized by a catalytic domain (classical nucleotide-binding Rossmann fold), two highly conserved motifs, i.e. HIGH and KMSKS. Class II aaRSs, on the other hand, are characterized by signature motifs (I, II, III), bent ATP morphology, and a connection via major groove. These two aaRS classes aminoacylate the tRNA in two ways. Class I enzymes carry out the reaction at the 2′OH, whereas class II enzymes at 3′OH of the cognate tRNA (with the exception of FRS) [15]. The established aaRS are multi-domain proteins consisting of multifarious and extensible structures. *Plasmodium* parasite aaRSs (~20) span across three active compartments – namely cytosol, mitochondria, and apicoplast thereby presenting an exceptional number of probable target sites. A wide range of structural and biochemical data are available for the aaRSs from *Pf* and *Pv*. Universal structural biology-based investigations complemented with drug-based programs have provided novel insights for a successful next-generation antimalarial.

The attachment of the aminoacyl group to the 3′ end, i.e. CCA of the tRNA molecule requires two steps as shown in Figure 8.1. First, the amino acid interacts with ATP and forms an intermediate aminoacyl adenylate, which is then transferred to the 3′ end of its corresponding tRNA so as to be used in protein synthesis. There are 36 aaRSs enzymes of 20 types in *Pf* with a complete set of tRNAs. Duplicate copies of aaRSs are due to active translating compartments as apicoplast and mitochondria, which being of bacterial origin are potent targets of antimalarials.

Figure 8.1 Two-step aminoacylation reaction catalyzed by aaRSs family of enzymes.

STEP 1: Activation

AA + ATP + aaRS ⇌ aaRS.AA-AMP + PPi

STEP 2: Transfer

aaRS.AA-AMP + tRNA → AA-tRNA + aaRS + AMP

Table 8.1 Structurally characterized aaRSs from *Plasmodium falciparum*.

aaRSs	PDB IDs
KRS	4H02, 4PG3, 4YCV, 5ZH2, 5ZH3, 5ZH4, 5ZH5, 6KCT, 6KAB, 6KA6, 6KBF, 6KCN, 6HCV, 6HCU, 6AGT
LRS	5FOC, 5FOD, 5FO4
PRS	4TWA, 5IFU, 4WI1, 4NCX, 4Q15, 4OLF, 4YDQ
RRS	5JLD
WRS	4JFA, 4J75, 4J76
YRS	3VGJ

Sixteen of these 36 aaRSs reside in the cytoplasm of the host, 15 in the apicoplastic. While four aaRSs (ARS, TRS, GRS, and CRS) are present as single-gene and shared between cytoplasm and apicoplast, one mitochondrial FRS (mFRS) is shared within the *Pf*. Of the characterized 36 *Pf*-aaRSs, a total of 30 three-dimensional crystal structures, co-crystallized with ligands and inhibitors are available. These are KRS (15), LRS (3), PRS (7), RRS (1), WRS (3), YRS (1) (Table 8.1). Several studies and research groups have detailed the structural comparisons among the active sites within the aaRSs enzymes from *Pf*/*Pv*. Despite the availability of the structures, there remain structurally unresolved gaps among the annotated sequences (Figure 8.2).

8.3 Aminoacyl-tRNA Synthetases as Druggable Targets

Inaccuracy in the translation machinery results in reduced protein synthesis, leading to pathogen mortality. Thus the development of various inhibitors of aaRSs has emerged as a powerful strategy for dealing with different infections. Strategies to inhibit aaRSs and utilize them to target various pathogens have been successfully exploited. Receptor-based drug discovery has helped develop aaRSs inhibitors, several of which are currently in clinical trials [16–18]. In 1967, furanomycin was discovered by Katagiri and coworkers and was found to inhibit IRS [19]. Another drug – mupirocin that is marketed as Bactroban™ against gram positive pathogens and is widely used for the treatment of *Staphylococcus aureus* infection also works by inhibiting the IRS [20]. Later in 1971, pseudomonic acid was discovered; both of these drugs were known to be effective against IRS [21, 22]. Among other aaRSs inhibitors are graniticin (LRS) [23], Ochratoxin A (FRS) [24], cispentacin (PRS) [25], borrelidin (TRS) [26], Ascamycin (FRS) [27], and indolmycin (WRS) [28]. A synthetic MRS inhibitor, REP8839, is used against *S. aureus* and various other gram-positive bacteria. A non-competitive inhibitor of LRS is AN2690, it contains fluorinated benzoxaborole and is effective against onychomycosis

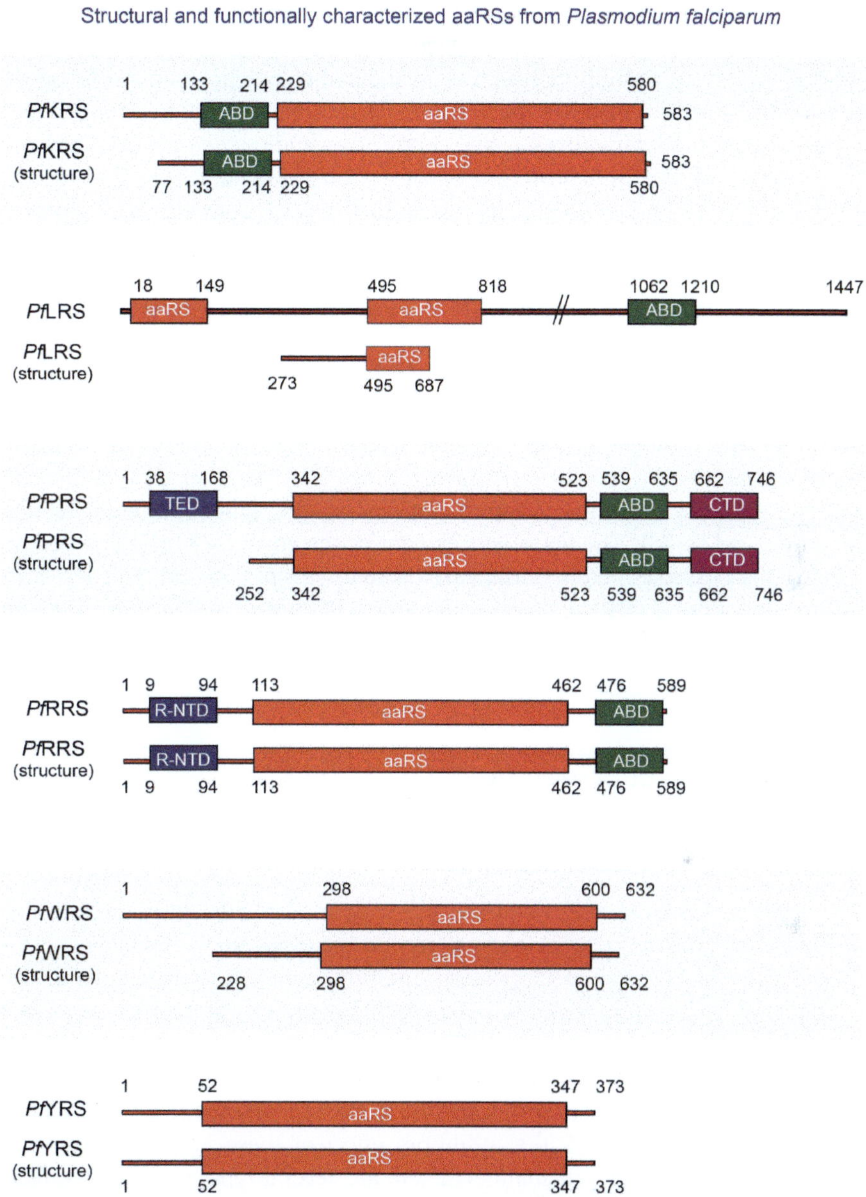

Figure 8.2 Structural and functionally characterized aminoacyl-tRNA synthetase from *Plasmodium falciparum*. The domain representation of the *Pf*-aaRSs in comparison with the structurally annotated *Pf*a-aaRSs is shown (KRS: Lysyl-tRNA synthetase; LRS: Leucyl-tRNA synthetase; PRS: Prolyl-tRNA synthetase; RRS: Arginyl-tRNA synthetase; WRS: Tryptophanyl-tRNA synthetase; YRS: Tyrosyl-tRNA synthetase).

[18]. AN2690 is currently undergoing phase 3 clinical trials. DWN12088 and T-3833261are inhibitors of PRS and are active against fibrosis [29, 30]. Further, 12 quinazolinone-based inhibitors have been validated as potent antiparasitic agents against PRS in several diseases including malaria. As new antimalarials, natural compounds and their derivatives have recently been studied to target aaRS [31–33]. The discovery of the utility of cladosporin (CLD) (fungal metabolite) against multiple stages of *Plasmodium* and its selectivity for *Pf* KRS has also been reported. CLD inhibits *Pf*KRS competitively by mimicking ATP's ribose and adenine moieties [31–33]. Borrelidin is also a fungal metabolite, which inhibits certain bacterial and eukaryotic TRS enzymes selectively as a non-competitive inhibitor [34]. It has recently been structurally and biochemically shown that a few CLD derivatives are highly specific for the *Plasmodium* spp. [35–37]. Mupirocin, or Bactroban, is another fungal metabolite. Mupirocin bound to IRS crystal [35] structures shows that mupirocin inhibits by blocking the Isoleucine–AMP interaction. Further mupirocin inhibits the growth of *Pf* in nM range [34]. Another example is from traditional Chinese medicine, *Dichroa febrifuga* shrub, which was used to treat malaria fevers [38–45]. The active component of the shrub is febrifugine (FF, an alkaloid) that possesses potent antimalarial activity *in vitro* [38–46]. The derivative of FF, Halofuginone (HF), a 7-bromo-6-chloro, has lower cell toxicity than FF [47–51]. HF is currently used as a coccidiostat against *Eimeria* and *Cryptosporidium* infections [52, 53].

8.4 Biochemical Screening of Drug Libraries

AaRSs have two step processes by which aminoacyl tRNAs are synthesized. The first step is accompanied by ATP in which amino acid is activated by formation of aminoacyl-adenylate (aa-AMP) and inorganic pyrophosphate (Ppi) is released. In the second step, the amino acid is transferred to the tRNA and aminoacyl-tRNA is released with AMP. Certain aaRSs possess the editing activity as well in order to keep the fidelity of tRNA aminoacylation. The specific hydrolysis of the incorrectly acylated products is achieved by these aaRSs either before or after the transfer process and is called pre-transfer or post-transfer editing, respectively. The importance of aaRSs makes them indispensable targets to generate antimalarial. Biochemical assays are required to check the inhibitory effect of these natural or synthetic inhibitors in high-throughput manner. There are several types of assays available for that which are described as follows.

8.4.1 Colorimetric Assays

The colorimetric assays are designed to be used in a high-throughput manner without using any radioactive compounds such as radiolabeled ATP or amino acid. In such assays, the aminoacylation reaction is coupled with inorganic pyrophosphatase (PPiase), which converts the PPi formed in the first step of aminoacylation to Pi (inorganic phosphate). Pi is detected with the help of malachite green. The reaction between Pi and malachite green changes the color of the solution from yellow to green. To measure this quantitatively, the absorbance is recorded at 620 nm using a spectrophotometer.

8.4.2 Enzyme-Coupled Assays

These enzyme-coupled assays require multiple enzymes to detect the activity of aaRS in a continuous manner. In these assays, the aminoacylation reaction is coupled to the oxidation reaction of NADH. This requires AMP to react with ATP to produce ADPs with the help of adenylate kinase, which is further used in pyruvate kinase reaction. This reaction is coupled with lactate dehydrogenase reaction and thus oxidation of NADH is monitored at 340 nm wavelength with the help of spectrophotometer [54]. In another assay, the Ppi formation is continuously monitored by coupling the aminoacylation reaction with inorganic pyrophosphatase. The phosphate produced is then coupled to phosphorolysis reaction of 2-amino 6-mercapto-7-methylpurine ribonucleoside (AMMR), which utilizes purine nucleoside phosphorylase enzyme to yield AMMP (2-amino 6-mercapto 7-methylpurine). The AMMP signal is observed at 360 nm wavelength for quantitative estimation [55]. These spectrophotometric assays have limitations of high background and a low signal-to-noise ratio due to multiple enzyme-coupled reactions.

8.4.3 Luciferase Assay

This assay measures the light emitted by the luciferase based on the relative amount of ATP utilized during the tRNA-aminoacylation reaction. This is based on the gene manipulation of luciferase enzyme by interrupting the sequence with a stop codon. A special tRNA containing the suppressor anticodon, which can translate this stop codon, is introduced, which is aminoacylated by the pathogenic aaRS. Inhibition of this specific pathogenic aaRS leads to decrease in luminescence produced as the gene does not get translated into luciferase. These three genes can be expressed in a human cell line, which can further be used for small compound libraries (reviewed in [56]).

8.4.4 Assay to Test Synthetic as Well as Proofreading Activity

This assay has been developed to ensure High throughput (HTP) detection of inhibitors against synthetic as well as editing activity of the aaRS enzymes. This assay incorporates two of the assays described above, which utilizes PPiase and purine nucleoside phosphorylase (PNPase). Non-cognate amino acids are used in this assay to produce mischarged AMP and tRNA, which needs to be hydrolyzed by the aaRS editing activity. This produces amino acid and tRNA, which can be used in additional cycles of aminoacylation leading to large production of PPi. PPiase converts PPi into Pi, Pi is subsequently used by PNPase to break down AMMR. The product of this reaction is quantifiable at 355 nm wavelength. This method can thus be used to identify inhibitors of both synthetic and editing sites of aaRS by observing the decrease in the rate of formation of PPi. The addition of PPiase prevents the reversal of the amino acid activation step and thus drives aminoacylation of both cognate and non-cognate amino acids [57].

8.5 Structurally Validated *Pf/Pv*-aaRSs as Drug Targets

8.5.1 Lysyl-tRNA Synthetase (KRS)

KRS is unique as it fits in both the classes of aaRSs family nomenclature. Class I KRS are present in bacteria and archaea, whereas most prokaryotes and eukaryotes show the presence of class II KRSs [58–60]. KRSs have been implicated in the synthesis of signaling molecules such as diadenosine polyphosphate (Ap4a). Ap4a

Table 8.2 Structurally characterized lysyl-tRNA synthetase from several pathogens is shown.

Lysyl-tRNA synthetase					
		PDB ID	Resolution (Å)	Ligands	Average B-factor
Homo sapiens	Holo – enzyme	3BJU	2.3	ATP, LYS	28.7
		4DPG	2.8	ALA, APC, LYS	42.4
		4YCU	2.1	LYS, CLD	31.6
		4YCW	2.9	LYS, CLD	62.4
		6CHD	2.5	KAA	52.8
Plasmodium falciparum	Apo	4H02	2.9	—	—
	Holo – enzyme	4PG3	2.7	LYS, CLD	—
		4YCV	3.4	KRS	58.4
		5ZH2	2.6	LYS, 9CU	48
		5ZH3	2.8	LYS, 9CF	102.6
		5ZH4	2.6	LYS, 9CC	66.2
		5ZH5	3.1	LYS, 9CX	93.5
		6KCT	3.2	LYS, D5O	60.8
		6KAB	2.9	LYS, D4U	—
		6KA6	1.9	LYS, D40	—
		6KBF	1.9	LYS, D4X	—
		6KCN	2.2	LYS, D5F	—
		6HCV	2.2	FYE	—
		6HCU	1.6	LYS, HIS, FYB	—
		6AGT	1.9	LYS, 9X0	—

Table 8.2 (Continued)

Lysyl-tRNA synthetase					
		PDB ID	Resolution (Å)	Ligands	Average B-factor
Cryptosporidium parvum	Apo	6C86	2.1		35.8
	Holo enzyme	5ELN	1.9	LYS	25.9
		5ELO	1.9	LYS, CLD	30.0
		6BNI	1.8	ADN	29.8
Loa loa	Holo	5HGQ	3.2	LYS, CLD	—

ADN: adenosine, ALA: alanine, APC: diphosphomethylphosphonic acid adenosyl ester, LYS: lysine, CLD: cladosporine, KAA: 54′-*O*-[(L-Lysylamino)sulfonyl]adenosine. 9CU: (3*R*)-6,8-dihydroxy-3-{[(2*R*,6*R*)-6-methyloxan-2-yl]methyl}-3,4-dihydro-1*H*-2-benzopyran-1-one, 9CF: (3*S*)-6,8-dihydroxy-3-{[(2*R*,6*R*)-6-methyloxan-2-yl]methyl}-3,4-dihydro-1*H*-2-benzopyran-1-one, 9CC: (3*R*)-6,8-dihydroxy-3-{[(2*S*,6*R*)-6-methyloxan-2-yl]methyl}-3,4-dihydro-1*R*-2-benzopyran -1-one, 9CX: (3*S*)-6,8-dihydroxy-3-{[(2*R*,6*S*)-6-methyloxan-2-yl]methyl}-3,4-dihydro-1*R*-2-benzopyran-1-one, D5O: 3-(cyclohexylmethyl)-6,8-bis(oxidanyl) isochromen-1-one, D4U: (3~{*S*})-3-(cyclohexylmethyl)-6,8-bis(oxidanyl)-3,4-dihydroisochromen-1-one, D4O: (3~{*S*}-3-[[(1~{*S*},3~{*S*})-3-methylcyclohexyl]methyl]-6,8-bis(oxidanyl)-3,4-dihydroisochromen-1-one, D4X: (3~{*S*})-3-[[1~{*S*},3~{*S*}-3-methylcyclohexyl]methyl]-6,8-bis(oxidanyl)-3,4-dihydro-2~{*H*}-isoquinolin-1-one, D4F: 3[[(1~{*S*},3~{*S*})-3-methylcyclohexyl]methyl]-6,8-bis(oxidanyl)isochromen-1-one, FYE: 6-fluoranyl~{*N*}-[(1-oxidanylcyclohexyl)methyl]-4-oxidanylidene-chromene-2-carboxamide, HIS: Histidine, FYB: ~{*N*}-[[4,4-bis(fluoranyl)-1-oxidanyl-cyclohexyl]methyl]-6-fluoranyl-4-oxidanylidene-chromene-2-carboxamide, 9X0: *N*-(cyclohexylmethyl)-4-oxo-4*H*-1-benzopyran-2-carboxamide.

is involved in several processes. For instance, DNA replication, regulation of ion channels, and gene expression [61]. The structural and biochemical attributes of KRS from several organisms including *Cryptosporidium parvum*, *Homo sapiens*, *Loa loa*, and *P. falciparum* have been elucidated in the context of CLD (IUPAC name is isocoumarin 3,4-dihydro-6,8-dihydroxy-3-(6-methyltetrahydropyran-2-ylmethyl)) and several of its derivatives (Table 8.2). CLD is a chiral complex molecule that is synthesized by fungi, such as *Aspergillus flavus* and *Cladosporium cladosporioides* [31]. The scaffold formed by the 6,8-dihydroxylisocoumarin and methyltetrahydropyrene (mTHP) group of CLD imitates the adenosine moiety, thereby competing with ATP (Figure 8.3a) [32, 33, 62]. CLD's discovery has opened new opportunities for targeting a plethora of eukaryotic parasites [63]. Initial cell-based screening detected CLD to inhibit *Pf* in the blood stages [31, 32]. Subsequently, the cytoplasmic *Pf*KRS (*Pf*KRS-cyto) was validated to be the CLD target based on biochemical investigations accompanied by structural analysis. The type II *Pf*KRS forms a homodimer consisting of monomers having 17 β-strands and 17 α-helices. The N-terminal and the C-terminal of the type II *Pf*KRS show the presence of OB-fold (anticodon-binding) and a catalytic domain, respectively (Figure 8.3b).

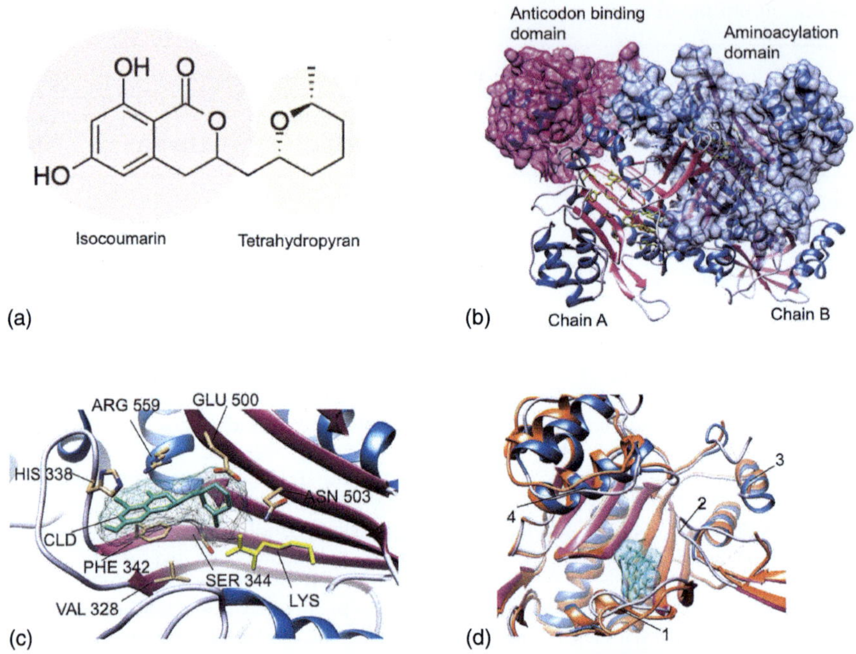

Figure 8.3 Cladosporin and its interactions with *Pf*KRS. (a) Cladosporin chemical structure – the rings tetrahydropyran (mTHP) and isocoumarin are highlighted in *yellow* and *orange* respectively. (b) Overview of the structure showing homodimer formed by chain A and B (PDB: 4PG3). The two domains, namely ABD (surface shown in *magenta)* and aminoacylation domain (surface shown in *cornblue*), are present on N- and C-terminal of the *Pf*KRS, respectively. (c) Interaction of Cladosporin with *Pf*KRS. The binding of Cladosporin (CLD, *cyan*) is shown in *Pf*KRS (PDB: 4PG3, color coded as described in Figure 8.2a) in the presence of lysine (*yellow*). The residues interacting with CLD in the aminoacylation binding site are shown as sticks (*beige*) and labeled (*black*). (d) Structural change in *Pf*KRSs driven by cladosporin (CLD) binding. In *Pf*KRS the interaction of CLD occurs by changes in three loops (numbered 1, 2, and 4) and an alpha helix (numbered 3). The binding induces closing in of loops 1 and 4 and further stabilization of loop 2 and of alpha helix 3. The CLD-free structure is colored in *orange* (PDB: 4H02) and the CLD-bound structure (PDB: 4PG3) is color coded as described in Figure 8.2a,b.

Binding affinity tests, thermal change, and micro-scale thermophoresis (MST) assays indicated minor increases in the stability of *Pf*KRS upon binding of natural substrate [32, 33]. On the contrary, CLD resulted in higher thermal stability of the *Pf*KRS–CLD complex with a higher melting temperature of around 16 °C. Binding assays for the AMPPNP and CLD revealed a KD value of approximately 4 μM and 14 nM, respectively. Biochemically, CLD exhibits selectivity to *Pf*KRS based on the two main residues, Val 328 and Ser 344 in close proximity to the ATP binding pocket of KRSs. These small residues make the enzyme CLD obligatory; however, the presence of bulkier groups such as Gln321 and Thr 337 as reported in *Hs*KRS hinders the CLD obligation (Figure 8.3c). Further, CLD restricts the *Pf* growth in blood and liver stages and is highly selective (>100 folds) when compared with *Hs*KRS. Upon CLD binding, three loops and one helix proximate to *Pf*KRS–CLD-binding pocket undergo key rearrangements and following the engagement of CLD the loops and alpha helix are closed and stabilized (Figure 8.3d) [64]. These changes result in CLD burial and are reminiscent of enzyme–drug interactions with the ligand-induced binding model. The KRSs–CLD complexes of other species, on the other hand, show little/no noticeable conformational improvement on CLD binding [64]. This is reinforced by the fact that secondary structural components do not have major global variations. It is important to remember that CLD can inhibit *Pf* growth in the liver and blood stages with IC50 below 100 nM [64]. However, owing to poor metabolic stability and low bioavailability, CLD is not compliant to be developed as a drug lead. CLD is a chiral complex, with three stereo-centers resulting in the possibility of eight stereoisomers [62]. A complete library of CLD stereoisomers has been developed and characterized using enzyme-, structure-, and parasite-based assays. Strikingly, the drug efficacy among these enantiomers shows ~500-fold difference. The structural characterization of the KRS bound CLD stereoisomers further revealed that alterations at C3 and C10 are detrimental to drug potency, whereas changes at C3 are sensed by rotameric flipping of Glu332 (Figure 8.3a) [62]. Currently, CLD-binding mechanisms have been best understood in the cyto-*Pf*KRS model. However, studying the eukaryotic parasites with highly conserved KRS active sites will be crucial for drug development. Further the most promising CLD-inspired inhibitors and its stereoisomers are worth further research.

8.5.2 Prolyl-tRNA Synthetase

All PRSs are defined by a catalytic domain, an anticodon-binding domain (ABD/HGTP-ABD); and a C-terminal zinc-binding domain (CTD) with a β–α–β–β motif. In contrast to *H. sapiens*, *Plasmodium* PRSs have an N-terminal tRNA editing domain capable of hydrolyzing non-cognate amino acids. Over the years, seven crystal structures of *Pf*PRS-cyto (4TWA, 4NCX, 4YDQ, 4Q15, 4WI1, 5IFU, and 4OLF) have been resolved (Table 8.1). Interestingly, no structural validation for a highly conserved (>50%) ~251 long N-terminal element has been reported out among the structurally annotated *Pf*PRS (seven PDBs) (Figure 8.2). This sub-structural fragment promises a strong structural implication for novel drug development. However, the structurally characterized fragment of the PRSs is among the most focused antimalarial target owing to a number of potent compounds that target the critical – ATP, amino acid, and tRNA-binding site (Table 8.2). The active component of *Dichroa febrifuga* (a Chinese herb) – FF and the highly potent derivative of FF – HF has demonstrated direct and strong binding to *Pf*PRS (Figure 8.4a) [46, 66, 67]. *Pf*PRS is a dimeric enzyme that localizes in the parasite's cytoplasm. The two domains of *Pf*PRS are joined by a linker separating an editing domain at the N-terminal from the canonical synthetase domain. Structural analysis of the *Pf*PRS has shown that there are at least four druggable subsites (Figure 8.4b) [65]. Biochemical and structural characterization of *Pf*PRS revealed that HF binds to PRS in ATP-dependent manner by mimicking the L-Proline and A76 of tRNA, where in the protein translation gets restored at saturating concentration of proline [46, 68]. Further, the structure determination of *Pf*PRS–HF–AMPPNP ternary

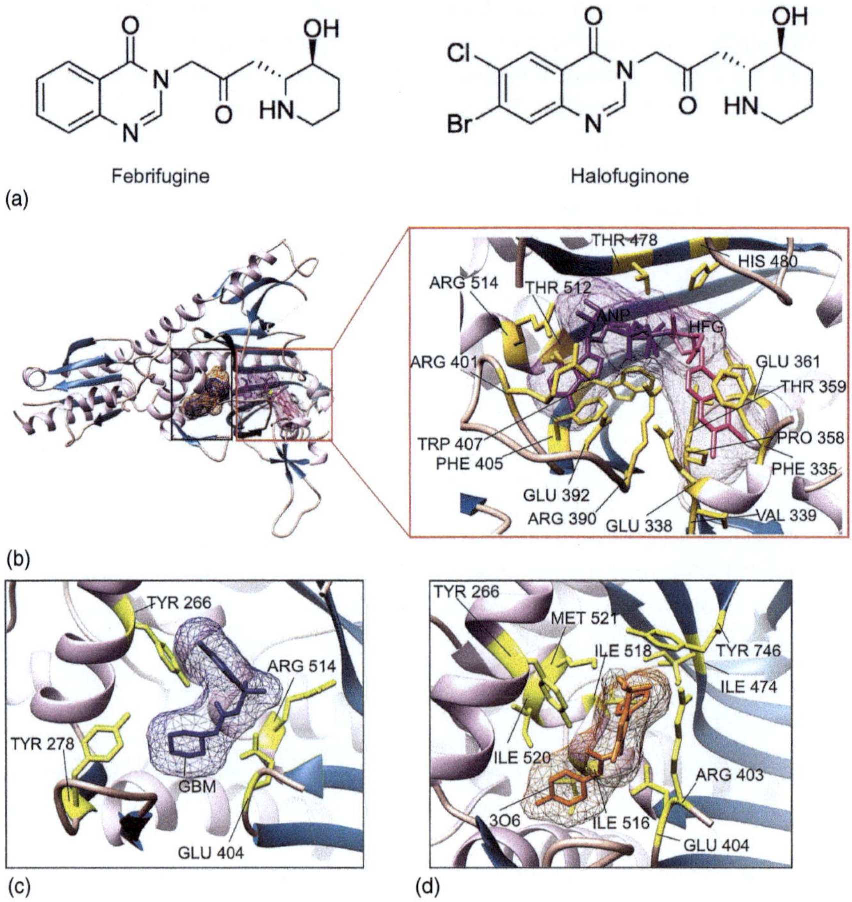

Figure 8.4 Structure of *Pf*PRS. (a) The chemical structure of febrifugine and its derivative, halofuginone is shown. (b) The overview of the crystal structure of *Pf*PRS with the four druggable sites (in *orange*, *blue*, *purple*, and *pink* mesh surface) is shown, where *Pf*PRS is color coded as helix: *pastel purple*, strand: d*eep blue* and loops: *beige*. The right panel (*red* box) shows the zoomed interactions of ANP (*purple*) and HFG (*pink*) with residues in *yellow* within <4 Å distance. (c) and (d) Represent the zoomed binding site (*black* box in Figure 8.4b) of GBM (*blue*) and 306 (*orange*), respectively. The residues interacting with GBM and 306 within <4 Å distance are highlighted in *yellow*. Source: Based on Jain et al. [65].

complex has proven the rationale behind the exquisite inhibitory properties of HF at a resolution of 2.3 Å. Additionally, the cell and enzyme-based inhibition assays to address have successfully addressed the drug-like properties of the four quinazolinone-based compounds, such as HF, FF, 6F-FF (6-fluoro febrifugine), and Th-FF (tetrahydro quinazolinone febrifugine) (Figure 8.4a). These drugs killed malaria parasites in the very first cycle of erythrocytic development, suggesting that the inhibitors targeted the cytoplasmic *Pf*PRS. The quinazolinone-based compounds (HF, FF, 6F-FF, and Th-FF) have a dose-dependent inhibition with EC50 (50% effective concentration) in subnanomolar range, i.e. 1–190 nM and IC50 of 9 nM (HF), 24 nM (FF), 13 nM (6F-FF), 352 nM (Th-FF), respectively against *Pf* [67, 69]. Further to this, AMPPNP increases the specificity, affinity, and stability of the drug–*Pf*PRS complex by ~30-fold (from ~300 to 9 nM) [67]. The HF and 6F-FF with halogen atoms substituted at the vulnerable aromatic protons increase the potency and activity of FF derivatives. In summary, PRS active site architecture demonstrates that HF-based leads present themselves direct focus in antimalarial drug development efforts.

8.6 Potential Drug Targets *Pf*/*Pv*-aaRSs

8.6.1 Leucyl-tRNA Synthetase (LRS)

The class-I aaRSs, LRS is 1447 residues long that is characterized by an N- and a C-terminal catalytic domain. In addition to these, there is an N-terminal connecting peptide (Rossmann fold) joining the N- and C-terminal catalytic domain as well as the C-terminal ABD (Figure 8.2). Additionally, the editing domain of the LRS is enclosed in the C-terminal catalytic domain. To date three crystal structures have been resolved for the *Pf*LRS structures (Table 8.3). The structural data is available partly for the *Pf*LRS, which is a monomeric enzyme with two monomers per asymmetric unit (ASU). The three-dimensional crystal structure is resolved for the ~414 residue that is part of the editing domain (273–687). In *Pf*LRS, the flexible loops residues 328–361 and 475–519 were deleted and not crystallized. The crystal structure of the editing domain docked with benzoxaboroles has been shown to effectively target the editing site of cyto-*Pf*LRS [70]. The same has been validated using two compounds, AN6426 and AN8432, with nanomolar *in vitro* activity. It is important to note that the structure for the catalytic and ABD remains to be validated.

8.7 Arginyl-tRNA Synthetase (RRS)

RRS belongs to the class I aaRSs and is a 590 residues long protein. It is characterized by an N-terminal domain (NTD) (residues 3–90, in pink), a catalytic domain (residues 105–410), and an ABD (residues 425–590, in blue) (Figures 8.2 and 8.5a). The cytoplasmic *P. falciparum* RRS (cyto-*Pf*RRS) not only plays an important role in protein translation, but the flagging of proteins with Arg also marks them for degradation via N-end rule [71–73]. The de novo heme synthesis pathway of the malaria parasite remains inactive during intraerythrocytic stages [74, 75]. Malaria parasites depend on host hemoglobin for amino acid supply. The heme produced during hemoglobin digestion is oxidized to hemin and subsequently to hemozoin. CQ acts by increasing the free hemin in the parasites. The increased levels of hemin result in protein misfolding, oxidation, and deregulation of redox/membrane potentials, resulting in cellular to toxicity. *Pf*RRS plays an important role during CQ treatment, wherein it senses the heme imbalance and alerts the parasite to evade toxic effects as a result of excess CQ-induced heme. On binding to the free hemin, the

Table 8.3 Structurally characterized prolyl-tRNA synthetase from several pathogens is shown.

Prolyl-tRNA synthetase					
		PDB ID	**Resolution (Å)**	**Ligands**	**Average B-factor**
Thermus thermophilus	Apo	1HC7	2.4	—	35.4
	Holo	1H4T	2.9	PRO	—
		1h4S	2.8	PSD	—
		1H4Q	3	ATP, PRI	—
Enterococcus faecalis	Holo	2J3M	2.3	ATP, PRI	21.8
		2J3L	2.3	P5A	29.5
Naegleria fowleri	Holo	6NAB	2.0	AMP, PRO	48
		6UYH	1.7	ANP, HFG	30.6
Leishmania major	Apo	5XIL	1.9	—	23.2
Giardia lambia	Holo	3IAL	2.2	PR8	34.6
Eimeria tenella	Holo	5XIP	3.1	ANP, HFG	58.8
Toxoplasma gondii	Apo	6AA0	3.2	—	76.6
		5XIF	2.5	—	44.6
	Holo	6A88	2.6	ANP, 9SF	46.2
		5XIQ	2.2	APC, HFG	44.4
		5XIG	2.4	87F, ANP	37.9
		5XII	2.2	86X, ANP	33.9
		5XIH	2.2	86U, ANP	31.5
		5XIK	2.5	ANP, 87C, 37.6	
		5XIJ	2.5	873, ANP	37.2
Plasmodium falciparum	Apo	4TWA	3.0	—	—
		4NCX	1.8	—	33.0
	Holo	5IFU	2.4	GBM	61.4
		4WI1	1.6	3O6	33.3
		4Q15	2.4	HFG	44.5
		4OLF	2.9	ANP	74.4
		4YDQ	2.3	ANP	44.8
Cryptosporidium parvum	Holo	5XIO	2.5	HFG	41.5

PRO: Proline, PSD: 5′-*O*-[*N*-(prolyl)-sulfamoyl]adenosine, ATP: Adenosine-5′-triphosphate, PRI: Pyrrolidine-2-carbaldehyde, P5A: '5'-*O*-(*N*-(L-prolyl)-sulfamoyl)adenosine, HFG: 7-bromo-6-chloro-3-{3-[(2*R*,3*S*)-3-hydroxy piperidin-2-yl]-2-oxopropyl}quinazolin-4-(3*H*)-one, ANP: Phosphpaminophophonic acid ester, PR8: 5′-*O*-[(*R*)-hydroxy{[(2*S*)-pyrrolidin-2-ylcarbonyl]oxy}phosphoryl]adenosine, 9SF: 3-{3-[(2*R*,3*S*)-3-hydroxypiperidin-2-yl]-2-oxopropyl} quinazolin-4(3*H*)-one, 87F: 3-[3-[(2*R*)-3-oxidanylidenepiperidin-2-yl]propyl]quinazolin-4-one, 86X: 6-chloranyl-7-fluoranyl-3-[3-[(2*R*)-3-oxidanylidenepiperidin-2-yl]propyl]quinazolin-4-one, 86U: 6,7-bis (fluoronyl)-3-[3-[(2*R*)-3-oxidanylidenepiperidin-2-yl]propyl]quinazolin-4-one, 87C: 3-[2-oxidanylidene-3-[(2*R*,3*R*)-3-oxidanylpiperidin-2-yl]propyl]-5-6,7,8-tetrahydroquinazoline-4-one, 873: 3-[(2*R*)-2-oxidanyl-3-[(2*R*,3*R*)-3-oxidanylpiperidin-2-yl]propyl]quinazolin-4-one, GBM: 5-chloro-*N*-(2-{4-[(cyclohexylcarbamoyl)sulfamoyl]phenyl}ethyl)-2-methoxybenzamide, 3O6: 1-(4-fluorophenyl)-3-[4-(4-fluorophenyl)-1-methyl-3-(trifluoromethyl)-1*H*-pyrazol-5-yl] urea.

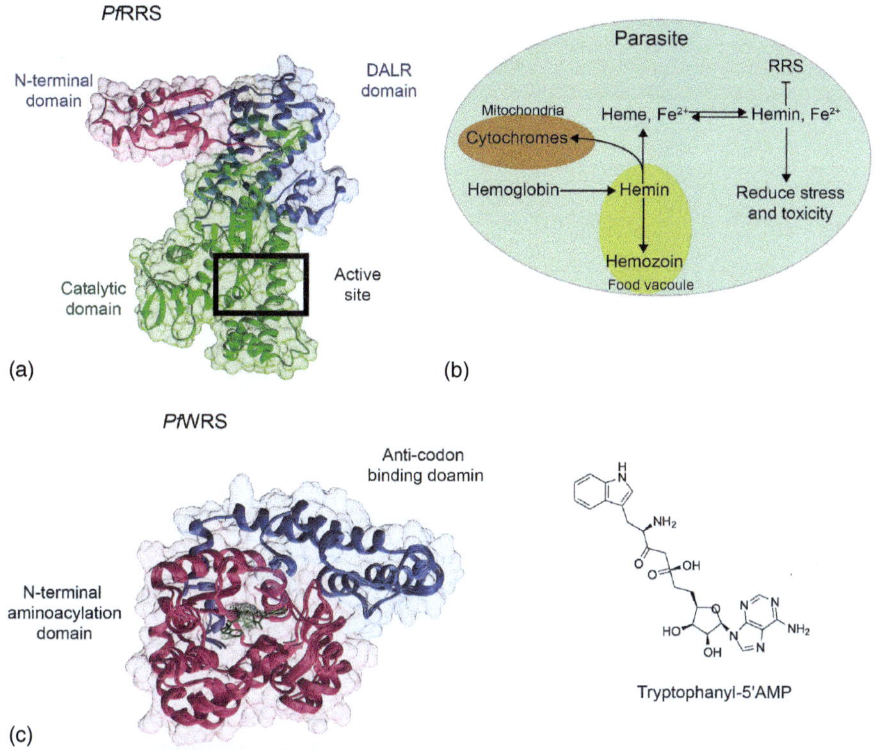

Figure 8.5 Structurally unannotated aaRSs: potential drug targets. (a) The three-dimensional crystal structure of *Pf*RRS is shown, with color-coded canonical domains of the enzyme. (b) Proposed model for *Pf*RRS action during heme stress is shown. (c) The surface view of the crystal structure with N-terminal aminoacylation and the anticodon domain is shown. The ligand – tryptophanyl-5′AMP (TYM) is in green.

cyto-*Pf*RRS is inactivated and undergoes dimerization. The dimerized *Pf*RRS fails to undergo aminoacylation reaction (Figure 8.5b). Heme-binding induced inhibition of *Pf*RRS and subsequent metabolic damping likely gives the parasite an ability to reach a dormancy-like state under drug stress conditions. In contrast to CQ's indirect hemin-mediated response, no new leads to directly target RRS have been validated.

8.7.1 Tryptophanyl-tRNA Synthetase (WRS)

To date, three crystal structures have been resolved for WRS. These are 4JFA, 4J75, and 4J76 (Table 8.4). The apo form of *Pf*WRS – 4J76 [76] and the holo-forms – 4J75, 4JFA [77] are co-crystallized with tryptophan (TRP) and tryptophanyl-adenylate (TYM), respectively. It is noteworthy that only the residues 228–662 have been detailed for both structural and biochemical assays, thereby representing only a fraction of WRS protein from *Pf* (Figure 8.2). While the non-crystallized NTD (1–227) is crucial for charging tRNAtrp and aminoacylation activity, the crystallized *Pf*WRS (PDB IDs: 4J76, 4J75, 4J76 – 229–632 residues) is indeed the catalytic domain of

Table 8.4 Structurally characterized potential drug targets aaRSs from *P. falciparum*.

		PDB ID	Resolution (Å)	Ligands	Average B-factor
LRS	Apo	5FOC	2.4	—	30.8
		5FOD	2.9	—	30.47
		5FOA	1.8	—	36.23
RRS	Apo	5JLD	2.2	—	61.2
WRS	Apo	4J76	2.3	—	61.2
	Holo	4J75	2.4	TYM	43.9
		4JFA	2.6	TRP	54.5
YRS	Holo	3VGJ	2.2	TYR, AMP	56.4

TYM: Tryptophanyl-5′AMP, TRP: Tryptophan, TYR: Tyrosine, AMP: Adenosine monophosphate.

the protein [76]. The residues comprise the complete eukaryote-specific N-terminal extension (ESE) (Ser229-His300), Rossmann-fold domain (Lys301-Thr520 and Thr611-Met632), and C-terminal helical domain (Asp521-Leu610). N-terminal aminoacylation domain spans from residue 228 to 496 (in hot pink, Figure 8.5c) and an ABD from residue 497 to 629 (in blue, Figure 8.5c). It has been validated that the apo-*Pf*WRS undergoes ligand-induced conformational changes on product formation. Molecules disrupting these conformational changes could be the key to developing inhibitors against the *Pf*RRS [77]. Despite the efforts to look for potential inhibitors employing structure-guided drug design [77], to date, the search for a lead to target WRS has been unfruitful, especially when looking at ligand-binding region.

8.7.2 Tyrosyl-tRNA Synthetase

YRS is ~373 residue long protein characterized by an N-terminal catalytic domain (18–260 residues, Rossmann fold) and an ABD (261–370 residues) [78, 79]. It is a homo-dimeric class-I enzyme with one homo-dimer ASU [80]. *Pf*YRS is a parasite-secreted protein with implications in pro-inflammatory host responses [81, 82]. The secreted *Pf*YRS exits into the infected red blood cell (iRBC) cytoplasm and is subsequently released into the extracellular medium upon the rupture/lysis of the infected RBCs [80]. The catalytic domain of *Pf*YRS is characterized by a tripeptide Glu-Leu-Arg (ELR) motif that is released into the extracellular medium on iRBC lysis. Further using this ELR motif, which it shares with IL-8, *Pf*YRS specifically binds to and internalizes into host macrophages, leading to enhanced secretion of the pro-inflammatory cytokines [83–88]. The *Pf*YRS ELR motif is surface exposed and significantly distal from aminoacylation sites. The implication of the *Pf*YRS in protein translation and triggering a pro-inflammatory cytokine release in the extracellular medium upon infected RBC lysis has highlighted the potential of this aaRSs as a potent target for antimalarial strategies. However, there have been no reports since and insights into the parasitic YRSs are needed.

8.8 Others

Several potential inhibitors of *Plasmodium* aaRSs have been screened based on in silico screening and enzyme-based assays. (i) Alanyl-tRNA synthetase (ARS) is a promising antimalarial drug target. It is localized in both the cytoplasm and the apicoplast of the *Pf*. *Pf*ARS potential inhibitor – A5 – {4-92-nitro-1-propenyl}1,2-benzenediol inhibits the parasite growth in μM range [33, 89, 90]. (ii) Isoleucyl-tRNA synthetase (IRS) binds to the Ile-AMP intermediate, thereby inhibiting the step of IRS aminoacylation. Further, IRS inhibits *Pf* in nM range [91, 92]. Due to reports on mutations in the apicoplastic IRS, and the detection of mupirocin-resistant parasites, IRS has not been explored against mupirocin. Additionally, based on cell-based assays in parasites and mammalian cells – thiaisoleucine has been shown to inhibit parasite growth as well as mammalian cells. Despite the drugs being ineffective, these observations have successfully established IRS as a suitable antimalarial. (iii) Threonyl-tRNA synthetase (TRS) in *Pf* is present in both cytoplasm and the apicoplast [93, 94]. Small-molecule compounds identified based on *in-silico* screening showed an inhibition in μM range [89] in *Pf in-vitro* culture. Independently, the drug borrelidin (an activator of proapoptotic mediators in endothelial cells and inhibits cyclin-dependent kinase in yeast) results in immediate parasite death. Further, the addition of L-threonine in *in-vitro* parasite culture reverses and abrogates the effects of the Borrelidin [94]. (iv) Methionyl-tRNA synthetase (MRS) from *Pf* is present in both cytoplasm and apicoplast. Further, the bacterial MRS inhibitors – REP3123 and REP8839 with an IC50 value in low μM range inhibit the protein synthesis pathway [95]. These four aaRSs provide novel targets to screen new compounds and investigate them as potential antimalarials employing various drug discovery strategies.

8.9 Conclusion: The Road Ahead

The crucial role of aaRS in the protein translation makes them essential for cell survival. Considering the variety of aaRSs present in any given organism, there are as many potential targets. In malaria parasites, the multistage targeting drugs are needed for current drug development strategies in which aaRSs can play an excellent role by stalling the protein production in all the three parasitic compartments. Among the 36 *P. falciparum* aaRSs, while ignoring 15 apicoplast aaRSs that show delayed-death phenotype, other 21 aaRSs are portent targets. The structural studies focusing on tRNA synthetase–inhibitor complexes have paved the way for structure-guided drug designing. Majority of the modern drugs have been supplied by natural compounds that have been used in traditional medicine. In the case of aaRSs' inhibitors, the theme has been followed where natural metabolites such as CLD and FF have been used. Crystal structures of *Pf*KRS in complex with CLD and *Pf*PRS in complex with HF have guided the discovery of their respective derivatives. Beside these two aaRSs (KRS and PRS), the other aaRSs (LRS, RRS, YRS, WRS) for which the three-dimensional crystal structure is available from the *P. falciparum* remain to be explored. For successful antimalarials, drug research pipelines need to concentrate on the *Plasmodium* proteome and biology for drug discovery.

References

1 WHO (2019). *World Malaria Report 2019*. Geneva: World Health Organization.

2 Contacos, P.G., Lunn, J.S., and Coatney, G.R. (1963). Drug-resistant falciparum malaria from Cambodia and Malaya. *Transactions of the Royal Society of Tropical Medicine and Hygiene* 57: 417–424. https://doi.org/10.1016/0035-9203(63)90074-9.

3 Alam, M.T., Vinayak, S., Congpuong, K. et al. (2011). Tracking origins and spread of sulfadoxine-resistant *Plasmodium falciparum* dhps alleles in Thailand. *Antimicrobial Agents and Chemotherapy* 55: 155–164. https://doi.org/10.1128/AAC.00691-10.

4 Gregson, A. and Plowe, C.V. (2005). Mechanisms of resistance of malaria parasites to antifolates. *Pharmacological Reviews* 57: 117–145. https://doi.org/10.1124/pr.57.1.4.

5 Dondorp, A.M., Nosten, F., Yi, P. et al. (2009). Artemisinin resistance in *Plasmodium falciparum* malaria. *The New England Journal of Medicine* 361: 455–467. https://doi.org/10.1056/NEJMoa0808859.

6 Gardner, M.J., Hall, N., Fung, E. et al. (2002). Genome sequence of the human malaria parasite *Plasmodium falciparum*. *Nature* 419: 498–511. https://doi.org/10.1038/nature01097.

7 Köhler, S., Delwiche, C.F., Denny, P.W. et al. (1997). A plastid of probable green algal origin in Apicomplexan parasites. *Science* 275: 1485–1489. https://doi.org/10.1126/science.275.5305.1485.

8 Conway, D.J. and Baum, J. (2002). In the blood – the remarkable ancestry of *Plasmodium falciparum*. *Trends in Parasitology* 18: 351–355. https://doi.org/10.1016/s1471-4922(02)02316-4.

9 Wilson, R.J., Gardner, M.J., Feagin, J.E. et al. (1991). Have malaria parasites three genomes? *Parasitology Today* 7: 134–136. https://doi.org/10.1016/0169-4758(91)90276-t.

10 Bhatt, T.K., Kapil, C., Khan, S. et al. (2009). A genomic glimpse of aminoacyl-tRNA synthetases in malaria parasite *Plasmodium falciparum*. *BMC Genomics* 10: 644. https://doi.org/10.1186/1471-2164-10-644.

11 Jeffries, A.C. and Johnson, A.M. (1996). The growing importance of the plastid-like DNAs of the Apicomplexa. *International Journal for Parasitology* 26: 1139–1150. https://doi.org/10.1016/s0020-7519(96)00098-7.

12 Baragaña, B., Hallyburton, I., Lee, M.C. et al. (2015). A novel multiple-stage antimalarial agent that inhibits protein synthesis. *Nature* 522: 315–320. https://doi.org/10.1038/nature14451.

13 Raphemot, R., Lafuente-Monasterio, M.J., Gamo-Benito, F.J. et al. (2015). Discovery of dual-stage malaria inhibitors with new targets. *Antimicrobial Agents and Chemotherapy* 60: 1430–1437. https://doi.org/10.1128/AAC.02110-15.

14 Ibba, M. and Soll, D. (2000). Aminoacyl-tRNA synthesis. *Annual Review of Biochemistry* 69: 617–650. https://doi.org/10.1146/annurev.biochem.69.1.617.

15 Moras, D. (1992). Structural and functional relationships between aminoacyl-tRNA synthetases. *Trends in Biochemical Sciences* 17: 159–164. https://doi.org/10.1016/0968-0004(92)90326-5.

16 De Jong, F.A., De Jonge, M.J., Verweij, J. et al. (2006). Role of pharmacogenetics in irinotecan therapy. *Cancer Letters* 234: 90–106. https://doi.org/10.1016/j.canlet.2005.04.040.

17 Koon, H.B., Fingleton, B., Lee, J.Y. et al. (2011). Phase II AIDS Malignancy Consortium trial of topical halofuginone in AIDS-related Kaposi sarcoma. *Journal of Acquired Immune Deficiency Syndromes* 56: 64–68. https://doi.org/10.1097/QAI.0b013e3181fc0141.

18 Rock, F.L., Mao, W., Yaremchuk, A. et al. (2007). An antifungal agent inhibits an aminoacyl-tRNA synthetase by trapping tRNA in the editing site. *Science* 316: 1759–1761. https://doi.org/10.1126/science.1142189.

19 Katagiri, K., Tori, K., Kimura, Y. et al. (1967). A new antibiotic. Furanomycin, an isoleucine antagonist. *Journal of Medicinal Chemistry* 10: 1149–1154. https://doi.org/10.1021/jm00318a035.

20 Nakama, T., Nureki, O., and Yokoyama, S. (2001). Structural basis for the recognition of isoleucyl-adenylate and an antibiotic, mupirocin, by isoleucyl-tRNA synthetase. *The Journal of Biological Chemistry* 276: 47387–47393. https://doi.org/10.1074/jbc.M109089200.

21 Fuller, A.T., Mellows, G., Woolford, M. et al. (1971). Pseudomonic acid: an antibiotic produced by *Pseudomonas fluorescens*. *Nature* 234: 416–417. https://doi.org/10.1038/234416a0.

22 Wuite, J., Davies, B.I., Go, M. et al. (1983). Pseudomonic acid: a new topical antimicrobial agent. *Lancet* 2: 394. https://doi.org/10.1016/s0140-6736(83)90358-6.

23 Ogilvie, A., Wiebauer, K., and Kersten, W. (1975). Inhibition of leucyl-transfer ribonucleic acid synthetase in *Bacillus subtilis* by Granaticin. *The Biochemical Journal* 152: 511–515. https://doi.org/10.1042/bj1520511.

24 Konrad, I. and Röschenthaler, R. (1977). Inhibition of phenylalanine tRNA synthetase from *Bacillus subtilis* by ochratoxin A. *FEBS Letters* 83: 341–347. https://doi.org/10.1016/0014-5793(77)81037-5.

25 Konishi, M., Nishio, M., Saitoh, K. et al. (1989). Cispentacin, a new antifungal antibiotic. I. Production, isolation, physico-chemical properties and structure. *Journal of Antibiotics (Tokyo)* 42: 1749–1755. https://doi.org/10.7164/antibiotics.42.1749.

26 Nass, G. and Poralla, K. (1976). Genetics of borrelidin resistant mutants of *Saccharomyces cerivisiae* and properties of their threonyl-tRNA-synthetase. *Molecular & General Genetics* 147: 39–43. https://doi.org/10.1007/BF00337933.

27 Isono, K., Uramoto, M., Kusakabe, H. et al. (1984). Ascamycin and dealanylascamycin, nucleoside antibiotics from *Streptomyces* sp. *Journal of Antibiotics (Tokyo)* 37: 670–672. https://doi.org/10.7164/antibiotics.37.670.

28 Werner, R.G., Thorpe, L.F., Reuter, W. et al. (1976). Indolmycin inhibits prokaryotic tryptophanyl-tRNA ligase. *European Journal of Biochemistry* 68: 1–3. https://doi.org/10.1111/j.1432-1033.1976.tb10758.x.

29 Park, J.S., Lee, C.H., Yoon, S. et al. (2017). Inhibition of prolyl-tRNA synthetase as a novel mediator of cardiac fibrosis. *Circulation* 136: A24036–A24036.

30 Shibata, A., Kuno, M., Adachi, R. et al. (2017). Discovery and pharmacological characterization of a new class of prolyl-tRNA synthetase inhibitor for anti-fibrosis therapy. *PLoS One* 12: e0186587. https://doi.org/10.1371/journal.pone.0186587.

31 Hoepfner, D., McNamara, C.W., Lim, C.S. et al. (2012). Selective and specific inhibition of the *Plasmodium falciparum* lysyl-tRNA synthetase by the fungal secondary metabolite cladosporin. *Cell Host & Microbe* 11: 654–663. https://doi.org/10.1016/j.chom.2012.04.015.

32 Khan, S., Garg, A., Camacho, N. et al. (2013a). Structural analysis of malaria-parasite lysyl-tRNA synthetase provides a platform for drug development. *Acta Crystallographica. Section D, Biological Crystallography* 69: 785–795. https://doi.org/10.1107/S0907444913001923.

33 Khan, S., Sharma, A., Belrhali, H. et al. (2014). Structural basis of malaria parasite lysyl-tRNA synthetase inhibition by cladosporin. *Journal of Structural and Functional Genomics* 15: 63–71. https://doi.org/10.1007/s10969-014-9182-1.

34 Pham, J.S., Dawson, K.L., Jackson, K.E. et al. (2014). Aminoacyl-tRNA synthetases as drug targets in eukaryotic parasites. *International Journal for Parasitology: Drugs and Drug Resistance* 4: 1–13. https://doi.org/10.1016/j.ijpddr.2013.10.001.

35 Fang, P., Yu, X., Jeong, S.J. et al. (2015). Structural basis for full-spectrum inhibition of translational functions on a tRNA synthetase. *Nature Communications* 6: 6402. https://doi.org/10.1038/ncomms7402.

36 Novoa, E.M., Camacho, N., Tor, A. et al. (2014). Analogs of natural aminoacyl-tRNA synthetase inhibitors clear malaria in vivo. *Proceedings of the National Academy of Sciences of the United States of America* 111: E5508–E5517. https://doi.org/10.1073/pnas.1405994111.

37 Teng, M., Hilgers, M.T., Cunningham, M.L. et al. (2013). Identification of bacteria-selective threonyl-tRNA synthetase substrate inhibitors by structure-based design. *Journal of Medicinal Chemistry* 56: 1748–1760. https://doi.org/10.1021/jm301756m.

38 Coatney, G.R., Cooper, W.C., Culwell, W.B. et al. (1950). Studies in human malaria. XXV. Trial of febrifugine, an alkaloid obtained from *Dichroa febrifuga* lour., against the Chesson strain of *Plasmodium vivax*. *Journal of the National Malaria Society* 9: 183–186.

39 Derbyshire, E.R., Mazitschek, R., and Clardy, J. (2012). Characterization of *Plasmodium* liver stage inhibition by halofuginone. *ChemMedChem* 7: 844–849. https://doi.org/10.1002/cmdc.201200045.

40 Kikuchi, H., Horoiwa, S., Kasahara, R. et al. (2014). Synthesis of febrifugine derivatives and development of an effective and safe tetrahydroquinazoline-type antimalarial. *European Journal of Medicinal Chemistry* 76: 10–19. https://doi.org/10.1016/j.ejmech.2014.01.036.

41 Kikuchi, H., Yamamoto, K., Horoiwa, S. et al. (2006). Exploration of a new type of antimalarial compounds based on febrifugine. *Journal of Medicinal Chemistry* 49: 4698–4706. https://doi.org/10.1021/jm0601809.

42 Kobayashi, S., Ueno, M., Suzuki, R. et al. (1999). Catalytic asymmetric synthesis of antimalarial alkaloids febrifugine and isofebrifugine and their biological activity. *The Journal of Organic Chemistry* 64: 6833–6841. https://doi.org/10.1021/jo990877k.

43 Koepfli, J.B., Mead, J.F., and Brockman, J.A. (1947). An alkaloid with high antimalarial activity from *Dichroa febrifuga*. *Journal of the American Chemical Society* 69: 1837. https://doi.org/10.1021/ja01199a513.

44 Samant, B.S. and Sukhthankar, M.G. (2009). Synthesis and comparison of antimalarial activity of febrifugine derivatives including halofuginone. *Medicinal Chemistry* 5: 293–300. https://doi.org/10.2174/157340609788185846.

45 Zhu, S., Wang, J., Chandrashekar, G. et al. (2010). Synthesis and evaluation of 4-quinazolinone compounds as potential antimalarial agents. *European Journal of Medicinal Chemistry* 45: 3864–3869. https://doi.org/10.1016/j.ejmech.2010.05.040.

46 Keller, T.L., Zocco, D., Sundrud, M.S. et al. (2012). Halofuginone and other febrifugine derivatives inhibit prolyl-tRNA synthetase. *Nature Chemical Biology* 8: 311–317. https://doi.org/10.1038/nchembio.790.

47 Elkin, M., Ariel, I., Miao, H.Q. et al. (1999). Inhibition of bladder carcinoma angiogenesis, stromal support, and tumor growth by halofuginone. *Cancer Research* 59: 4111–4118.

48 Halevy, O., Nagler, A., Levi-Schaffer, F. et al. (1996). Inhibition of collagen type I synthesis by skin fibroblasts of graft versus host disease and scleroderma patients: effect of halofuginone. *Biochemical Pharmacology* 52: 1057–1063. https://doi.org/10.1016/0006-2952(96)00427-3.

49 Mcgaha, T., Kodera, T., Phelps, R. et al. (2002). Effect of halofuginone on the development of tight skin (TSK) syndrome. *Autoimmunity* 35: 277–282. https://doi.org/10.1080/0891693021000001235.

50 Pines, M. and Nagler, A. (1998). Halofuginone: a novel antifibrotic therapy. *General Pharmacology* 30: 445–450. https://doi.org/10.1016/s0306-3623(97)00307-8.

51 Pines, M., Snyder, D., Yarkoni, S. et al. (2003). Halofuginone to treat fibrosis in chronic graft-versus-host disease and scleroderma. *Biology of Blood and Marrow Transplantation* 9: 417–425. https://doi.org/10.1016/s1083-8791(03)00151-4.

52 Linder, M.R., Heckeroth, A.R., Najdrowski, M. et al. (2007). (2*R*,3*S*)-(+)- and (2*S*,3*R*)-(−)-Halofuginone lactate: synthesis, absolute configuration, and activity against *Cryptosporidium parvum*. *Bioorganic & Medicinal Chemistry Letters* 17: 4140–4143. https://doi.org/10.1016/j.bmcl.2007.05.053.

53 Ryley, J.F. and Wilson, R.G. (1975). Laboratory studies with some recent anticoccidials. *Parasitology* 70: 203–222. https://doi.org/10.1017/s0031182000049672.

54 Wu, M.X. and Hill, K.A. (1993). A continuous spectrophotometric assay for the aminoacylation of transfer RNA by alanyl-transfer RNA synthetase. *Analytical Biochemistry* 211: 320–323. https://doi.org/10.1006/abio.1993.1276.
55 Lloyd, A.J., Thomann, H.U., Ibba, M. et al. (1995). A broadly applicable continuous spectrophotometric assay for measuring aminoacyl-tRNA synthetase activity. *Nucleic Acids Research* 23: 2886–2892. https://doi.org/10.1093/nar/23.15.2886.
56 Saint-Léger, A. and Ribas De Pouplana, L. (2017). A new set of assays for the discovery of aminoacyl-tRNA synthetase inhibitors. *Methods* 113: 34–45. https://doi.org/10.1016/j.ymeth.2016.10.011.
57 Grube, C.D. and Roy, H. (2018). A continuous assay for monitoring the synthetic and proofreading activities of multiple aminoacyl-tRNA synthetases for high-throughput drug discovery. *RNA Biology* 15: 659–666. https://doi.org/10.1080/15476286.2017.1397262.
58 Ibba, M., Losey, H.C., Kawarabayasi, Y. et al. (1999). Substrate recognition by class I lysyl-tRNA synthetases: a molecular basis for gene displacement. *Proceedings of the National Academy of Sciences of the United States of America* 96: 418–423. https://doi.org/10.1073/pnas.96.2.418.
59 Ibba, M., Morgan, S., Curnow, A.W. et al. (1997). A euryarchaeal lysyl-tRNA synthetase: resemblance to class I synthetases. *Science* 278: 1119–1122. https://doi.org/10.1126/science.278.5340.1119.
60 O'donoghue, P. and Luthey-Schulten, Z. (2003). On the evolution of structure in aminoacyl-tRNA synthetases. *Microbiology and Molecular Biology Reviews* 67: 550–573. https://doi.org/10.1128/mmbr.67.4.550-573.2003.
61 Sharma, A. and Yogavel, M. (2016). Structural and functional attributes of malaria parasite diadenosine tetraphosphate hydrolase. *Scientific Reports* 6: 19981. https://doi.org/10.1038/srep19981.
62 Das, P., Babbar, P., Malhotra, N. et al. (2018). Specific stereoisomeric conformations determine the drug potency of cladosporin scaffold against malarial parasite. *Journal of Medicinal Chemistry* 61: 5664–5678. https://doi.org/10.1021/acs.jmedchem.8b00565.
63 Sharma, A., Sharma, M., and Yogavel, M. (2016). Protein translation enzyme lysyl-tRNA synthetase presents a new target for drug development against causative agents of loiasis and schistosomiasis. *PLoS Neglected Tropical Diseases* 10: e0005084. https://doi.org/10.1371/journal.pntd.0005084.
64 Chhibber-Goel, J. and Sharma, A. (2019). Side chain rotameric changes and backbone dynamics enable specific cladosporin binding in *Plasmodium falciparum* lysyl-tRNA synthetase. *Proteins* 87: 730–737. https://doi.org/10.1002/prot.25699.
65 Jain, V., Yogavel, M., Kikuchi, H. et al. (2017). Targeting prolyl-tRNA synthetase to accelerate drug discovery against malaria, leishmaniasis, toxoplasmosis, cryptosporidiosis, and coccidiosis. *Structure* 25: 1495.e6–1505.e6. https://doi.org/10.1016/j.str.2017.07.015.
66 Jain, V., Kikuchi, H., Oshima, Y. et al. (2014). Structural and functional analysis of the anti-malarial drug target prolyl-tRNA synthetase. *Journal of Structural and Functional Genomics* 15: 181–190. https://doi.org/10.1007/s10969-014-9186-x.

67 Jain, V., Yogavel, M., Oshima, Y. et al. (2015). Structure of prolyl-tRNA synthetase-halofuginone complex provides basis for development of drugs against malaria and toxoplasmosis. *Structure* 23: 819–829. https://doi.org/10.1016/j.str.2015.02.011.

68 Zhou, H., Sun, L., Yang, X.L. et al. (2013). ATP-directed capture of bioactive herbal-based medicine on human tRNA synthetase. *Nature* 494: 121–124. https://doi.org/10.1038/nature11774.

69 Kelly-Hope, L., Ranson, H., and Hemingway, J. (2008). Lessons from the past: managing insecticide resistance in malaria control and eradication programmes. *The Lancet Infectious Diseases* 8: 387–389. https://doi.org/10.1016/S1473-3099(08)70045-8.

70 Sonoiki, E., Palencia, A., Guo, D. et al. (2016). Antimalarial benzoxaboroles target *Plasmodium falciparum* leucyl-tRNA synthetase. *Antimicrobial Agents and Chemotherapy* 60: 4886–4895. https://doi.org/10.1128/AAC.00820-16.

71 Hu, R.G., Wang, H., Xia, Z. et al. (2008). The N-end rule pathway is a sensor of heme. *Proceedings of the National Academy of Sciences of the United States of America* 105: 76–81. https://doi.org/10.1073/pnas.0710568105.

72 Sriram, S.M., Kim, B.Y., and Kwon, Y.T. (2011). The N-end rule pathway: emerging functions and molecular principles of substrate recognition. *Nature Reviews. Molecular Cell Biology* 12: 735–747. https://doi.org/10.1038/nrm3217.

73 Tasaki, T., Sriram, S.M., Park, K.S. et al. (2012). The N-end rule pathway. *Annual Review of Biochemistry* 81: 261–289. https://doi.org/10.1146/annurev-biochem-051710-093308.

74 Ke, H., Sigala, P.A., Miura, K. et al. (2014). The heme biosynthesis pathway is essential for *Plasmodium falciparum* development in mosquito stage but not in blood stages. *The Journal of Biological Chemistry* 289: 34827–34837. https://doi.org/10.1074/jbc.M114.615831.

75 Sigala, P.A., Crowley, J.R., Henderson, J.P. et al. (2015). Deconvoluting heme biosynthesis to target blood-stage malaria parasites. *eLife* 4: https://doi.org/10.7554/eLife.09143.

76 Khan, S., Garg, A., Sharma, A. et al. (2013b). An appended domain results in an unusual architecture for malaria parasite tryptophanyl-tRNA synthetase. *PLoS One* 8: e66224. https://doi.org/10.1371/journal.pone.0066224.

77 Koh, C.Y., Kim, J.E., Napoli, A.J. et al. (2013). Crystal structures of *Plasmodium falciparum* cytosolic tryptophanyl-tRNA synthetase and its potential as a target for structure-guided drug design. *Molecular and Biochemical Parasitology* 189: 26–32. https://doi.org/10.1016/j.molbiopara.2013.04.007.

78 Burbaum, J.J. and Schimmel, P. (1991). Structural relationships and the classification of aminoacyl-tRNA synthetases. *The Journal of Biological Chemistry* 266: 16965–16968.

79 Eriani, G., Delarue, M., Poch, O. et al. (1990). Partition of tRNA synthetases into two classes based on mutually exclusive sets of sequence motifs. *Nature* 347: 203–206. https://doi.org/10.1038/347203a0.

80 Bhatt, T.K., Khan, S., Dwivedi, V.P. et al. (2011). Malaria parasite tyrosyl-tRNA synthetase secretion triggers pro-inflammatory responses. *Nature Communications* 2: 530. https://doi.org/10.1038/ncomms1522.

81 Bhatt, T.K., Yogavel, M., Wydau, S. et al. (2010). Ligand-bound structures provide atomic snapshots for the catalytic mechanism of D-amino acid deacylase. *The Journal of Biological Chemistry* 285: 5917–5930. https://doi.org/10.1074/jbc.M109.038562.

82 Yogavel, M., Khan, S., Bhatt, T.K., et al. (2010). Structure of D-tyrosyl-tRNATyr deacylase using home-source Cu Kα and moderate-quality iodide-SAD data: structural polymorphism and HEPES-bound enzyme states. *Acta Crystallographica Section D: Biological Crystallography,* 66: 584–592. https://doi.org/10.1107/S0907444910006062

83 Kapoor, M., Otero, F.J., Slike, B.M. et al. (2009). Mutational separation of aminoacylation and cytokine activities of human tyrosyl-tRNA synthetase. *Chemistry & Biology* 16: 531–539. https://doi.org/10.1016/j.chembiol.2009.03.006.

84 Wakasugi, K. and Schimmel, P. (1999). Two distinct cytokines released from a human aminoacyl-tRNA synthetase. *Science* 284: 147–151. https://doi.org/10.1126/science.284.5411.147.

85 Wakasugi, K., Slike, B.M., Hood, J. et al. (2002). Induction of angiogenesis by a fragment of human tyrosyl-tRNA synthetase. *The Journal of Biological Chemistry* 277: 20124–20126. https://doi.org/10.1074/jbc.C200126200.

86 Yang, X.L., Kapoor, M., Otero, F.J. et al. (2007). Gain-of-function mutational activation of human tRNA synthetase procytokine. *Chemistry & Biology* 14: 1323–1333. https://doi.org/10.1016/j.chembiol.2007.10.016.

87 Yang, X.L., Skene, R.J., Mcree, D.E. et al. (2002). Crystal structure of a human aminoacyl-tRNA synthetase cytokine. *Proceedings of the National Academy of Sciences of the United States of America* 99: 15369–15374. https://doi.org/10.1073/pnas.242611799.

88 Zhao, X., Town, J.R., Li, F. et al. (2009). ELR-CXC chemokine receptor antagonism targets inflammatory responses at multiple levels. *Journal of Immunology* 182: 3213–3222. https://doi.org/10.4049/jimmunol.0800551.

89 Khan, S., Sharma, A., Jamwal, A. et al. (2011). Uneven spread of cis- and trans-editing aminoacyl-tRNA synthetase domains within translational compartments of *P. falciparum*. *Scientific Reports* 1: 188. https://doi.org/10.1038/srep00188.

90 Lee, J.W., Beebe, K., Nangle, L.A. et al. (2006). Editing-defective tRNA synthetase causes protein misfolding and neurodegeneration. *Nature* 443: 50–55. https://doi.org/10.1038/nature05096.

91 Istvan, E.S., Dharia, N.V., Bopp, S.E. et al. (2011). Validation of isoleucine utilization targets in *Plasmodium falciparum*. *Proceedings of the National Academy of Sciences of the United States of America* 108: 1627–1632. https://doi.org/10.1073/pnas.1011560108.

92 Liu, J., Istvan, E.S., Gluzman, I.Y. et al. (2006). *Plasmodium falciparum* ensures its amino acid supply with multiple acquisition pathways and redundant proteolytic enzyme systems. *Proceedings of the National Academy of Sciences of the United States of America* 103: 8840–8845. https://doi.org/10.1073/pnas.0601876103.

93 Jackson, K.E., Pham, J.S., Kwek, M. et al. (2012). Dual targeting of aminoacyl-tRNA synthetases to the apicoplast and cytosol in *Plasmodium falciparum*. *International Journal for Parasitology* 42: 177–186. https://doi.org/10.1016/j.ijpara.2011.11.008.

94 Otoguro, K., Ui, H., Ishiyama, A. et al. (2003). In vitro and in vivo antimalarial activities of a non-glycosidic 18-membered macrolide antibiotic, borrelidin, against drug-resistant strains of Plasmodia. *Journal of Antibiotics (Tokyo)* 56: 727–729. https://doi.org/10.7164/antibiotics.56.727.

95 Hussain, T., Yogavel, M., and Sharma, A. (2015). Inhibition of protein synthesis and malaria parasite development by drug targeting of methionyl-tRNA synthetases. *Antimicrobial Agents and Chemotherapy* 59: 1856–1867. https://doi.org/10.1128/AAC.02220-13.

9

Natural Products as a Source for Antimalarial Drug Development Process – An Overview

Uma R. Lal[1] *and Snigdha Lal*[2]

[1]*National Institute of Pharmaceutical Education and Research (NIPER), Department of Natural Products, Ahmedabad, Opposite Air Force Head Quarters, Palaj, Gandhinagar, Gujarat 382355, India*
[2]*Ram Lakhan Singh Yadav College, Department of Chemistry, Bettiah, Bihar 845438, India*

9.1 Introduction

Malaria is a parasitic disease, geographically restricted to tropical regions where climate is suitable for transmission. As per World Malaria Report, 2020, there were 228 million infections and 405 000 deaths cited for 2017 [1]. Africa is the most burdened among all, which accounts for more than a total of 50% deaths and cases. However, in recent years, it has reduced (thanks to natural product-based therapy) [2]. A number of drugs have been developed, but the mainstay is artemisinin-based combination therapy. Due to the development of resistance of *Plasmodium* parasite to the existing antimalarial drugs and also of the mosquito vector against the insecticides, there is a dire need to search for novel and more efficacious drugs.

Antimalarial chemotherapy is linked with the history of herbal medicinal products. Natural products, such as artemisinin and quinine, sourced from medicinal plants are most effective antimalarial agents. From Quinine came the classical 4-aminoquinolines and amino alcohols, such as chloroquine, amodiaquine, and mefloquine. The natural product naphthoquinone lapachol also identified as the active ingredient in tree bark, formed the basis for Lapinone, which provided atovaquone, a component of Malarone. These have been the mainstay of malarial treatment over the last century. Artemisinin and its synthetic derivatives, which are the basis of the next generation of therapies, are active against artemisinin-resistant malaria (Figure 9.1).

Thus the research and development process for remains the same whereby initial identification of natural product, followed by their modification for clinical use. Not only plants could be potential sources for potent antimalarial remedies but we also need to focus on traditional usage of plant material in the formulations (the way they are processed) in the traditional system of medicine. This will accelerate the drug development process. Natural products have multiple stereo centers, flexible conformations, and the presence of heteroatoms, which makes them eligible to have

Drug Development for Malaria: Novel Approaches for Prevention and Treatment, First Edition.
Edited by Pravin Kendrekar.

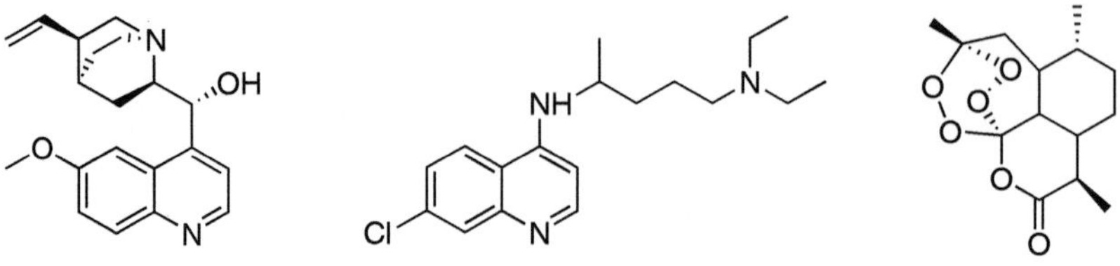

(1) (2) (3)

Figure 9.1 Structures of compounds (**1**–**3**).

multiple targets and/or new targets. It is important to focus on the other potential advantages of natural products.

- Natural products represent a source of potential new pharmacophores.
- Herbal medicinal products are often perceived by the patient community as being safe, and many have been used by communities in disease endemic countries for generations.
- Exploration of ethnopharmacological heritage to identify new medicines to combat malaria using documented herbal medicinal products is one of the areas where researchers from disease endemic countries can have a large impact.
- Herbal medicinal products used by the community have anecdotal evidence.

The success with natural products can be improved by starting with extracts which have associated ethnopharmacology data; those suggested to be active by the local traditional healers. Studies should be performed where the plant extract is the preferred treatment. The present article reviews the literature on natural products with antiplasmodial activity from 2015 onward and is organized according to structural types of compounds. There are 124 structures in present review, which suggest that medicinal plants are still the most comprehensively explored source for antiplasmodial compounds. Regardless of the *in vitro* assay method, in this review, only compounds with $IC_{50} \leq 3.0\,\mu M$ were considered to be of interest for further studies.

9.2 Phytochemicals as Antimalarial Agents: Recent Developments

9.2.1 Alkaloids

The naphthylisoquinolines are a unique class of polyketide-derived biaryls of natural origin. These compounds are found exclusively in the Ancistrocladaceae and Dioncophyllaceae families and are biosynthetically derived from the acetate-polymalonate pathway. C-6 oxygenated alkaloids with an *S*-configuration at C-3 are produced mostly by Ancistrocladaceae (Ancistrocladaceae-type), whereas the alkaloids of Dioncophyllaceae (Dioncophyllaceae-type) exclusively have an *R* configuration at C-3 and lack oxygenation at C-6 [3]. The *N*-methylated 5,1′-coupled ancistrocline (**4**) from the twigs of *Ancistrocladus tectorius* showed encouraging antiplasmodial activity against the K1 and NF54 strains. It had low cytotoxicity against L6 cells and was two to three times more active against chloroquine-resistant K1 than the chloroquine-sensitive NF54 strain [4]. Dioncophyllines C2 (**5**) and F (**6**), and ancistrocladisine A (**9**) and 5′-*O*-methyldioncophylline D (**7**) isolated from the root bark of Congolese *Ancistrocladus ileboensis*, and 7,8′-coupled dioncophylline D2 (**8**) from the leaves of *A. ileboensis* were found to be active against the NF54 strain. Interestingly, **6** displayed double the activity against the K1 over the NF54 strain. And, all new compounds were non-toxic to L6 cells with selectivity index (SI) values ranging from 61 to 586 [3] (Figure 9.2). Dimeric naphthylisoquinolines Shuangancistrotectorines (**10–14**) isolated from *A. tectorius* displayed antiplasmodial activity superior to chlroquine. These compounds revealed submicromolar antiplasmodial activity against the K1 strain coupled with low toxicity against L6

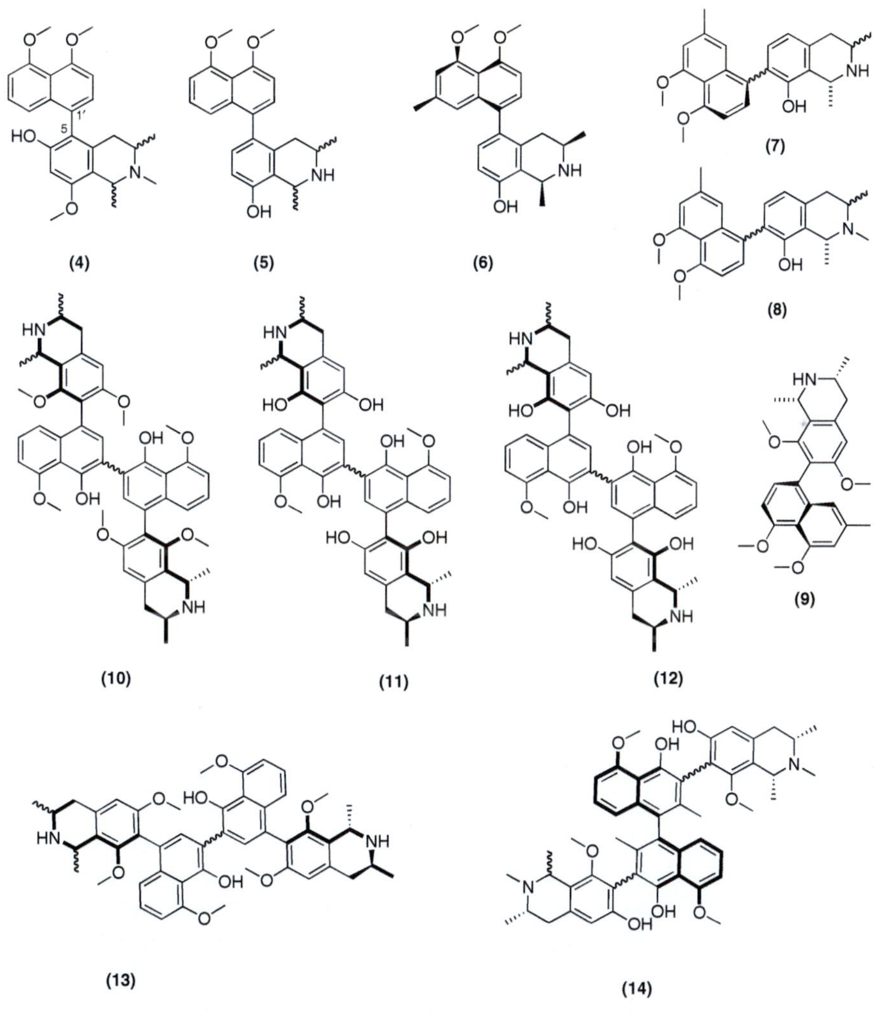

Figure 9.2 Structures of compounds (**4–14**).

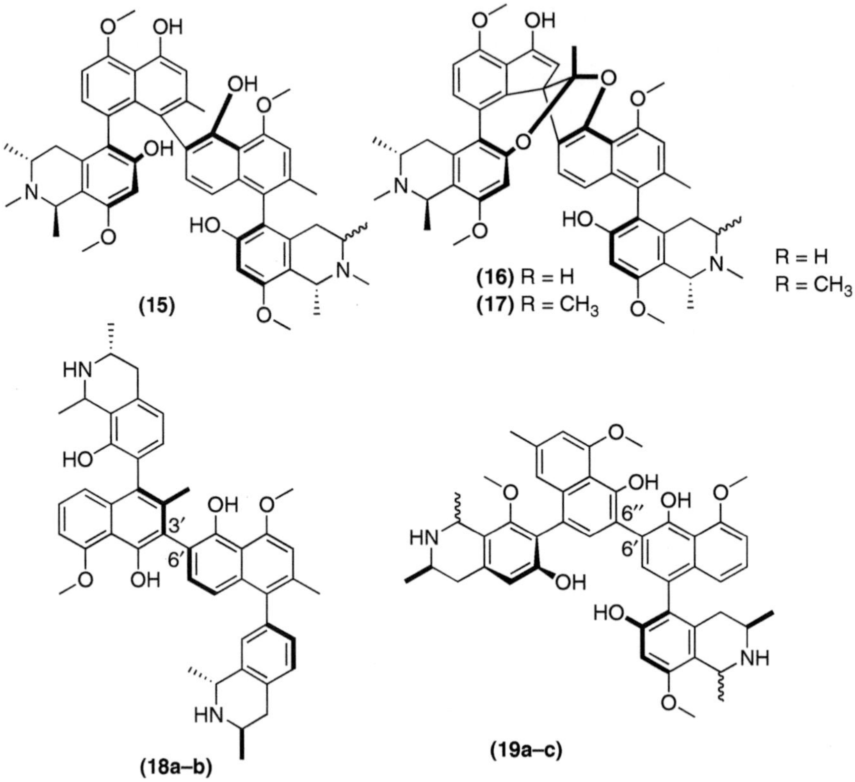

Figure 9.3 Structures of compounds (**15**–**19**).

cells (SI = 99.8–610.6), with compounds **10**, **11**, and **14**, in particular, displaying antiplasmodial activity superior to that of chloroquine [5]. Mbandakamine B2 (**15**) pirombandakamines A1 (**16**) and A2 (**17**) isolated from Congolese *Ancistrocladus* sp. exhibited nanomolar antiplasmodial activity against both the K1 and NF54 parasite strains. The structural comparison revealed that cyclization is not beneficial to activity [6]. Jozilebomines A (**18a**) and B (**18b**), 3,6″-coupled dimers isolated from the root extract of the Congolese *A. ileboensis*, exhibited selective antiplasmodial activity against NF54 *Plasmodium falciparum* strain, with weak toxicity toward L6 cells (SI = 160 and 52.3, respectively) (Figure 9.3). However, this activity was lower than the related symmetrically coupled jozimine A2 [3]. Heterodimeric naphthylisoquinolines Ealapasamines A–C (**19**$_{\mathbf{a\text{-}c}}$) isolated from the leaf of *Ancistrocladus ealensis* were active against *P. falciparum* (K1 and NF54) with low nanomolar IC_{50} values and low toxicity to L6 cells [7]. Bioassay-guided fractionation of *Stephania venosa* tubers yielded the aporphine alkaloids stephanine (**20**), crebanine (**21**), and *O*-methylbulbocapnine (**22**) as antiplasmodial principles. The most active alkaloid against 3D7 and W2 parasites, stephanine (**20**), was found to be cytotoxic to cancerous and non-cancerous cell lines [8]. Another compound **23** in combination with chloroquine resulted in a 44-fold potentiation of parasite killings showing resistance-reversal effect with *Plasmodium* species [9].

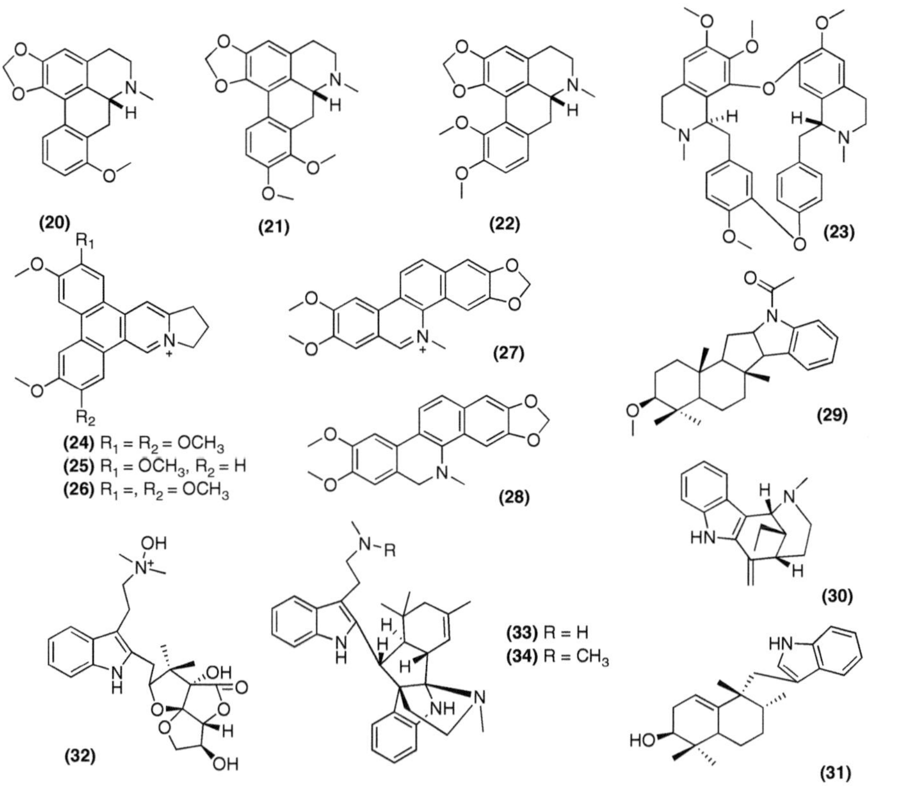

Figure 9.4 Structures of compounds (**20–34**).

Bioassay-guided fractionation of the chloroform fraction of the active methanol extract of *Ficus septica* (Moraceae) twigs led to the isolation of the known compounds, dehydrotylophorine (**24**), dehydroantofine (**25**), and tylophoridicine (**26**) (Figure 9.4). These phenanthroindolizidine alkaloids inhibited the 3D7 strain with submicromolar IC_{50} and had low cytotoxicity [10]. Compound **27**, dihydronitidine (**28**), isolated from *Zanthoxylum heitzii* bark displayed a slow-acting drug effect against 3D7 parasites [11]. The poor water solubility of **28** might also limit its viability as an antimalarial lead. The monoterpenoid indole alkaloid uleine (**29**) (Figure 9.4) isolated from the stem bark of the Brazilian tree *Aspidosperma parvifolium* (Apocynaceae) was more active against the W2 than the 3D7 strain, with low cytotoxicity against the Hep G2A16 and Vero cell lines [12]. Traditionally, *Greenwayodendron suaveolens* (Annonaceae) is used by Nkundo people in the DR Congo malaria. And, it has been seen that some species of monkeys chew the bitter leaves, presumably for zoopharmacognostic purposes. Sesquiterpenyl indole alkaloids, *N*-acetylpolyveoline (**30**), and polyalthenol (**31**) (Figure 9.4), isolated from the root bark of *G. suaveolens*, were active against the K1 strain [13]. Pimentelamine C (**32**), the known borreverine (**33**), and 4-methylborreverine (**34**), isolated from *Flindersia pimenteliana*, were reported to be active against *P. falciparum* 3D7 and Dd2 with low toxicity to HEK-293 cells. Compound **32** (isolated as the trifluoroacetate salt) is one of three new indole alkaloids incorporating an ascorbic acid moiety. The other two analogues without a polar *N*-oxide moiety on the ethylamine unit attached to the indole skeleton were inactive [14]. New bisindole alkaloids, 3′,4′,5′,6′-tetradehydrogeissospermine (**33**) and geissolosimine (**34**), isolated from *Geissospermum laeve* (Apocynaceae) exhibited non-selective antiplasmodial activity against FcB1 parasites [15]. The indole-quinazoline alkaloid tryptoquivaline (**35**), obtained from the culture broth of *Neosartorya spinosa* KKU-1NK1 (sexual state of *Aspergillus* fungus species), was active against K1 parasites. The compound was slightly cytotoxic to Vero cells (SI = 25) but was inactive against a panel of cancer cell lines [16]. However, the glucoside derivative of previously isolated β-carboline indole alkaloid hyrtiosulawesine (**36**) was only half as active as it is an aglycone [17]. The chloroform fraction of an extract from the combined twigs, leaves, and fruits of *Buxus cochinchinensis* afforded a number of bioactive triterpenoids, including the cycloartane alkaloid, *N*-benzoyldihydrocyclomicrophylline F (**37**). This compound inhibited both Dd2 *P. falciparum* and HT-29 human colon cancer cells, suggesting non-selective activity [18].

Pregnane-type steroidal alkaloids, mokluangin A (**38**) and irehline (**39**), isolated from the root of *Holarrhena pubescens* (Apocynaceae), were found to be active against K1 *P. falciparum* with low cytotoxicity against NCI-H187 lung cancer cells (IC_{50} = 30.6 and 27.7 μM, respectively) [19]. Macrocyclic lactams cripowellin A–D (**40–43**) (Figure 9.5), isolated from *Crinum erubescens* (Amaryllidaceae), inhibited the Dd2 strain (IC_{50} in nanometer) but were cytotoxic against cancerous A2780 cells. The 1,3,5-trioxepane-ring in **40** and **43** correlated with improved activity [20]. Another bioassay-guided fractionation of *Crinum firmifolium* leaf extract led to the isolation of the new 2-alkylquinolinones **44**, **45**, and the known **46**, having activity against the 3D7 and Dd2 strains with mild cytotoxicity. Structure-activity relationship (SAR) revealed that branching of the alkyl side chain is beneficial to potency [21]. Marine sponge *Monanchora unguiculata* (Madagascar) afforded four new guanidine alkaloids ptilomycalins E–H (**47–50**), along with the known crambescidin 800 (**51**) and fromiamycalin (**52**) (Figure 9.6) with submicromolar antiplasmodial activity against the 3D7 strain but were cytotoxic [22]. The decalin-tetramic acid metabolite phomasetin (**53**) obtained from the culturing of the *Pyrenochaetopsis* sp. RK10-F058 fungus was active against *P. falciparum* 3D7 with moderate cytotoxicity against cancerous HeLa, HL-60, and srcts-NRK cells. The same culture broth yielded two more decalin metabolites, possessing a cyclopentanone-fused decalin skeleton and a serine-derived *N*-methylated amino acid instead of the tetramic acid moiety. However, they were >21 times less active than **53**, indicating that the cyclized tetramic acid group might be crucial for potent activity [23].

Allonorsecurinine (**54**), previously reported as a synthetic compound, was isolated with *ent*-norsecurinine (**55**) from the antiplasmodial plant *Phyllanthus fraternus* (Phyllanthaceae) (methanol extract IC_{50} = 0.44 μg/ml against 3D7) [24]. The two securinega alkaloids were more active against chloroquine-resistant W2 than against chloroquine-sensitive 3D7 parasites. No cytotoxicity was observed against human umbilical vein endothelial cells at the highest concentration of 100 μM [25].

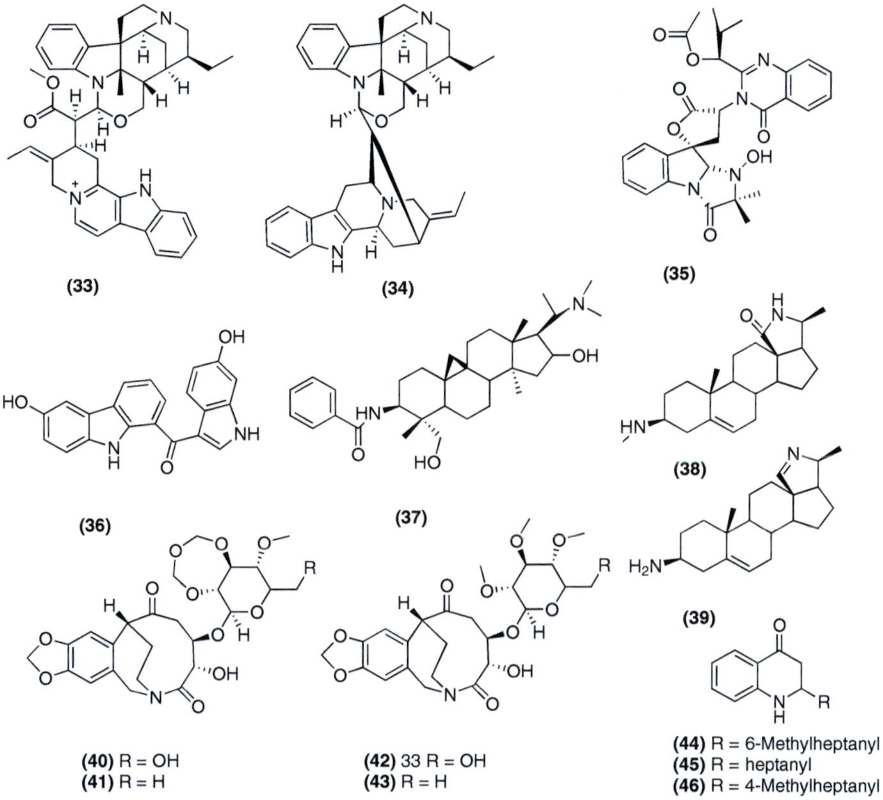

Figure 9.5 Structures of compounds (**33–46**).

9.2.2 Terpenes

The eremophilane sesquiterpenoid sporogen-AO1 (**56**), produced by the soil fungus *Penicillium copticola* PSURSPG138, not only inhibited K1 parasites but was also cytotoxic against human oral epidermoid carcinoma (KB) and Vero cells [26]. The Australian nudibranch *Phyllidia ocellata* afforded three new isonitrile sesquiterpenes, 2-isocyanoclovene (**57**), 2-isocyanoclovane (**58**), and 4,5-*epi*-10-isocyanoisodauc-6-ene (**59**), having selective antiplasmodial activity against the 3D7 and Dd2 strains. Isonitrile functionality was found to be crucial for the potent activity of isonitrile terpenes [27]. In support to this, β-hematin inhibition assay of six terpenoid isonitriles also proved it, in which inhibition of heme crystallization was seen at different levels by isonitriles [28].

9.2.2.1 Sesquiterpene Lactones

Lindenane-type sesquiterpenoid monomers and dimers isolated from different *Chloranthus* species and *Sarcandra glabra* (Chloranthaceae) were assayed for antiplasmodial activity. Compounds with $IC_{50} \leq 100\,nM$ were also assessed for cytotoxicity on embryonic lung tissue (WI-38) cells, and some compounds, e.g. fortunilide A (**60**), sarglabolide J (**61**), and chlorajaponilide C (**62**), had potencies

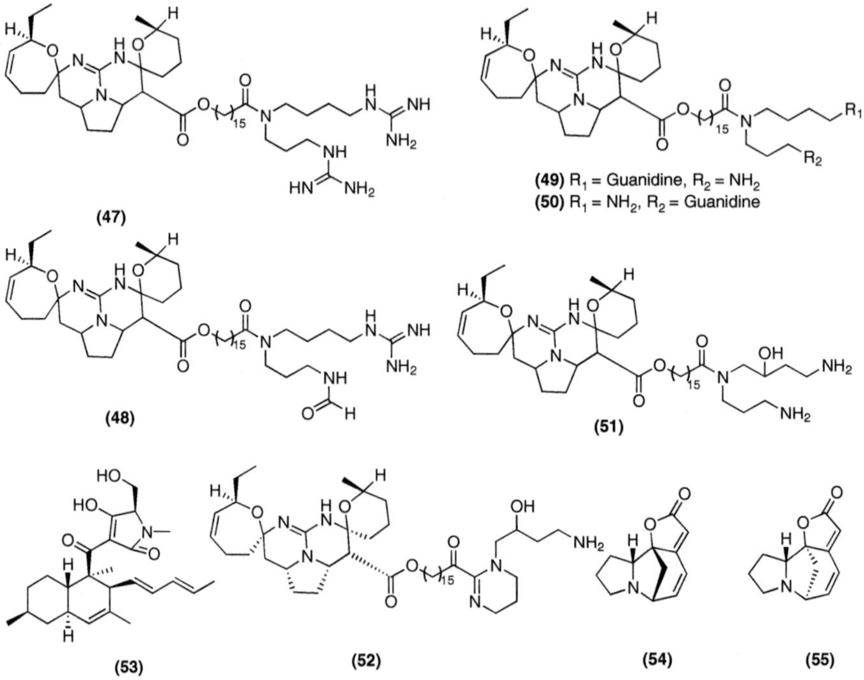

Figure 9.6 Structures of compounds (**47–55**).

comparable to that of artemisinin and were not cytotoxic. SAR observations indicated that all the active compounds were dimers, had a Δ4 double bond and a hydroxy group at C-4′, and contain a (*Z*)-5-hydroxy-4-oxopent-2-enoate ester. The presence and nature of the ester groups at C-13′ and C-15′ affected the antiplasmodial activity, suggesting that these ester groups could be manipulated to optimize potency [29]. Bioassay guided fractionation of the dichloromethane extract of *Trichospira verticillata* (Asteraceae) afforded the new germacranolide trichospirolide A (**63**) (Figure 9.7) as the most active constituent. However, it was also toxic to A2780 ovarian cancer and HEK293 cells [30]. The bioactivities of sesquiterpene lactones have been ascribed to the presence of an α-methylene-γ-lactone moiety in the structures. SAR studies around this enigmatic functionality to make sesquiterpene lactones more selective are essential if these compounds are to enjoy further development as antimalarial scaffolds.

9.2.2.2 Diterpenes

Three new cassane diterpenes (Figure 9.8) were isolated from chloroform extract of *Caesalpinia sappan* (Fabaceae) seeds (IC_{50} = 0.38 μg/ml against K1), namely caesalsappanins G–I (**64–66**), which inhibited K1 *P. falciparum*. Cytotoxicity studies against a panel of cancer cell lines showed moderate selectivity for the parasite (SI = 10.5–17.6). Structural comparison revealed that active compounds had a hydroxy group at C-12, whereas compounds lacking the C-12 hydroxy were less active [31]. The dichloromethane extract of *Caesalpinia bonducella* root showed

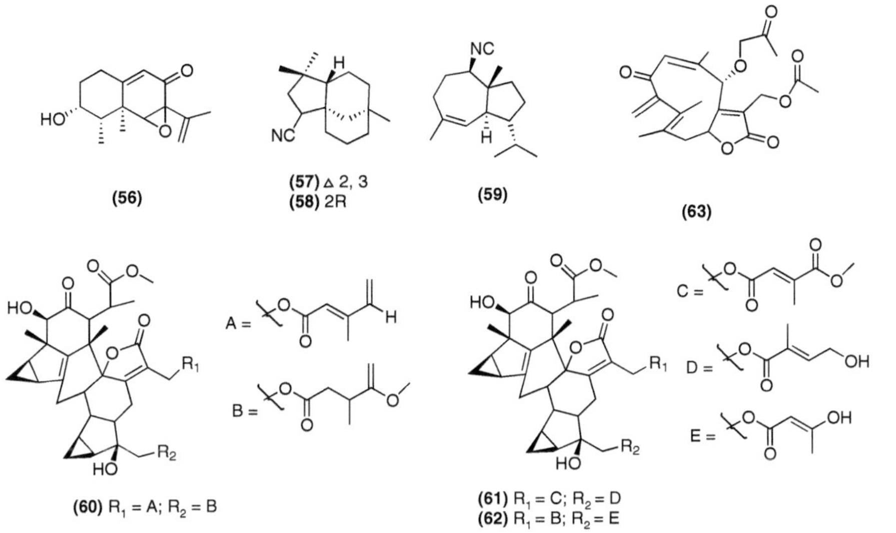

Figure 9.7 Structures of compounds (**56–62**).

in vivo dose-dependent antiplasmodial activity [32]. A phytochemical investigation of the root afforded norcaesalpin D (**67**) as the antiplasmodial component. No cytotoxicity was observed against mammalian LLCMK2 cells at the highest concentration (200 μg/ml) tested [33]. The leaf extract of *Aphanamixis grandifolia* (Meliaceae) afforded the diterpenoid lactones amphadilactones A–F and H–I (**68–75**) (Figure 9.8), exhibiting antiplasmodial activity by inhibiting *Pf*DGAT [34]. The serrulatane diterpenoid **76**, isolated from the aerial parts of *Eremophila microtheca* (Scrophulariaceae), was not active, but a semi-synthetic amide derivative **77** exhibited antiplasmodial activity against the 3D7 and Dd2 strains without being cytotoxic to HEK293 cells at 80 μM [35]. Two new pre-segetane and jatrophane diterpenoids euphorbesulins A (**78**) and G (**79**) (Figure 9.8), isolated from the twigs of *Euphorbia esula* (Euphorbiaceae), had shown activity against the *P. falciparum* Dd2 strain [29, 36]. Isonitrile amphilectanes, monamphilectines B (**80**) and C (**81**), were isolated from the Caribbean marine sponge *Svenzea flava* (Puerto Rico). These new metabolites were first marine natural products with an α-substituted monocyclic β-lactam ring. The compounds were active against the 3D7 parasites with nanomolar IC_{50} values. Interestingly, 8,15-diisocyano-11(20)-amphilectene (**82**), which differs from the new compound by the absence of the substituted β-lactam moiety, was also active, suggesting that the β-lactam moiety may not contribute to antiplasmodial potency and confirming the crucial role of the isonitrile functionality [37]. Pustulosaisonitrile-1 (**83**), isolated from the Australian nudibranch *Phyllidiella pustulosa*, exhibited antiplasmodial activity against 3D7 and Dd2 *P. falciparum* strains. Diastereoisomers of **83**, obtained by enantio- and stereoselective total synthesis, were not only as active as the natural compound but also showed cross-resistance [38]. A new linear diterpenoid, bifurcatriol (**84**), was isolated from the Irish brown alga *Bifurcaria bifurcata* and had activity against K1 *P. falciparum* with negligible cytotoxicity against L6 cells [39]. The phenanthrenone

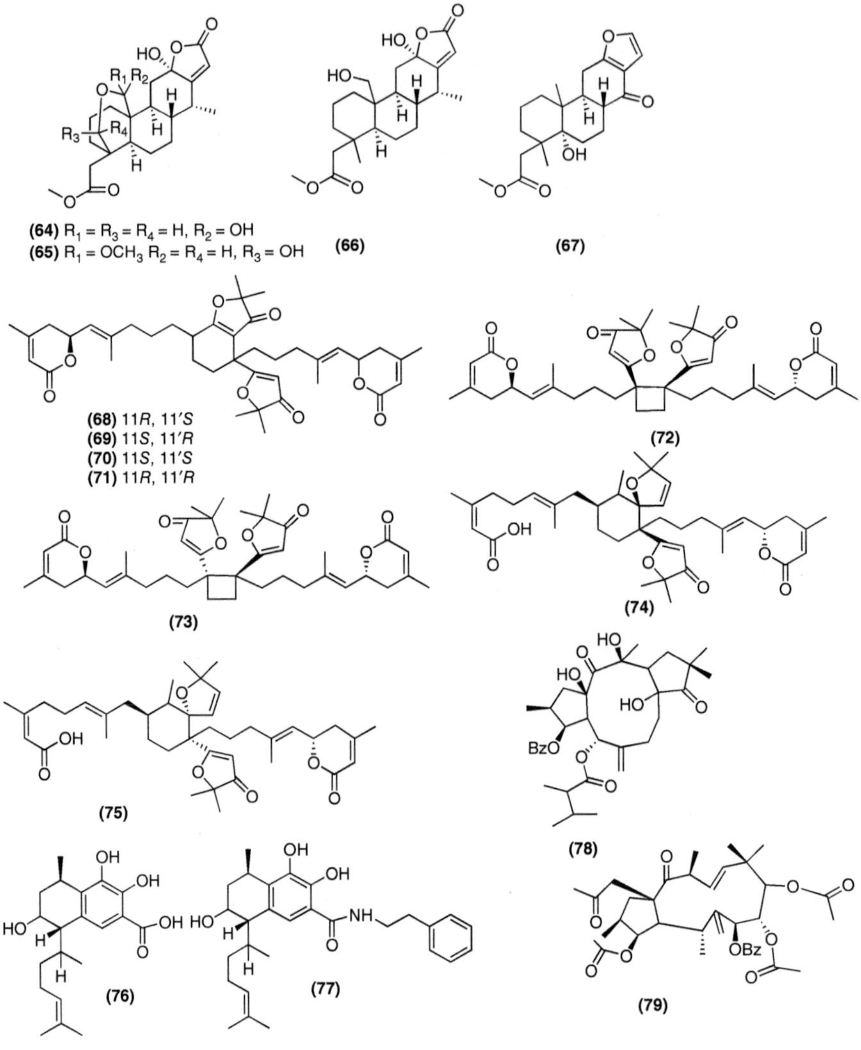

Figure 9.8 Structures of compounds (**64–79**).

derivatives fimbricalyx A (**85**) and B (**86**), isolated from *Strophioblachia fimbricalyx* (Euphorbiaceae) root, also inhibited *P. falciparum* K1.

9.2.2.3 Triterpenes

The chloroform extract of *B. cochinchinensis* (Buxaceae) leaves, twigs, and fruits yielded five betulin coumaroyl esters (Figure 9.9) [18]. The lupane esters **87**, **88**, and **89** were also isolated from the methanolic supercritical fluid extract of *Buxus sempervirens* together with five other new coumaroyl and feruloyl esters of betulin (**90–94**) [40]. The esters were active against *P. falciparum* Dd2, HB3, and NHP1337 strains without cytotoxicity against HeLa cells. **90**, with an *E*-feruloyl group attached

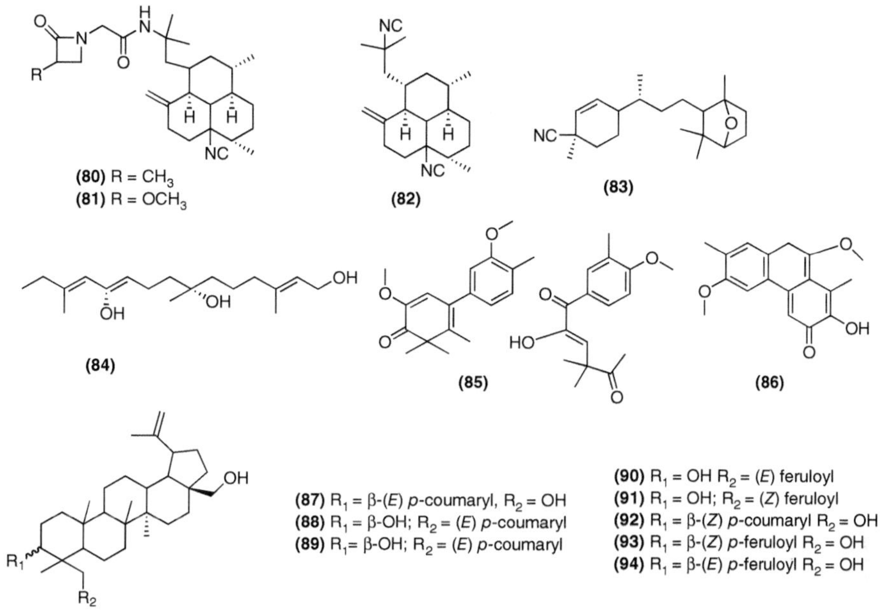

Figure 9.9 Structures of compounds (**80–94**).

at C-23, was the most active with submicromolar IC_{50} values, whereas analogues with *E* or *Z* coumaroyl or *Z*-feruloyl at C-23 were slightly less active. The esterified betulin derivatives were more active than betulin and 23-hydroxybetulin, and the diacetate ester was inactive [18, 40]. The compounds displayed antiplasmodial activity against NF54 *P. falciparum* strain with varying levels of toxicity to L6 cells (SI = 4–107). Triterpenoid **96**, with a submicromolar IC_{50} value, was the most selective against the parasite [41]. Compounds **96** and **97** differ only in the orientation of the hydroxy group at C-24 and presence or absence of acetylation at C-7 of ring B. A tirucallane triterpenoid, isoflindissone lactone (**98**), isolated from the dichloromethane extract of *Boswellia serrata* (Burseraceae) oleo-gum resin inhibited *P. falciparum* with IC_{50} = 2.6 μg/ml. Compound **98** also had low toxicity against L6 cells (IC_{50} = 40 μM) [42]. Thus, for bulky groups, monoesterification is optimal for activity, whereas diesterification is favored for the smaller groups. The root bark of *G. suaveolens* (Annonaceae) afforded polycarpol (**99**) as one of the active metabolites against K1 *P. falciparum* but was also cytotoxic [13]. Azadironolide (**100**) was isolated as the most active antiplasmodial compound from the plant stem bark with moderate cytotoxicity against Vero cells [43]. Three new triterpenoid saponins, maesargentoside I, III, IV (**101–103**) from the leaf extract of *Maesa argentea* (Myrsinaceae), have displayed nonselective antiplasmodial activity against K1 *P. falciparum* [44]. The antiplasmodial activity of squalene (**104**), isolated from *Uapaca paludosa* (Euphorbiaceae) trunk bark extract, was reported for the first time. However, it was also cytotoxic against KB and Vero cells [45].

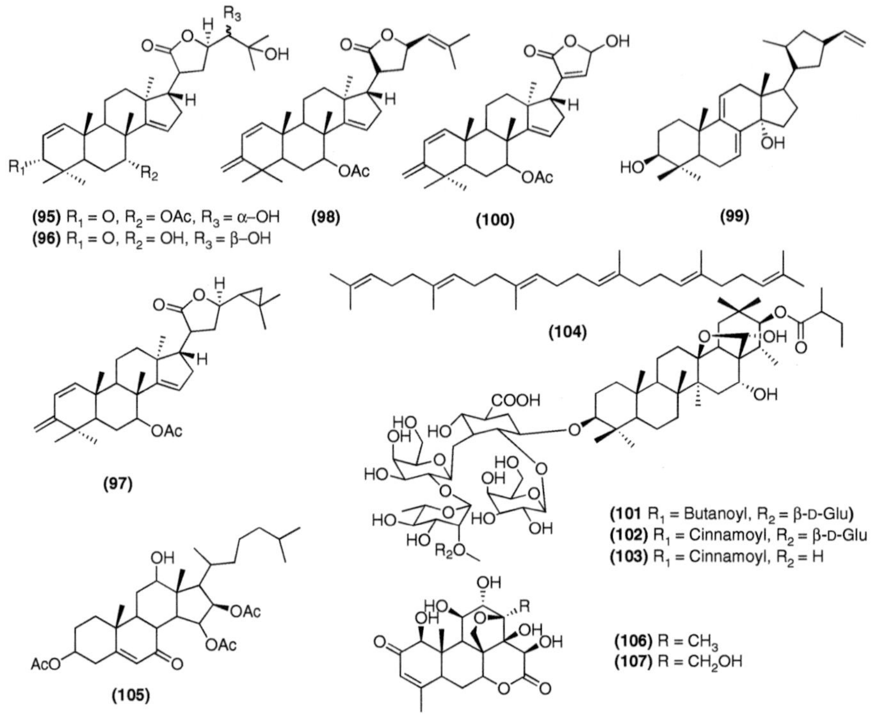

Figure 9.10 Structures of compounds (**95–107**).

9.2.2.4 Steroids and Others

The marine red alga *Halymenia floresii* afforded a new steroid, halymeniaol (**105**), inhibited 3D7 *P. falciparum* and was not cytotoxic [46]. It has been suggested that the antiplasmodial activity of limonoids has been attributed to the presence of the α,β-unsaturated carbonyl moiety in the structures, which may be involved in Michael-type addition reactions [47]. The acetone extract of *Brucea javanica* (Simaroubaceae) stem afforded antiplasmodial quassinoids bruceine D (**106**) and H (**107**) (Figure 9.10). Bruceine D has also been isolated from the roots of the same plant. Both compounds inhibited *P. falciparum* K1 strain, but bruceine D was cytotoxic against cancerous human KB and NCI-H187 cells. The bioactivity of quassinoids has been correlated with the presence of an α,β-unsaturated ketone in ring A. Quassinoids possessing an oxymethylene bridge joining C-8 and C-13 have also shown pronounced activity [48].

9.2.3 Polyphenols

9.2.3.1 Biflavonoids

Bioassay-guided fractionation led to the isolation of three biflavanones GB1a (**108**), GB1 (**109**), and GB2 (**110**) from the 70% ethanolic extract of the seed that inhibited *P. falciparum* by 87% (Figure 9.11). These compounds exhibited submicromolar

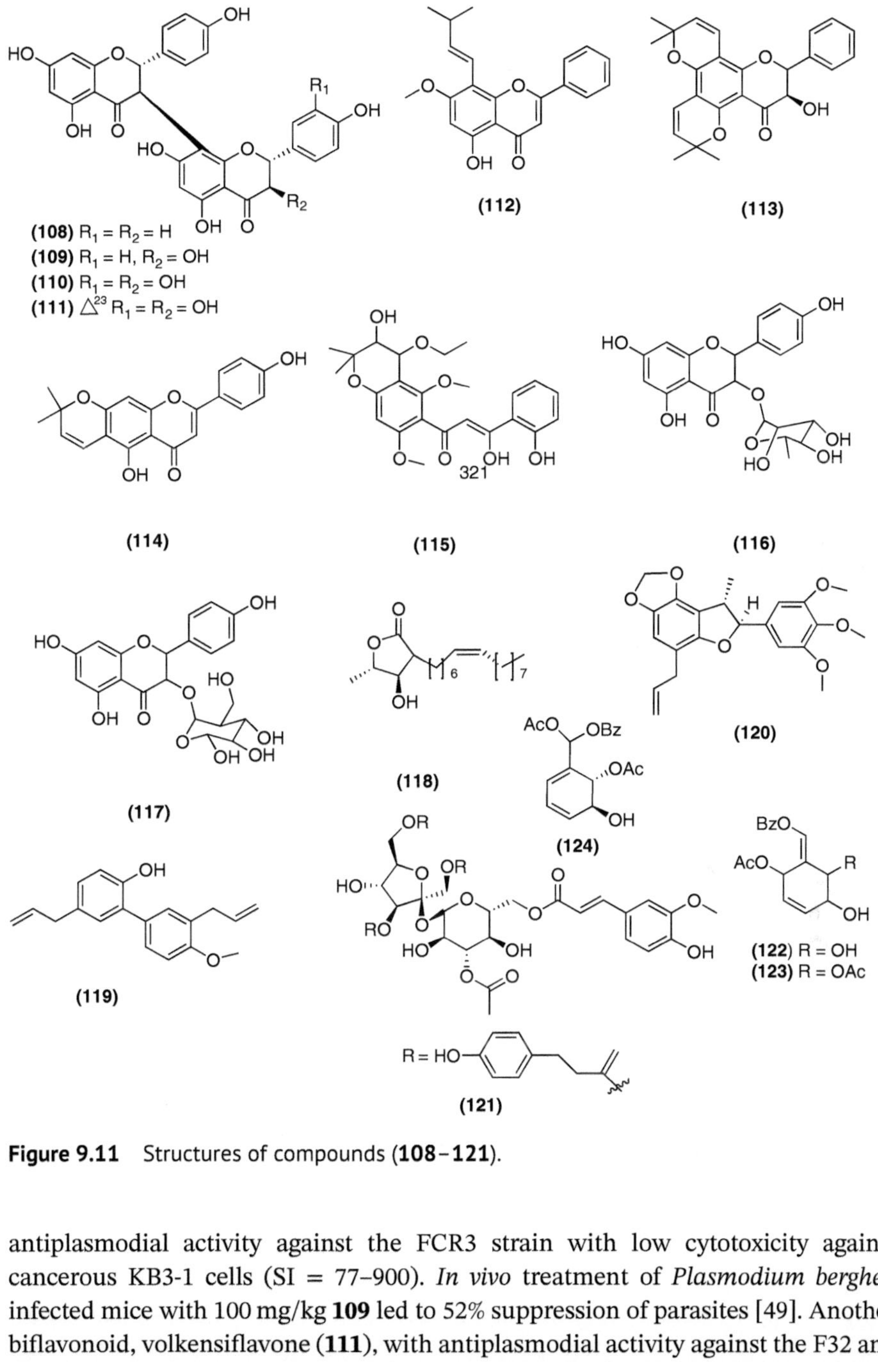

Figure 9.11 Structures of compounds (**108–121**).

antiplasmodial activity against the FCR3 strain with low cytotoxicity against cancerous KB3-1 cells (SI = 77–900). *In vivo* treatment of *Plasmodium berghei*-infected mice with 100 mg/kg **109** led to 52% suppression of parasites [49]. Another biflavonoid, volkensiflavone (**111**), with antiplasmodial activity against the F32 and FcM29 *P. falciparum* strains, was isolated from *Allanblackia floribunda* (Clusiaceae). Two structural analogues of **111** with an additional hydroxy at C-3′ on the lower flavone unit were >10 times less active, suggesting a SAR that could be further exploited [50].

9.2.3.2 Prenylated Flavonoids

Tephrosia purpurea subsp. *leptostachya* afforded a new antiplasmodial prenylflavone, (*E*)-5-hydroxytephrostachin (**112**) (Figure 9.11). It was not cytotoxic to cancerous HepG2 cells at 100 μM while being moderately cytotoxic against noncancerous human cells, indicating selectivity against D6 parasites [51]. The prenylated flavonoid MS-II (**113**) from the active extract inhibited the 3D7, KSM 009, and artemisinin-sensitive F32-TEM strains. The compound was not cytotoxic against Hep2 and Vero cells at 247.5 μM [52]. The root extract of *Tephrosia aequilata*, which inhibited 3D7 *P. falciparum* by 100% at 10 μg/ml, afforded new aequichalcone C (**114**) that it inhibited the 3D7 strain without being cytotoxic against HEK-293 cells up to 40 μM [51]. Another prenylated flavonoid, carpachromene (**115**), isolated from *F. pimenteliana* (Rutaceae) as one of the antiplasmodial principles, was not cytotoxic against HEK-293 cells at 40 μM [14].

9.2.3.3 Other Flavonoids

Methanol supercritical fluid extraction yielded four kaempferol 3-*O*-rhamnosides (**116**) from *Platanus occidentalis* (Platanaceae) and three kaempferol 3-*O*-glucosides (**117**) from *Quercus laceyi* (Fagaceae). The glucosides were also cytotoxic against HeLa cells, whereas rhamnosides were more selective against HB3 parasites (SI = 6–34) [40]. (−)-Epigallocatechin-3-gallate (EGCG), the major polyphenol in green tea (*Camellia sinensis*, Theaceae), displayed antiplasmodial activity against 3D7 *P. falciparum*. It also inhibited chaperone and ATPase functions by targeting *Pf*Hsp70-1 and *Pf*Hsp70-z [53]. The active dichloromethane extract of *Malleastrum* sp. (Meliaceae) afforded a new butanolide lactone, malleastrumolide A (**118**), and was not only found to inhibit Dd2 parasites but it was also cytotoxic against A2780 cancer cells [54]. A new gallic acid ester, 2,3,4-trihydroxy-2-methylbutyl gallate, with activity against D6 and W2 *P. falciparum*, was isolated from the aerial parts of *Limonium leptophyllum* (Plumbaginaceae). The compound was almost twice as active against the chloroquine-resistant W2 strain as against the chloroquine-sensitive D6 strain [55]. The active ethyl acetate fraction of *Magnolia grandiflora* (Magnoliaceae) fruit and twig extracts afforded known 4′-*O*-methylhonokiol (**119**) bioactive neolignans against the Dd2 strain. Honokiol, which is structurally similar to **119** but is not methoxylated, was six times less active (IC_{50} = 16.5 μM). A new dihydrobenzofuranoid neolignan, ococymosin (**120**), was obtained from the antiplasmodial hexane stem extract (IC_{50} = 1.25 μg/ml) of *Ocotea cymosa* (Lauraceae) as the most active metabolite against the Dd2 strain [56]. The phenylpropanoid glycoside vanicoside F (**121**), isolated as a major constituent of *Polygonum hydropiper* (Polygonaceae) aerial parts, inhibited *P. falciparum* D6 and W2 strains without cytotoxicity against Vero cells [57]. A phytochemical reinvestigation of *Cleistochlamys kirkii* (Annonaceae) leaf extract led to the isolation of new polyoxygenated cyclohexenones cleistodienediol (**122**), cleistodienol B (**123**), and the known cleistodienol A (**124**) (Figure 9.11). All three compounds inhibited 3D7 and Dd2 *P. falciparum* strains but were also cytotoxic against noncancerous HEK-293 and cancerous MDA-MB-231 cells [58].

9.3 Traditional System of Medicine and Malaria

Malaria cases in India are mainly reported from West Bengal, Jharkhand, Chhattisgarh, Odisha, Madhya Pradesh, Uttar Pradesh, and Gujarat. India currently accounts for only 3% of the total malaria cases and 2% of malaria deaths across the globe [1]. Health measures in downtrodden society are purely dependent on the traditional knowledge system (TKS) of herbal plants. These people mainly use herbal plants possessing potential remedy even for some incurable disease. The plant parts used, their preparation method of medicine from it, and administration vary geographically. Many ancient texts mention about various aspects of malaria and its linkage with bites of insects and mosquitoes. Several plants are used in traditional medicine for the treatment of malaria and fever in many parts of the world. The relevance of traditional knowledge for local health treatments has not diminished despite of the deeper penetration in the modern aspect of medicine system. Malaria had been prevalent in African countries, and it spreads along travel/shipping routes to Europe, India, China, and Indonesia.

It is an amazing fact that Malaria was considered as a Deity, in Greek mythology, who lives in marshes. Later on, Hippocrates, father of medicine in Greece, had argued that the stagnant water is the very reason for the birth of mosquito and is root cause of malaria. He also explored on ill effects of stagnant water, as those who drink it have hard, thin, hot stomachs and large, stiff spleens, while their collarbones, faces, and shoulders are thin. In India, Dhanvantari (800 BCE) claimed that bites of mosquitoes could cause diseases such as fever and shivering which is malaria symptom. Later, Charaka Samhita (300 BCE) classified the fevers into five different categories which were further confirmed that there is relationship of different types of fever with the insect bites by Susruta Samhita (100 BCE). Ronald Ross in later demonstrated that *Anopheles* mosquito was the vector for primarily responsible for malaria [59]. Presently, national institutions like National Vector Borne Disease Control Program (NVBDCP) and National Institute of Malaria Research (NIMR), New Delhi are playing an important role in eradication of malaria. There is a historical aspect of disease treatment in Ancient India, hidden in customs and practices Indian societies primarily based on the traditional knowledge system. We need to derive meaning from ancient literature to prepare road map for modern challenges and current medication system especially millennium most fatal disease of malaria which is killing millions of people every year.

9.3.1 Plants/Formulations Used in Malaria Treatment in Ayurvedic System of Medicine

Some very common Ayurvedic herbs to cure malaria are *Vernonia cinerea, Adina cordifolia, Gentiana kurroo, Momordica charantia, Momordica cochinchinensis, Alstonia scholaris, C. bonducella, Leucas cephalotes, Ocimum sanctum*, and *Swertia chirata*. Other herbs like *Aloe barbadensis, Argemone mexicana, Tinospora cordifolia, Datura stramonium, Andrographis paniculata, Calotropis procera, Piper longum, Euphorbia lancifolia, Aconitum ferox, Eclipta prostrata, and Zingiber officinale* are having antimalarial properties. Some herbal medicines that are useful for malaria and are free from any side effects are absolutely safe to use (mentioned in *Bhav Prakasha*). Such medicines are *Sudarshan Ghanvati, Maha Sudarshan Churna, Sudarshan Churna, Saptpam Ghan Vati, Nimbashava Nimbadi Chrna, Amritrista, Kalmegha Shava, and Guruchi Ghanstava Vati.*

9.4 Conclusions

At present, there is an urgent requirement of discovering new antimalarial agents especially in view of emerging resistance to existing drugs as well as increase in cases of coinfection with other tropical diseases. Exploration of natural sources taking clues from traditional knowledge holds great promise for finding new leads, as has been clear from successes of such studies in the past. This is particularly meaningful today as huge strides have been made in understanding the biology of malaria cycle disease parasites, and more biochemical targets are known today. This coupled with advances in technology for isolation, structure elucidation, and biological evaluation makes the search for novel agents from natural sources even more exciting. Exploration of traditional formulation, i.e. the way plant materials are used in the formulations, also needs to be taken care of as it will only tell the hidden truth.

References

1 WHO (2019). *World Malaria Report 2019*. Geneva: World Health Organization. https://www.who.int/malaria/publications/en/ (accessed 22 October 2021).

2 Snow, R.W., Sartorius, B., Kyalo, D. et al. (2017). The prevalence of *Plasmodium falciparum* in sub-Saharan Africa since 1900. *Nature* 550: 515–518. https://doi.org/10.1038/nature24059.

3 Li, J., Seupel, R., Feineis, D. et al. (2017). Dioncophyllines C_2, D_2, and F and related naphthylisoquinoline alkaloids from the Congolese liana *Ancistrocladus ileboensis* with potent activities against *Plasmodium falciparum* and against multiple myeloma and leukemia cell lines. *Journal of Natural Products* 80: 443–458. https://doi.org/10.1021/acs.jnatprod.6b00967.

4 Bringmann, G., Seupel, R., Feineis, D. et al. (2017). Antileukemic ancistrobenomine B and related 5,1′-coupled naphthylisoquinoline alkaloids from the Chinese liana *Ancistrocladus tectorius*. *Fitoterapia* 121: 76–85. https://doi.org/10.1016/j.fitote.2017.07.001.

5 Xu, M., Bruhn, T., Hertlein, B. et al. (2010). Shuangancistrotectorines A-E, dimeric naphthylisoquinoline alkaloids with three chiral biaryl axes from the Chinese plant *Ancistrocladus tectorius*. *Chemistry – A European Journal* 16: 4206–4216. https://doi.org/10.1002/chem.200903247.

6 Lombe, B.K., Bruhn, T., Feineis, D. et al. (2017). Antiprotozoal spiromban-dakamines A1 and A2, fused naphthylisoquinoline dimers from a Congolese

Ancistrocladus plant. *Organic Letters* 19: 6740–6743. https://doi.org/10.1021/acs.orglett.7b00209.

7 Tshitenge, D.T., Feineis, D., Mudogo, V. et al. (2017). Antiplasmodial ealapasamines A–C, 'mixed' naphthylisoquinoline dimers from the Central African liana *Ancistrocladus ealaensis. Scientific Reports* 7: 5767. https://doi.org/10.1038/s41598-017-05719-w.

8 Le, P.M., Srivastava, V., Nguyen, T.T. et al. (2017). Stephanine from *Stephania venosa* (Blume) Spreng showed effective antiplasmodial and anticancer activities, the latter by inducing apoptosis through the reverse of mitotic exit. *Phytotherapy Research* 31: 1357–1368. doi: 10.1002/ptr.5861.

9 Ye, Z. and van Dyke, K. (2015). Antimalarial activity of various bisbenzylisoquinoline and aporphine-benzylisoquinoline alkaloids and their structure-activity relationships against chloroquine—sensitive and resistant *Plasmodium falciparum* malaria *in vitro. Malaria Control and Elimination* 5: 1. https://doi.org/10.4172/2470-6965.1000137.

10 Kubo, M., Yatsuzuka, W., Matsushima, S. et al. (2016). Antimalarial phenanthroindolizine alkaloids from *Ficus septica. Chemical & Pharmaceutical Bulletin* 64: 957–960. https://doi.org/10.1248/cpb.c16-00181.

11 Goodman, C.D., Austarheim, I., Mollard, V. et al. (2016). Natural products from *Zanthoxylum heitzii* with potent activity against the malaria parasite. *Malaria Journal* 15: 481. https://doi.org/10.1186/s12936-016-1533-x.

12 Dolabela, M.F., Póvoa, M.M., Brandão, G.C. et al. (2015). *Aspidosperma* species as sources of anti-malarials: uleine is the major anti-malarial indole alkaloid from *Aspidosperma parvifolium* (Apocynaceae). *Malaria Journal* 14: 498. https://doi.org/10.1186/s12936-015-0997-4.

13 Muganza, D.M., Fruth, B., Nzunzu, J.L. et al. (2016). *In vitro* antiprotozoal activity and cytotoxicity of extracts and isolated constituents from *Greenwayodendron suaveolens. Journal of Ethnopharmacology* 193: 510–516. https://doi.org/10.1016/j.jep.2016.09.051.

14 Robertson, L.P., Dufy, S., Wang, Y. et al. (2017). Pimentelamines A-C, indole alkaloids isolated from the leaves of the Australian tree *Flindersia pimenteliana. Journal of Natural Products* 80: 3211–3217. https://doi.org/10.1021/acs.jnatprod.7b00587.

15 Fox Ramos, A.E., Alcover, C., Evanno, L. et al. (2017). Revisiting previously investigated plants: a molecular networking-based study of *Geissospermum laeve. Journal of Natural Products* 80: 1007–1014. https://doi.org/10.1021/acs.jnatprod.

16 Rajachan, O.-A., Kanokmedhakul, K., Sanmanoch, W. et al. (2016). Chevalone C analogues and globoscinic acid derivatives from the fungus *Neosartorya spinosa* KKU-1NK1. *Phytochemistry* 132: 68–75. https://doi.org/10.1016/j.phytochem.2016.09.008.

17 Pereira, M.D., da Silva, T., Aguiar, A.C.C. et al. (2017). Chemical composition, antiprotozoal and cytotoxic activities of indole alkaloids and benzofuran neolignan of *Aristolochia cordigera. Planta Medica* 83: 912–920. https://doi.org/10.1055/s-0043-104776.

18 Pan, L., Acuña, U.M., Chai, H. et al. (2015). New bioactive lupane triterpene coumaroyl esters isolated from *Buxus cochinchinensis*. *Planta Medica* 81: 1133–1140. https://doi.org/10.1055/s-0035-1546118.

19 Cheenpracha, S., Boapun, P., Limtharakul, T. et al. (2017). Antimalarial and cytotoxic activities of pregnene-type steroidal alkaloids from *Holarrhena pubescens* roots. *Natural Product Research* 33 (6): 782–788. https://doi.org/10.1080/14786419.2017.1408108.

20 Presley, C.C., Krai, P., Dalal, S. et al. (2016). New potently bioactive alkaloids from *Crinum erubescens*. *Bioorganic & Medicinal Chemistry* 24: 5418–5422. https://doi.org/10.1016/j.bmc.2016.08.058.

21 Presley, C.C., Du, Y., Dalal, S. et al. (2017). Isolation, structure elucidation, and synthesis of antiplasmodial quinolones from *Crinum firmifolium*. *Bioorganic & Medicinal Chemistry* 25: 4203–4211. https://doi.org/10.1016/j.bmc.2017.06.017.

22 Campos, P.-E., Wolfender, J.-L., Queiroz, E.F. et al. (2017). Unguiculin A and ptilomycalins E–H, antimalarial guanidine alkaloids from the marine sponge *Monanchora unguiculata*. *Journal of Natural Products* 80: 1404–1410. https://doi.org/10.1021/acs.jnatprod.6b01079.

23 Nogawa, T., Kato, N., Shimizu, T. et al. (2018). Wakodecalines A and B, new decaline metabolites isolated from a fungus *Pyrenochaetopsis* sp. RK10-F058. *The Journal of Antibiotics* 71: 123. https://doi.org/10.1038/ja.2017.103.

24 Komlaga, G., Cojean, S., Dickson, R.A. et al. (2016). Antiplasmodial activity of selected medicinal plants used to treat malaria in Ghana. *Parasitology Research* 115: 3185–3195. https://doi.org/10.1007/s00436-016-5080-8.

25 Komlaga, G., Genta-Jouve, G., Cojean, S. et al. (2017). Antiplasmodial *Securinega* alkaloids from *Phyllanthus fraternus*: discovery of natural (+)-allonorsecurinine. *Tetrahedron Letters* 58: 3754–3756. https://doi.org/10.1016/j.tetlet.2017.08.045.

26 Daengrot, C., Rukachaisirikul, V., Tansakul, C. et al. (2015). Eremophilane sesquiterpenes and diphenyl thioethers from the soil fungus *Penicillium copticola* PSURSPG138. *Journal of Natural Products* 78: 615–622. https://doi.org/10.1021/np5005328.

27 White, A.M., Pierens, G.K., Skinner-Adams, T. et al. (2015). Antimalarial isocyano and isothiocyanato sesquiterpenes with tri- and bicyclic skeletons from the nudibranch *Phyllidia ocellata*. *Journal of Natural Products* 78: 1422–1427. https://doi.org/10.1021/acs.jnatprod.5b00354.

28 Young, R.M., Adendorff, M.R., Wright, A.D., and Davies-Coleman, M.T. (2015). Antiplasmodial activity: the first proof of inhibition of heme crystallization by marine isonitriles. *European Journal of Medicinal Chemistry* 93: 373–380. https://doi.org/10.1016/j.ejmech.2015.02.011.

29 Zhou, B., Wu, Y., Dalal, S. et al. (2016). Nanomolar antimalarial agents against chloroquine-resistant *Plasmodium falciparum* from medicinal plants and their structure–activity relationships. *Journal of Natural Products* 80: 96–107. https://doi.org/10.1021/acs.jnatprod.6b00744.

30 Du, Y., Pearce, K.C., Dai, Y. et al. (2017). Antiplasmodial sesquiterpenoid lactones from *Trichospira verticillata*: structure elucidation by spectroscopic

methods and comparison of experimental and calculated ECD data. *Journal of Natural Products* 80: 1639–1647. https://doi.org/10.1021/acs.jnatprod.7b00247.

31 Ma, G., Wu, H., Chen, D. et al. (2015). Antimalarial and antiproliferative cassane diterpenes of *Caesalpinia sappan*. *Journal of Natural Products* 78: 2364–2371. https://doi.org/10.1021/acs.jnatprod.5b00317.

32 Nondo, R.S., Erasto, P., Moshi, M.J. et al. (2016). *In vivo* antimalarial activity of extracts of Tanzanian medicinal plants used for the treatment of malaria. *Journal of Advanced Pharmaceutical Technology & Research* 7: 59. https://doi.org/10.4103/2231-4040.179748.

33 Nondo, R.S.O., Moshi, M.J., Erasto, P. et al. (2017). Anti-plasmodial activity of norcaesalpin D and extracts of four medicinal plants used traditionally for treatment of malaria. *BMC Complementary and Alternative Medicine* 17: 167. https://doi.org/10.1186/s12906-017-1673-8.

34 Zhang, X.-Q., Spadafora, C., Pineda, L.M. et al. (2017). Discovery, semisynthesis, antiparasitic and cytotoxic evaluation of 14-membered resorcylic acid lactones and their derivatives. *Scientific Reports* 7: 11822. https://doi.org/10.1038/s41598-017-12336-0.

35 Kumar, R., Duffy, S., Avery, V.M. et al. (2017). Synthesis of antimalarial amide analogues based on the plant serrulatane diterpenoid 3,7,8-trihydroxyserrulat-14-en-19-oic acid. *Bioorganic & Medicinal Chemistry Letters* 27: 4091–4095. https://doi.org/10.1016/j.bmcl.2017.07.039.

36 Zhou, B., Wu, Y., Dalal, S. et al. (2016). Euphorbesulins A–P, structurally diverse diterpenoids from *Euphorbia esula*. *Journal of Natural Products* 79: 1952–1961. https://doi.org/10.1021/acs.jnatprod.6b00205.

37 Avilés, E., Prudhomme, J., Le Roch, K.G., and Rodríguez, A.D. (2016). Structures, semisyntheses, and absolute configurations of the antiplasmodial α-substituted β-lactam monamphilectines B and C from the sponge *Svenzea flava*. *Tetrahedron* 71: 487–494. https://doi.org/10.1016/j.tet.2014.11.060.

38 White, A.M., Dao, K., Vrubliauskas, D. et al. (2017). Catalyst-controlled stereoselective synthesis secures the structure of the antimalarial isocyanoterpene pustulosaisonitrile-1. *The Journal of Organic Chemistry* 82: 13313–13323. https://doi.org/10.1021/acs.joc.7b02421.

39 Smyrniotopoulos, V., Merten, C., Kaiser, M., and Tasdemir, D. (2017). Bifurcatriol, a new antiprotozoal acyclic diterpene from the brown alga *Bifurcaria bifurcata*. *Marine Drugs* 15: 245. https://doi.org/10.3390/md15080245.

40 Cai, S., Risinger, A.L., Nair, S. et al. (2015). Identification of compounds with efficacy against malaria parasites from common North American plants. *Journal of Natural Products* 79: 490–498. https://doi.org/10.1021/acs.jnatprod.5b00874.

41 Happi, G.M., Kouam, S.F., Talontsi, F.M. et al. (2015). Minor secondary metabolites from the bark of *Entandrophragma congoense* (Meliaceae). *Fitoterapia* 102: 35–40. https://doi.org/10.1016/j.fitote.2015.01.018.

42 Greve, H.L., Kaiser, M., Brun, R., and Schmidt, T.J. (2017). Terpenoids from the oleo-gum-resin of *Boswellia serrata* and their antiplasmodial effects in vitro. *Planta Medica* 83: 1214–1226. https://doi.org/10.1055/s-0043-116943.

43 Irungu, B.N., Adipo, N., Orwa, J.A. et al. (2015). Antiplasmodial and cytotoxic activities of the constituents of *Turraea robusta* and *Turraea nilotica*. *Journal of Ethnopharmacology* 174: 419–425. https://doi.org/10.1016/j.jep.2015.08.039.

44 Foubert, K., Gorella, T., Faizal, A. et al. (2016). Triterpenoid saponins from *Maesa argentea* leaves. *Planta Medica* 82: 1568–1575. https://doi.org/10.1055/s-0042-1181896b01013.

45 Banzouzi, J., Soh, P.N., Ramos, S. et al. (2015). Samvisterin, a new natural antiplasmodial betulin derivative from *Uapaca paludosa* (Euphorbiaceae). *Journal of Ethnopharmacology* 173: 100–104. https://doi.org/10.1016/j.jep.2015.07.023.

46 Meesala, S., Gurung, P., Karmodiya, K. et al. (2017). Isolation and structure elucidation of halymeniaol, a new antimalarial sterol derivative from the red alga *Halymenia floresii*. *Journal of Asian Natural Products Research* 20 (4): 391–398. https://doi.org/10.1080/10286020.2017.1342636.

47 Sidjui, L.S., Nganso, Y.O., Toghueo, R.M. et al. (2018). Kostchyienones A and B, new antiplasmodial and cytotoxicity of limonoids from the roots of *Pseudocedrela kotschyi* (Schweinf.) Harms. *Zeitschrift für Naturforschung - Section C Journal of Biosciences* 73: 153–160. https://doi.org/10.1515/znc-2017-0102.

48 Chumkaew, P. and Srisawat, T. (2017). Antimalarial and cytotoxic quassinoids from the roots of *Brucea javanica*. *Journal of Asian Natural Products Research* 19: 247–253. https://doi.org/10.1080/10286020.2016.1205040.

49 Konziase, B. (2015). Protective activity of biflavanones from *Garcinia kola* against *Plasmodium* infection. *Journal of Ethnopharmacology* 172: 214–218. https://doi.org/10.1016/j.jep.2015.06.038.

50 Azebaze, A.G.B., Teinkela, J.E.M., Nguemfo, E.L. et al. (2015). Antiplasmodial activity of some phenolic compounds from Cameroonians *Allanblackia*. *African Health Sciences* 15: 835–840. https://doi.org/10.4314/ahs.v15i3.18.

51 Atilaw, Y., Muiva-Mutisya, L., Ndakala, A. et al. (2017). Four prenylflavone derivatives with antiplasmodial activities from the stem of *Tephrosia purpurea* subsp. *leptostachya*. *Molecules* 22: 1514. https://doi.org/10.3390/molecules22091514.

52 Muiva-Mutisya, L.M., Atilaw, Y., Heydenreich, M. et al. (2018). Antiplasmodial prenylated flavanonols from *Tephrosia subtriflora*. *Natural Product Research* 32 (12): 1407–1414. https://doi.org/10.1080/14786419.2017.1353510.

53 Zininga, T., Ramatsui, L., Makhado, P.B. et al. (2017). (−)-Epigallocatechin-3-gallate inhibits the chaperone activity of *Plasmodium falciparum* Hsp70 chaperones and abrogates their association with functional partners. *Molecules* 22: 2139. https://doi.org/10.3390/molecules22122139.

54 Du, Y., Abedi, A.K., Valenciano, A.L. et al. (2017). Isolation of the new antiplasmodial butanolide, malleastrumolide A, from *Malleastrum* sp. (Meliaceae) from Madagascar. *Chemistry & Biodiversity* 14: e1700331. https://doi.org/10.1002/cbdv.201700331.

55 Gadetskaya, A.V., Mohamed, S.M., Tarawneh, A. et al. (2017). Phytochemical characterization and biological activity of secondary metabolites from three

Limonium species. *Medicinal Chemistry Research* 26: 2743–2750. https://doi.org/10.1007/s00044-017-1973-z.

56 Latif, A., Du, Y., Dalal, S.R. et al. (2017). Bioactive neolignans and other compounds from *Magnolia grandiflora* L.: isolation and antiplasmodial activity. *Chemistry & Biodiversity* 14 (9): e1700209. https://doi.org/10.1002/cbdv.201700209.

57 Xiao, H., Rao Ravu, R., Tekwani, B.L. et al. (2017). Biological evaluation of phytoconstituents from *Polygonum hydropiper*. *Natural Product Research* 31: 2053–2057. https://doi.org/10.1080/14786419.2016.1269094.

58 Upegui, Y., Robledo, S.M., Gil Romero, J.F. et al. (2015). In vivo antimalarial activity of α-mangostin and the new xanthone δ-mangostin. *Phytotherapy Research* 29: 1195–1201. https://doi.org/10.1002/ptr.5362.

59 Gupta, A., Singh, A.K., and Qayum, A. (2014). Evaluating ancient Indian history and culture towards malaria control measures based on traditional knowledge system. *International Journal of Interdisciplinary and Multidisciplinary Studies (IJIMS)* 1 (8): 181–190.

10

Mushroom-Derived Products as an Alternative Antimalarial Therapeutics: A Review

Senzosenkosi S. Mkhize[1], Kgothatso E. Machaba[1], Mthokozisi B. C. Simelane[2], and Ofentse J. Pooe[1]

[1] *University of KwaZulu-Natal, Discipline of Biochemistry, Westville Campus, Private Bag X54001, Durban 4000, South Africa*
[2] *University of Johannesburg, Department of Biochemistry, P.O. Box 524, Auckland Park 2006, South Africa*

10.1 Introduction

Mushrooms are an interesting natural food source, containing a large number of biomolecules with both nutritional and medicinal properties [1]. By definition, mushrooms are said to be 'fleshy fungi', which can be characterized by an umbrella-shaped cap consisting of a stalk [2]. Mushrooms belong to *Agaricomycetes*, a class of fungi in the division Basidiomycota. To date, over 16 000 species of mushrooms have been classified, with approximately 2000 known pharmacological properties [3]. Extracts of mushrooms contain, amongst other components, polysaccharides, proteins, phenolics, lectins, glycol and non-glycosylated proteins, lipid components (ergosterol), terpenoids, and alkaloids [4]. These substances contribute to some of the well-known medicinal properties (Figure 10.1) displayed by mushroom extracts such as nematicidal, anti-inflammatory, immunomodulatory, anticancer, antibacterial, antileishmanial, and antimalarial properties [2–7] (Figure 10.1). Thus, the purpose of this chapter is to cover the antimalarial properties of mushroom extract and compounds. It further highlights the potential of mushrooms as a natural antimalarial agent, bioactive compounds isolated from mushrooms for antimalarial activity, the mechanism of both mushroom compounds and extract in eliminating malaria and further stipulates the potential of various mushrooms in eliminating malaria pandemic.

10.2 Biological Roles of Mushrooms

10.2.1 Malarial History and Impact

Parasite-borne infections such as malaria, leishmaniases, and toxoplasmosis are of major concern as they have global impact [8]. Combined these neglected tropical

Drug Development for Malaria: Novel Approaches for Prevention and Treatment, First Edition.
Edited by Pravin Kendrekar.

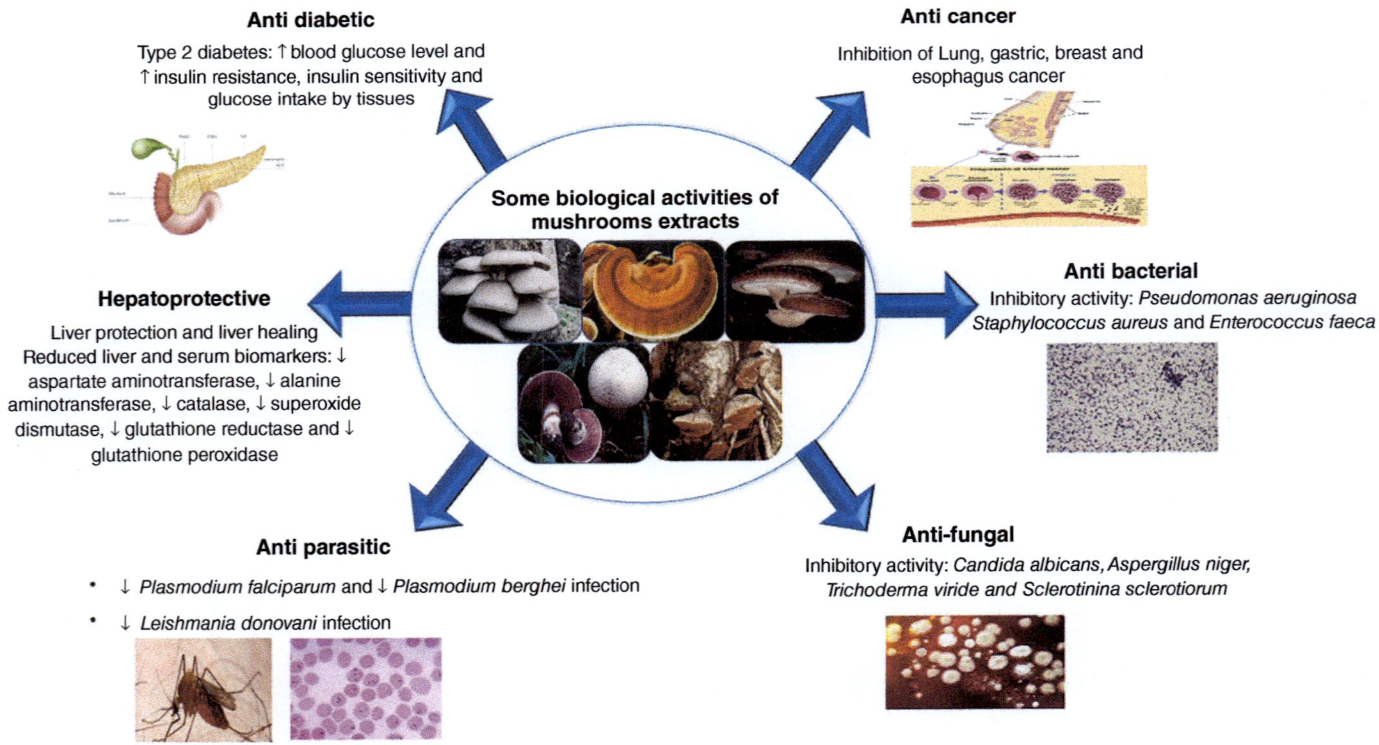

Figure 10.1 Some medicinal properties of edible mushrooms found in nature. '↓' represents reduction, whereas '↑' increase.

diseases (NTDs) infect at least two million people annually in poverty stricken regions worldwide [9, 10]. Treatment options for NTDs are financially burdensome in poor communities [11]. To date, malaria is still regarded as a major public health problem across the world. Malaria, in particular, has undoubtedly had a great impact on world history than most infectious diseases. In 2017, approximately 219 million cases of malaria were recorded worldwide, with half a million mortality cases [12]. Even though malaria has been eradicated in certain parts of the world, it is still a major problem across most tropical regions. Five parasite species of the *Plasmodium* genus, *P. vivax, P. ovale, P. malariae, P. knowlesi,* and *P. falciparum,* are known to cause malaria in humans [13, 14]. Of these, *P. falciparum* is responsible for at least 90% of all malaria infections and mortalities across the globe [15]. The *P. falciparum* is majorly dominant in tropics and subtropics especially in African continent, whereas *P. vivax* and *P. malariae* are found all over tropical regions of the world, *P. ovale* found in Western Africa, and *P. knowlesi* found in Southeast Asia [16]. The *Plasmodium* spp. exhibit a heterogeneous life cycle involving a stint in the vertebrate host and a phase in an arthropod vector. *Anopheles funestus* and *Anopheles gambiae* are the most prominent malaria parasite vectors [12, 17]. Malaria parasites are transmitted from one host to another mostly through an insect vector. Upon infecting the human host, sporozoites invade the hepatocyte cells inside the liver, where they develop into merozoites. These merozoites ultimately rupture from the hepatocytes and enter the bloodstream where they invade erythrocytes and begin a continuous asexual cycle [18]. The continual development and discovery of novel antimalarial drugs inhibiting the sexual and asexual stages of the *Plasmodium* spp. parasite is fundamental in the eradication strategies of malaria.

10.2.2 Antimalarial Activity of Mushroom Extracts

To date, there is still ambiguity about the mechanism of action of most antimalarials and about their stage-specific targets in the malaria life cycle. Furthermore, most antimalarials were primarily designed to alleviate symptoms of the diseases malaria in the blood stage. However, some drugs such as artemisinin [19], artemisinin combination therapies (ACTs) [17, 20], and primaquine [21] have been shown to effectively reduce gametocyte carriage. Antimalarial drugs, such as pyronaridine and atovaquone, have been shown to target liver and sexual stages along with the asexual blood stages in the *P. falciparum* life cycle [18]. The continual discovery of nontoxic therapeutics with reliable multistage-targeting capabilities is pivotal to the continued and effective malaria control. Animal studies demonstrated that treatment with *Agaricus blazei* water extracts (100 mg/kg) displayed antioxidant activity, reduced weight loss, and significant malaria control on *Plasmodium berghei*-infected mice [6]. Val et al. [6] directly demonstrated that treatment with *Ag. blazei* reduced parasitaemia by disrupting the erythrocytic stage of malaria parasites [6]. Previous studies by Adam et al. [22], have indicated that the ethyl

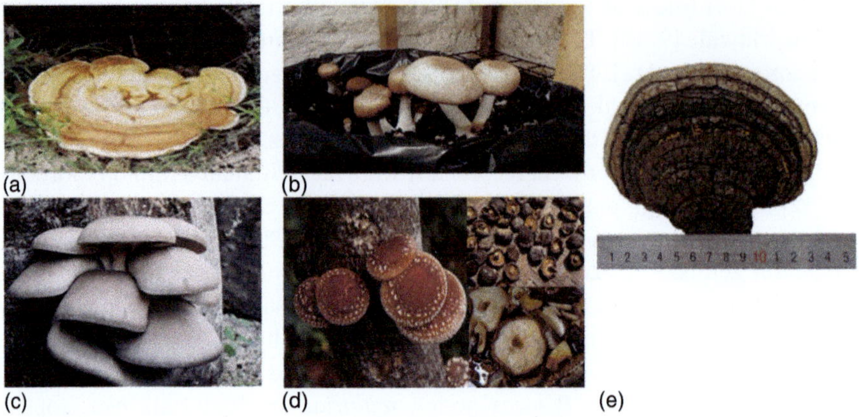

Figure 10.2 Some mushrooms with known antimalarial activity. (a) *G. lucidum*. Source: Photo Courtesy of University of Namibia Zeri project. (b) *A. blazei*. Source: Photo Courtesy of Andrej Gregori, Marija Gregori, Andrej Piltaver, Tamara Korošec. (c) *Pl. ostreatus*. Source: Photo Courtesy of Andrej Gregori, Marija Gregori, Andrej Piltaver, Tamara Korošec. (d) *Lentinula edodes*. Source: Photo Courtesy of Hyde Kevin. (e) *Phellinus linteus*. Source: Photo Courtesy of Wenhua Chen.

acetate extract of *Ganoderma lucidum* mushroom (Figure 10.2) demonstrated the antiplasmodial activity as it showed 79% inhibition of plasmodium at a minimum concentration of 4.9 μg/ml. Oluba et al. [23] demonstrated the antimalarial and liver-protective effects of crude ethanolic extract, *G. lucidum* mushrooms, in *P. berghei*-infected mice [23].

Although mushrooms are promising in fights against malaria, however, there are several mushroom species which have not been evaluated as the possible treatment of malaria. To date, at least 126 medicinal activities, including antimicrobial, anti-fungal, antiviral, and mostly antiparasitic activities, have been reported from isolates derived from mushrooms and fungi [23]; some of these are highlighted in Table 10.1. Previous studies on anti-malarial mushrooms and plants have mainly focussed on their antiparasitic activity but rarely investigate other mechanisms that may play a role in the killing the parasite. A number of studies have reported a synergistic parasite killing action, when crude extracts are administered with anti-malaria drugs [32]. Plant crude extracts are likely to contain phenolics, terpenoids amongst other components [33]. Some researchers have speculated that phenolics from plant extracts such as *Artemisia annua* may also inhibit enzymes involved in metabolism and thus, elevating the action of artemisinin, *in vivo* [34–36]. Little research has been conducted to evaluate mushroom extract-to-drug interactions. However, it is plausible that other components in the extract may influence the bioavailability and metabolism of the antimalarials drugs. On the other hand, some researcher has reported clinical evidence indicating that some herbs may have side effects and adverse events may occur due to herb-to-drug interactions [37]. Thus, more research and assays are required to adequately investigate potential interactions between herbal medicines, mushroom extracts, and prescribed drugs.

Table 10.1 Biological properties of different mushrooms found in nature.

Mushroom species	Biological activity	Type of crude extract	References
Phellinus linteus	Antimalarial (*Plasmodium falciparum*): IC_{50} of 3.15 μg/ml	Methanol (MEOH)	[5]
Lactifluus piperatus	Antimicrobial activity (*Enterococcus faecalis*): MIC of 1.25–5 mg/ml	Acetone extract	[24]
Pleurotus ostreatus	Antimicrobial activity (*Candida albicans*, *Pseudomonas aeruginosa*, and *Staphylococcus aureus*)	Water (H_2O)	[25]
Pl. ostreatus and *Pl.* var florida	Antifungal (*Trichoderma harzianum*): 16 mm inhibition at 2 mg/disc	Water (H_2O)	[26]
Pl. ostreatus	Antiparasitic/antimalarial (*Plasmodium berghei*)	Ethanol and water	[27]
Pl. ostreatus	Antiparasitic/antimalarial (*P. falciparum*)	*n*-Hexane extract	[28]
Agaricus bisporus	Antifungal activity (*Candida* spp.)	MEOH	[29]
Ganoderma lucidum	Antifungal activity (*Trichoderma viride*, *Aspergillus fumigatus*, *Aspergillus versicolor*, and *Aspergillus niger*): MIC of 0.005–1.5 mg/ml	MEOH	[30]
G. lucidum	Antiparasitic/antimalarial (*P. berghei*)	Ethanol extract (EtOH)	[23]
G. lucidum	Antiparasitic/antimalarial (*P. falciparum*): IC_{50} of 6.0–20 μM	MEOH and EtOAc	[22]
Terfezia pfeilii	Antimalarial (*P. falciparum* 3D7, chloroquine-sensitive strain): 5, 10, and 50 μg/ml	Water (H_2O)	[31]

10.2.3 Bioactive Molecules Found Within Mushrooms

Mushrooms form part of the human diet due to their taste, aroma, and texture. In fact, ever since ancient period's mushrooms have been utilized by people for their nutritional and medicinal value. Medicinal properties of mushrooms stem from their wide variety of secondary metabolites, with potent activity against protozoan parasites [1, 4]. Some of these secondary metabolites are classified as alkaloids, terpeneoids, flavonoids, limonoids, peptides, calkon, santon, and coumarin [38]

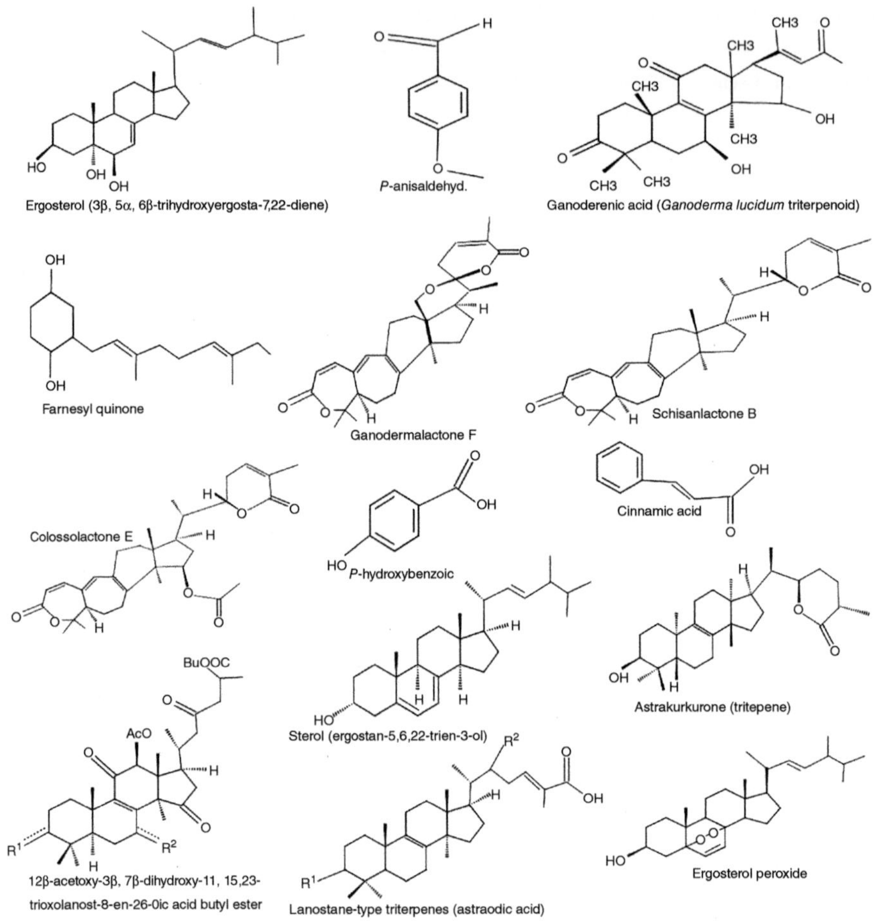

Figure 10.3 Type of biological active compounds found in different mushrooms.

(Figure 10.3). Mushrooms produce diverse number of terpenoids that have several biological actions such as antiplasmodial, antioxidant, antitumor, antibacterial, antifungal, anti-inflammatory, antimicrobial, antiviral, and cytotoxic actions [29]. Table 10.2 stipulates the biological activity of some mushroom-derived compounds. Majority of the triterpenes that are produced by the basidiomycete fungi (oyster mushrooms) are known as lanostane, which also have different biological activity such as anticancer and antiparasitic activity [45]. Adams et al. [22] presented evidence that basidiomycetes have antiparasitic activity as they have managed to demonstrate that mushroom *G. lucidum* produces a compound named triterpene lanostanes which is effective against *P. falciparum* [22]. Edible mushrooms from the *Pleurotus* genus, such as *Pl. sajor-caju*, also consist of compounds such as triterpenes, sterols, alkaloids, flavonoids, tannins, proteins, vitamins, minerals, and fatty acids that have previously been reported to present biological activity [11]. Mushrooms have been reported to be a very efficient source of new antibiotics and antiparasitic drugs [40, 46]. Mushrooms are effective since they mostly produce triterpenoids

Table 10.2 Antiparasitic activity of compounds derived from different mushrooms spp.

Mushroom species	Reported active compound	Reported biological activity	References
Pleurotus pulmonarius	*p*-Anisaldehyde	Antiparasitic (*Caenorhabditis elegans*)	[39]
Ganoderma sp.	Ganoderma Triterpenes (farnesyl quinone)	Antimicrobial and antiparasitic	[40]
Ganoderma sp. KM01	Triterpenes (ganodermalactone F (1), schisanlactone B (2), and colossolactone E (3))	Antiparasitic (*Plasmodium falciparum*): 6–10 μm	[41]
Ganoderma lucidum	Phenolic acids (*p*-hydroxybenzoic (1) and cinnamic acid (2))	Antifungal (*Aspergillus fumigatus, Aspergillus versicolor, Trichoderma viride, Penicillum funiculosum*): MIC of 0.003–0.12 and 0.007–0.03 mg/ml	[42]
Pleurotus ostreatus	Ergostane 5α,8α epidioxy-22*E*-ergosta-6,22-dien-3 β-ol	Antiparasitic (*Trypanosoma cruzi*): IC_{50} of 6.74 μg/ml	[43]
Pl. ostreatus	Sterol (ergostan-5,6,22-trien-3-ol)	Antiparasitic (*Anti-plasmodial*)	[28]
Astraeus hygrometricus	Astrakurkurone (tritepene)	Antileishmanial activity (*Leishmania donovani*)	[44]

Source: Based on Öztürk et al. [29].

which are known as antiparasitic agents [11]. Other studies have also indicated that *Pleurotus ostreatus* mushrooms produced the compound namely ergostane 5α,8α-epidioxy-22 *E*-ergosta-6,22-dien-3β-ol which showed to be effective against parasite *Trypanosoma cruzi* as it was observed that it had the IC_{50} of 6.74 μg/ml [43]. The *Leishmania* parasites were also reported in previous studies to be inhibited by *Pl. ostreatus* alcoholic extract which caused apoptosis of the parasites with IC_{50} of 160 μg/ml [47]. The study conducted by Haque et al. [48] proved that *Pleurotus high-king* mushrooms had potent anthelmintic activity in comparison to the standard drugs which are usually used. Besides the above-mentioned antiparasitic activity of mushrooms, some other researchers such as Adams et al. [22], have stipulated that mushrooms like *G. lucidum* produce compound called triterpene lanostanes which has proven to be very active against the deadly malaria parasite (*P. falciparum*).

10.2.4 Phytochemical Properties of Mushroom Derived Antimalarial Products

Mushrooms such as *Pl. ostreatus* and *G. lucidum* have shown to suppress malaria parasites *in-vivo*; however, the actual mechanism contributing to the antiplasmodial activity of mushrooms remains unclear even though there is some increasing evidence that suggest that changes in lipid content of tissues might be involved in the mechanism of anti-malarial activity [23, 49]. The malaria infection activates the immune system by stimulating the release of reactive oxygen species (ROS) and reactive nitrogen species (RNS), which are associated with oxidative stress resulting in the development of systemic complications [50]. Hydroxyl radicals ($OH^{\cdot}$) and H_2O_2 are produced during infection within the liver and erythrocytes leading to oxidative stress and apoptosis [51]. Furthermore, the malaria parasites have been shown to be induce high production of phospholipids and cholesterol within infected cells [51]. Over the years, mushrooms such as *G. lucidum* [52, 53], *Pl. ostreatus* [54], and *Agaricus bisporus* [55] have been recognized for their medicinal properties which include cholesterol lowering activity. Oluba et al. [56] stipulated extracts of the *G. lucidum* mushroom reduced malarial infection by reducing liver and serum lipoprotein cholesterol [56]. Kadhila [15], also demonstrated that mushrooms namely *G. lucidum* and *Terfezia pfeilii* from Namibia possessed various compounds including anthraquinones, flavonoids, and steroids and attributed their high antimalarial activity to their ability to elevate the oxidation of red blood cells [31].

Moreover, mushrooms also consist of phenolic compounds which possess antiplasmodial activity by counteracting the oxidative damages caused malaria and also inhibiting the synthesis of parasite's protein together with increasing oxidation of red blood cell (Figure 10.4). The process of protein kinases inhibition by mushroom's phenolic acids and flavonoids has been reported to play major role in breaking the cycle of protozoa (*Toxoplasma gondii* and *P. falciparum*) since these enzymes especially calcium-dependent protein kinases (CDPKs) largely control survival, motility, replication, attachment, and egression of protozoa in host cells [57–61]. Figure 10.4 describes some of the known antimalarial/antiprotozoan mechanism of action utilized by mushrooms, it is likely that there are many other antimalarial/antiprotozoan mechanism yet to be discovered.

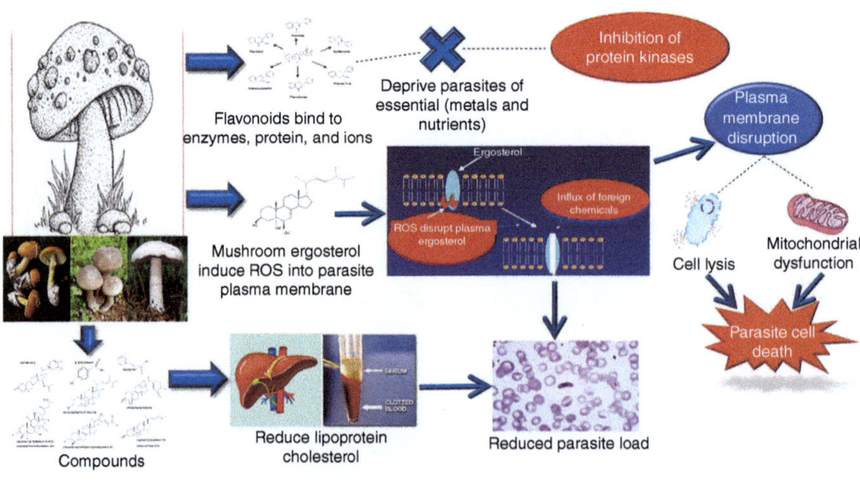

Figure 10.4 Anticipated antimalarial mode of action of mushroom compounds. Source: Adopted Abugri et al. [47].

10.2.5 Immunomodulatory Properties of Mushrooms

The activation of innate immune system is important in controlling the replication and spread of the parasite; hence, this might contribute to the elimination of malaria infection [62]. However, it has been noted that the response of immune system towards the parasites is complicated and not thoroughly understood especially since it is both stage- and species-dependent [63]. Some studies have indicated that malaria activates immune system within the body, which therefore triggers the release of ROS and RNS that usually degrade the haemoglobin [64]. This is probably due to abnormal activation of macrophage, pro-inflammatory, and anti-inflammatory cytokines which elevate malaria disease by stimulating factors such as reactive nitrogen intermediates (NOI) and reactive oxygen intermediates (ROI) [65]. The protective immunity is only mediated by early pro-inflammatory cytokines, whereas late responses cause the pathology towards malaria infection. Therefore, this suggest that unbalanced response causes severe disease caused by malaria; hence, anti-inflammatory cytokines such as interleukin 4, transforming growth factor (TGF), and interleukin 10 play the role of downregulating pro-inflammatory response [65]. Furthermore, some authors have also supported this concept as they had also demonstrated that some T helper 1 (Th1) cytokines (IFN, TNF, and lymphotoxin) caused immunopathological processes which then cause cerebral malaria, but some Th2 cytokines (IL 10, TGF) inhibited the immunopathological process [66]. Mushrooms have been described to have immunomodulatory properties especially since a single mushroom could produce both stimulatory and inhibitory effect towards immune system [67]. Mushrooms consist of various bioactive compounds (1,6-branched 1,3-β-glucans) that stimulate the immune system to activate natural killer (NK) cells, T cells, macrophages, and produce cytokines [68]. Some studies have also indicated the effectiveness of mushrooms in preventing the severity of malaria infection as observed during *P. berghei* infection that upon administration of *Ag. blazei* mushroom extract/purified fraction resulting in the reduced production of pro-inflammatory cytokines within spleen (IFN-γ, IL-17, and IL-6) and brain (TNF, IL-1β, and IL-6) [69]. This suggest that mushrooms have synergistic effect, for example, a research by Davis et al. [70], proved that mushroom induced multiple cytokines with both pro- and anti-inflammatory activity; hence, the induction of anti-inflammatory cytokines such as IL-1 assisted a lot in moderating and resolving immune defense caused by pro-inflammatory responses [70].

10.3 Conclusion

Mushrooms have proven to the potential source of various medicinal compounds which could be beneficial in the ongoing battle with malaria. The continued development of drug resistance underscores the need for the development of new antimalarials, thus highlighting mushrooms as a potential hub in the search for novel therapeutics. Albeit the physiopathology of malaria is yet to be fully elucidated, we can appreciate that its pathogenesis is multifactorial and extremely intricate; hence, new therapeutic approaches must focus on developing a 'multi-target, multidrug' strategies as opposed to the 'one target, one drug' approach. Furthermore, it must be noted that compounds highlighted in this chapter, regardless of their antiplasmodium potency status, can be used as probes in the development and synthesis of new antimalarial drug targets and may also be used as scaffolds for novel lead structures and drugs.

Acknowledgements

Authors would like to acknowledge sponsors such National Research Foundation (NRF) for their financial support. Further acknowledgements go to the University of KwaZulu-Natal for very support provide by the staff.

References

1 Bala, N., Aitken, E.A.B., Fechner, N. et al. (2011). Evaluation of antibacterial activity of Australian basidiomycetous macrofungi using a high-throughput 96-well plate assay. *Pharmaceutical Biology* 49: 492–500. https://doi.org/10.3109/13880209.2010.526616.

2 Chang, S.T. and Miles, P.G. (2004). *Mushrooms: Cultivation, Nutritional Value, Medicinal Effect, and Environmental Impact*, 2e. CRC Press; ISBN 9780203492086.

3 Wasser, S.P. (2010). Medicinal mushroom science: history, current status, future trends and unsolved problems. *International Journal of Medicinal Mushrooms* 12: 1–16. https://doi.org/10.1615/IntJMedMushr.v12.i1.10.

4 Soares, A.A., De Sá-Nakanishi, A.B., Bracht, A. et al. (2013). Hepatoprotective effects of mushrooms. *Molecules* 18: 7609–7630. https://doi.org/10.3390/molecules18077609.

5 Samchai, S., Seephonkai, P., Sangdee, A. et al. (2009). Antioxidant, cytotoxic and antimalarial activities from crude extracts of mushroom *Phellinus linteus*. *Journal of Biological Sciences* 9: 778–783. https://doi.org/10.3923/jbs.2009.778.783.

6 Val, C.H., Brant, F., Miranda, A.S. et al. (2015). Effect of mushroom *Agaricus blazei* on immune response and development of experimental cerebral malaria. *Malaria Journal* 14: 1–13. https://doi.org/10.1186/s12936-015-0832-y.

7 Fatima, N., Muhammad, S.A., Qazi, M.A. et al. (2017). Fungal metabolites and antimalarial drug discovery; a review. *Acta Poloniae Pharmaceutica. Drug Research* 74: 1327–1341.

8 Secrieru, A., Costa, I.C.C., O'Neill, P.M., and Cristiano, M.L.S. (2020). Antimalarial agents as therapeutic tools against toxoplasmosis – a short bridge between two distant illnesses. *Molecules* 25 (7): 1574. https://doi.org/10.3390/molecules25071574.

9 Ben-Harari, R.R., Goodwin, E., and Casoy, J. (2017). Adverse event profile of Pyrimethamine-based therapy in toxoplasmosis: a systematic review. *Drugs in R&D* 17: 523–544. https://doi.org/10.1007/s40268-017-0206-8.

10 Osorio, J.C.C. and García, A.M.G. (2019). Antiparasitic phytotherapy perspectives, scope and current development. *Infection* 23: 189–204. https://doi.org/10.22354/in.v23i2.777.

11 Lenzi, J., Costa, T.M., Alberton, M.D. et al. (2018). Medicinal fungi: a source of antiparasitic secondary metabolites. *Applied Microbiology and Biotechnology* 102: 5791–5810. https://doi.org/10.1007/s00253-018-9048-8.

12 Talapko, J., Škrlec, I., Alebić, T. et al. (2019). Malaria: the past and the present. *Microorganisms* 7: 179. https://doi.org/10.3390/microorganisms7060179.

13 Watts, K.R., Tenney, K., and Crews, P. (2010). The structural diversity and promise of antiparasitic marine invertebrate-derived small molecules. *Current Opinion in Biotechnology* 21: 808–818. https://doi.org/10.1016/j.copbio.2010.09.015.

14 Krečmerová, M., Dračínský, M., Hocková, D. et al. (2012). Synthesis of purine *N*9-[2-hydroxy-3-*O*-(phosphonomethoxy)propyl] derivatives and their side-chain modified analogs as potential antimalarial agents. *Bioorganic and Medicinal Chemistry* 20: 1222–1230. https://doi.org/10.1016/j.bmc.2011.12.034.

15 Kadhila, N. P. (2007). Evaluation of indigenous Namibian mushrooms and plants for antimalarial properties. A dissertation submitted in fulfilment of the requirements for the degree of Doctor of Philosophy the University of Namibia; University of Namibia.

16 Singh, B. and Daneshvar, C. (2013). Human infections and detection of *Plasmodium knowlesi*. *Clinical Microbiology Reviews* 26: 165–184. https://doi.org/10.1128/CMR.00079-12.

17 Stepniewska, K., Price, R.N., Sutherland, C.J. et al. (2008). *Plasmodium falciparum* gametocyte dynamics in areas of different malaria endemicity. *Malaria Journal* 7: 1–22. https://doi.org/10.1186/1475-2875-7-249.

18 Delves, M., Plouffe, D., Scheurer, C. et al. (2012). The activities of current antimalarial drugs on the life cycle stages of *Plasmodium*: a comparative study with human and rodent parasites. *PLoS Medicine* 9: https://doi.org/10.1371/journal.pmed.1001169.

19 Piyaphanee, W., Krudsood, S., Tangpukdee, N. et al. (2006). Emergence and clearance of gametocytes in uncomplicated *Plasmodium falciparum* malaria. *American Journal of Tropical Medicine and Hygiene* 74: 432–435. https://doi.org/10.4269/ajtmh.2006.74.432.

20 Group, W. G. S (2016). Gametocyte carriage in uncomplicated *Plasmodium falciparum* malaria following treatment with artemisinin combination therapy: a systematic review and meta-analysis of individual patient data. *BMC Medicine* 14: 79. https://doi.org/10.1186/s12916-016-0621-7.

21 Bousema, T., Okell, L., Shekalaghe, S. et al. (2010). Revisiting the circulation time of *Plasmodium falciparum* gametocytes: molecular detection methods to estimate the duration of gametocyte carriage and the effect of gametocytocidal drugs. *Malaria Journal* 9: 136. https://doi.org/10.1186/1475-2875-9-136.

22 Adams, M., Christen, M., Plitzko, I. et al. (2010). Antiplasmodial lanostanes from the *Ganoderma lucidum* mushroom. *Journal of Natural Products* 73: 897–900. https://doi.org/10.1021/np100031c.

23 Oluba, O. M.; Olusola, A. O.; Fagbohunka, B. S.; Onyeneke, E. C. Antimalarial and hepatoprotective effects of crude ethanolic extract of Lingzhi or Reishi medicinal mushroom, *Ganoderma lucidum* (W. Curt.: Fr.) P. Karst. (higher basidiomycetes), in *Plasmodium berghei*-infected mice. *International Journal of Medicinal Mushrooms* 2012, 14(5):459-66, https://doi.org/10.1615/intjmedmushr.v14.i5.30.

24 Kosanic, M., Rankovic, B., and Dasic, M. (2013). Antioxidant and antimicrobial properties of mushrooms. *Bulgarian Journal of Agricultural Science* 19: 1040–1046.

25 Wolff, E.R.S., Wisbeck, E., Silveira, M.L.L. et al. (2008). Antimicrobial and antineoplasic activity of *Pleurotus ostreatus. Applied Biochemistry and Biotechnology* 151: 402–412. https://doi.org/10.1007/s12010-008-8208-1.

26 Owaid, M.N., Al-Saeedi, S.S.S., and Al-Assaffii, I.A.A. (2017). A actividade anti-fúngica de cogumelos de ostra cultivada em várias agro-resíduos. *Summa Phytopathologica* 43: 9–13. https://doi.org/10.1590/0100-5405/2069.

27 Omoya, O.F., Momoh, A.O., and Adegoke, O.A. (2017). In vivo evaluation of the antiplasmodial property of ethanol and hot water extracts of *Pleurotus ostreatus* mushroom. *Science Journal of Public Health* 5: 178–185. https://doi.org/10.11648/j.sjph.20170503.14.

28 Afieroho, O.E., Noundou, X.S., Onyia, C.P. et al. (2019). Antiplasmodial activity of the *n*-hexane extract from *Pleurotus ostreatus* (Jacq. Ex. Fr) P. Kumm. *Turkish Journal of Pharmaceutical Sciences* 16: 37–42.

29 Öztürk, M., Duru, M.E., Kivrak, Ş. et al. (2011). In vitro antioxidant, anticholinesterase and antimicrobial activity studies on three *Agaricus* species with fatty acid compositions and iron contents: a comparative study on the three most edible mushrooms. *Food and Chemical Toxicology* 49: 1353–1360. https://doi.org/10.1016/j.fct.2011.03.019.

30 Heleno, S.A., Ferreira, I.C.F.R., Esteves, A.P. et al. (2013). Antimicrobial and demelanizing activity of *Ganoderma lucidum* extract, *p*-hydroxybenzoic and cinnamic acids and their synthetic acetylated glucuronide methyl esters. *Food and Chemical Toxicology* 58: 95–100. https://doi.org/10.1016/j.fct.2013.04.025.

31 El Enshasy, H., Elsayed, E.A., Aziz, R., and Wadaan, M.A. (2013). Mushrooms and truffles: historical biofactories for complementary medicine in Africa and in the middle East. *Evidence-based Complementary and Alternative Medicine* 2013: https://doi.org/10.1155/2013/620451.

32 Mallard, B., Leach, D.N., Wohlmuth, H., and Tiralongo, J. (2019). Synergistic immuno-modulatory activity in human macrophages of a medicinal mushroom formulation consisting of Reishi, Shiitake and Maitake. *PLoS One* 14: 1–14. https://doi.org/10.1371/journal.pone.0224740.

33 Ayeni, G., Pooe, O.J., Singh, M. et al. (2019). Cytotoxic and antioxidant activities of selected South African medicinal plants. *Pharmacognosy Journal* 11: https://doi.org/10.5530/PJ.2019.11.234.

34 Ashraf, A., Sarfraz, R.A., and Mahmood, A. (2017). Phenolic compounds' characterization of *Artemisia rutifolia* spreng from *Pakistani flora* and their relationships with antioxidant and antimicrobial attributes. *International Journal of Food Properties* 20: 2538–2549. https://doi.org/10.1080/10942912.2016.1243556.

35 Skowyra, M., Gallego, M.G., Segovia, F., and Almajano, M.P. (2014). Antioxidant properties of *Artemisia annua* extracts in model food emulsions. *Antioxidants* 3: 116–128. https://doi.org/10.3390/antiox3010116.

36 Ferreira, J.F.S., Luthria, D.L., Sasaki, T., and Heyerick, A. (2010). Flavonoids from *Artemisia annua* L. as antioxidants and their potential synergism with artemisinin against malaria and cancer. *Molecules* 15: 3135–3170. https://doi.org/10.3390/molecules15053135.

37 Izzo, A.A. (2012). Interactions between herbs and conventional drugs: overview of the clinical data. *Medical Principles and Practice* 21: 404–428. https://doi.org/10.1159/000334488.

38 Saxena, A.K., Saxena, S., and Chaudhaery, S.S. (2010). Molecular modelling and docking studies on heat shock protein 90 (Hsp90) inhibitors. *SAR and QSAR in Environmental Research* 21: 1–20. https://doi.org/10.1080/10629360903560504.

39 Stadler, M., Mayer, A., Anke, H., and Sterner, O. (1994). Fatty acids and other compounds with nematicidal activity from cultures of basidiomycetes. *Planta Medica* 60: 128–132. https://doi.org/10.1055/s-2006-959433.

40 Basnet, B.B., Liu, L., Bao, L., and Liu, H. (2017). Current and future perspective on antimicrobial and anti-parasitic activities of *Ganoderma* sp.: an update. *Mycology* 8: 111–124.

41 Lakornwong, W., Kanokmedhakul, K., Kanokmedhakul, S. et al. (2014). Triterpene lactones from cultures of *Ganoderma* sp. KM01. *Journal of Natural Products* 77: 1545–1553. https://doi.org/10.1021/np400846k.

42 Alves, M.J., Ferreira, I.C.F.R., Dias, J. et al. (2012). A review on antimicrobial activity of mushroom (Basidiomycetes) extracts and isolated compounds. *Planta Medica* 78: 1707–1718.

43 Ramos-Ligonio, A., Lõpez-Monteon, A., and Trigos, Á. (2012). Trypanocidal activity of ergosterol peroxide from *Pleurotus ostreatus*. *Phytotherapy Research* 26: 938–943. https://doi.org/10.1002/ptr.3653.

44 Lai, T.K., Biswas, G., Chatterjee, S. et al. (2012). Leishmanicidal and anticandidal activity of constituents of Indian edible mushroom *Astraeus hygrometricus*. *Chemistry & Biodiversity* 9: 1517–1524. https://doi.org/10.1002/cbdv.201100272.

45 Kayser, O., Kiderlen, A.F., and Croft, S.L. (2003). Natural products as antiparasitic drugs. *Parasitology Research* 90: 55–62. https://doi.org/10.1007/s00436-002-0768-3.

46 De Silva, D.D., Rapior, S., Sudarman, E. et al. (2013). Bioactive metabolites from macrofungi: ethnopharmacology, biological activities and chemistry. *Fungal Diversity* 62: 1–40. https://doi.org/10.1007/s13225-013-0265-2.

47 Abugri, D.A., Ayariga, J.A., Tiimob, B.J. et al. (2019). Medicinal mushrooms as novel sources for new antiparasitic drug development. In: *Medicinal Mushrooms* (ed. Dinesh Chandra Agrawal and Muralikrishnan Dhanasekaren), 251–273. Singapore: Springer.

48 Haque, M.A., Sarker, A.K., Paul, R.K. et al. (2015). Screening for antiparasitic activity of crude extracts of *Pleurotus highking*, a Bangladeshi edible mushroom. *Bangladesh Pharmaceutical Journal* 18: 38–41. https://doi.org/10.3329/bpj.v18i1.23512.

49 Oluba, O.M. (2019). *Ganoderma* terpenoid extract exhibited anti-plasmodial activity by a mechanism involving reduction in erythrocyte and hepatic lipids in *Plasmodium berghei* infected mice. *Lipids in Health and Disease* 18: 1–9. https://doi.org/10.1186/s12944-018-0951-x.

50 Percário, S., Moreira, D.R., Gomes, B.A.Q. et al. (2012). Oxidative stress in malaria. *International Journal of Molecular Sciences* 13: 16346–16372. https://doi.org/10.3390/ijms131216346.

51 Kumar, S. and Bandyopadhyay, U. (2005). Free heme toxicity and its detoxification systems in human. *Toxicology Letters* 157: 175–188.

52 Khan, I., Saeed, K., and Khan, I. (2019). Nanoparticles: properties, applications and toxicities. *Arabian Journal of Chemistry* 12: 908–931.

53 Kabir, Y., Klmura, S., and Tamura, T. (1988). Dietary effect of *Ganoderma lucidum* mushroom on blood pressure and lipid levels in Spontaneously Hypertensive Rats (SHR). *Journal of Nutritional Science and Vitaminology* 34: 433–438.

54 Cheung, P.C.K. and Lee, M.Y. (2000). Fractionation and characterization of mushroom dietary fiber (nonstarch polysaccharides) as potential nutraceuticals from sclerotia of *Pleurotus tuber-regium* (fries) singer. *Journal of Agricultural and Food Chemistry* 48: 3148–3151. https://doi.org/10.1021/jf000382s.

55 Fukushima, M., Nakano, M., Morii, Y. et al. (2000). Hepatic LDL receptor mRNA in rats is increased by dietary mushroom (*Agaricus bisporus*) fiber and sugar beet fiber. *The Journal of Nutrition* 130: 2151–2156. https://doi.org/10.1093/jn/130.9.2151.

56 Oluba, O.M., Olusola, A.O., Eidangbe, G.O. et al. (2012). Modulation of lipoprotein cholesterol levels in *Plasmodium berghei* malarial infection by crude aqueous extract of *Ganoderma lucidum*. *Cholesterol* 2012: https://doi.org/10.1155/2012/536396.

57 Ghartey-Kwansah, G., Yin, Q., Li, Z. et al. (2020). Calcium-dependent protein kinases in malaria parasite development and infection. *Cell Transplantation* 29: 1–12. https://doi.org/10.1177/0963689719884888.

58 Debarry, J.D. and Kissinger, J.C. (2011). Jumbled genomes: missing apicomplexan synteny. *Molecular Biology and Evolution* 28: 2855–2871. https://doi.org/10.1093/molbev/msr103.

59 Sibley, L.D. (2004). Intracellular parasite invasion strategies. *Science* 304: 248–253. https://doi.org/10.1126/science.1094717.

60 Wernimont, A.K., Artz, J.D., Finerty, P. et al. (2010). Structures of apicomplexan calcium-dependent protein kinases reveal mechanism of activation by calcium. *Nature Structural and Molecular Biology* 17: 596–601. https://doi.org/10.1038/nsmb.1795.

61 Kadian, K., Gupta, Y., Kempaiah, P. et al. (2017). Calcium dependent protein kinases (CDPKs): key to malaria eradication. *Current Topics in Medicinal Chemistry* 17: https://doi.org/10.2174/1568026617666170130112714.

62 Urban, B.C., Ing, R., and Stevenson, M.M. (2005). Early interactions between blood-stage *Plasmodium* parasites and the immune system. *Current Topics in Microbiology and Immunology* 297: 25–70. https://doi.org/10.1007/3-540-29967-x_2.

63 Stevenson, M.M. and Riley, E.M. (2004). Innate immunity to malaria. *Nature Reviews Immunology* 4: 169–180. https://doi.org/10.1038/nri1311.

64 Nsiah, K., Bahaah, B., Oppong Afranie, B. et al. (2019). Oxidative stress and hemoglobin level of complicated and uncomplicated malaria cases among children: a cross-sectional study in Kumasi Metropolis, Ghana. *Journal of Tropical Medicine* 2019: https://doi.org/10.1155/2019/8479076.

65 Malaguarnera, L. and Musumeci, S. (2002). The immune response to *Plasmodium falciparum* malaria. *Lancet Infectious Diseases* 2: 472–478. https://doi.org/10.1038/nri1311.

66 Lin, C.S., Chang, C.J., Lu, C.C. et al. (2014). Impact of the gut microbiota, prebiotics, and probiotics on human health and disease. *Biomedical Journal* 37: 259–268. https://doi.org/10.4103/2319-4170.138314.

67 Dong, C.H. and Yao, Y.J. (2011). On the reliability of fungal materials used in studies on *Ophiocordyceps sinensis*. *Journal of Industrial Microbiology and Biotechnology* 38: 1027–1035. https://doi.org/10.1007/s10295-010-0877-4.

68 Roupas, P., Keogh, J., Noakes, M. et al. (2012). The role of edible mushrooms in health: evaluation of the evidence. *Journal of Functional Foods* 4: 687–709. https://doi.org/10.1016/j.jff.2012.05.003.

69 Blumfield, M., Abbott, K., Duve, E. et al. (2020). Examining the health effects and bioactive components in *Agaricus bisporus* mushrooms: a scoping review. *Journal of Nutritional Biochemistry* 84: 108453. https://doi.org/10.1016/j.jnutbio.2020.108453.

70 Davis, R., Taylor, A., Nally, R. et al. (2020). Differential immune activating, anti-inflammatory, and regenerative properties of the aqueous, ethanol, and solid fractions of a medicinal mushroom blend. *Journal of Inflammation Research* 13: 117–131. https://doi.org/10.2147/JIR.S229446.

11

Discovery and Trends of 8-Aminoquinoline and 4-Aminoquinoline Classes of Antimalarials

Meenakshi Jain, Samarpita Das, and Rahul Jain

National Institute of Pharmaceutical Education and Research (NIPER), Department of Medicinal Chemistry, Sector 67, S. A. S. Nagar, Mohali, Punjab 160062, India

11.1 Introduction

Malaria is one of the most crucial, life-threatening, vector-borne diseases caused by parasites of *Plasmodium* sp., especially *Plasmodium falciparum* and *Plasmodium vivax*, which has afflicted mankind since time immemorial and refuses to perish. It is caused by infection with protozoan parasites transmitted by female *Anopheles* mosquitoes [1]. Malaria is an extremely contagious disease claiming approximately 405 000 lives worldwide in 2018 [2]. Children under the age of five and pregnant women are mostly susceptible to the risk of morbidity and mortality as posed by malaria, accounting for nearly 90% of the fatalities in the sub-Saharan regions of Africa [3].

Concerted efforts and increased funding, over the past decade, have substantially reduced the malaria burden, and since 2000, these numbers have decreased by about 37% worldwide. However, recent reports have suggested that this level is eventually plateauing, thereby emphasizing on the complacency with the current therapeutic strategies. Moreover, lack of a highly effective malaria vaccine and the emergence of existing drug-resistant parasites continue to contribute to the ongoing challenges toward the control and gradual eradication of the disease (Figure 11.1) [4, 5].

11.1.1 History

Chloroquine (**1**), the classical drug of the 4-aminoquinoline class of antimalarials, was first chemically synthesized as a substitute of quinine in the year 1934 and has been the mainstay for the treatment of malaria caused by *P. falciparum* for at least five decades and still remains the drug of choice for treating *P. vivax* induced uncomplicated malaria [3]. Apart from chloroquine, the long-standing success of other members of the 4-aminoquinoline class of antimalarials, such as amodiaquine, piperaquine, and other conjugates, having comparable efficacy, safety, and cost-effectivity relative to the parent molecule, is also worthy of mention.

Drug Development for Malaria: Novel Approaches for Prevention and Treatment, First Edition.
Edited by Pravin Kendrekar.

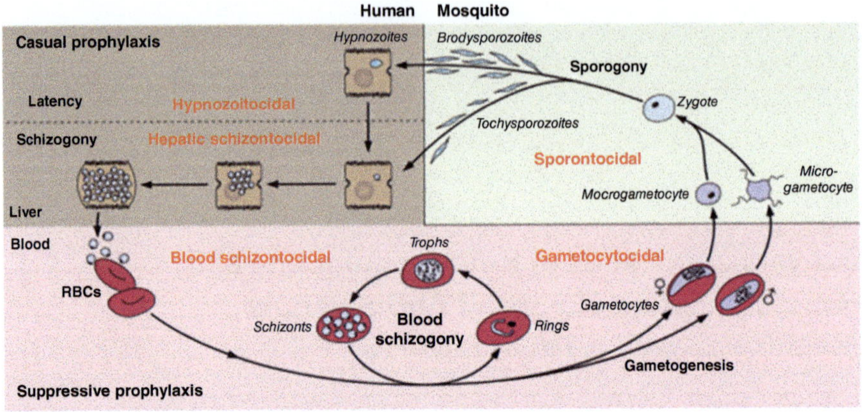

Figure 11.1 Life cycle of *Plasmodium* sp. inside both hosts: humans and mosquitoes.

These drugs mainly act as blood-stage schizonticidal agents. However, the misuse of chloroquine in terms of discontinuation of the treatment and administration of the drug as a prophylactic has added to the emergence and development of chloroquine-resistant *P. falciparum* and *P. vivax*-resistant strains [4]. The usage of the other drugs is also affected by the large diffusion of cross-resistance to amodiaquine (**2**) and mefloquine (**3**). In absence of the drug pressure in some of the malaria-burdened countries, the chloroquine-resistant *P. falciparum* strains have been replaced by chloroquine sensitive isolates, thus keeping the research and development of chloroquine analogs as multispecies antimalarial agents, still alive and regularly reviewed. The increased cases of chloroquine resistance could be overcome to some extent by chemical modification in the side chain of 4-aminoquinolines, such as chain lengthening or introduction of basic bulky groups. Several compounds showcasing these features, such as ferroquine, have been synthesized and successfully evaluated against chloroquine-resistant strains. Apart from that, the antimalarial target profiles have recently been scrutinized, thereby suggesting the importance of developing molecules with good absorption, distribution, metabolism, excretion- pharmacokinetics (ADME-PK) profiles that can target different parasitic species at different stages of their life cycle, which can be relevant for combination therapies [6].

Most of the antimalarials are the outcomes of several wars fought in the tropics in the early nineteenth century and as a matter of fact, the 8-aminoquinolines are no exception to that. In the 1920s, pamaquine (**4**), the oldest 8-aminoquinoline antimalarial drug, was synthesized in Germany and was introduced during the Burma conflict by the British and Indian armies in addition to quinine for the large-scale treatment of malaria. As a potent gametocytocidal agent, it could be utilized as a prophylactic agent to lower the incidence of malaria, but owing to its frequent adverse reactions like dose-related methemoglobinemia and severe hemolytic reactions, its use was limited. Moreover, the advent of the 4-aminoquinoline and quinacrine classes of antimalarials forced the research progress of 8-aminoquinolines to take a backseat for sometimes, until renewed research resulted in the invention of primaquine (**5**) during the later stages of Second World War in the late 1940s. Dawned with all the advantages of pamaquine, primaquine was found to be more potent than the earlier. Mass administration of primaquine in conjunction with chloroquine, during the Korean War, helped in aborting late relapses of *P. vivax*-induced malaria in military personnel. This drug attacks the hypnozoite stage of the *P. vivax* parasites in the human liver and acts as a gametocytocidal agent in *P. falciparum* malaria. However, the incidence of hemolytic anemia caused by glucose-6-phosphate dehydrogenase (G6PD) deficiency, predominantly in African-Americans, hindered the increased use of primaquine. G6PD deficiency is an X-chromosome linked disorder, hence predominant in males. However, X-chromosome inactivation in heterozygous women may also lead to development of clinically significant hemolysis after exposure to primaquine. Qualitative and quantitative G6PD activity assays provide a temporary solution for such cases, but further studies are required for traveler population as these tests require significant turnover time and pose a risk to prescribe to persons traveling on short notice. Besides G6PD deficiency, pharmacodynamics of the drug also contributes to its failure. The drug is dependent on the activity of cytochrome P_{450}2D6 (CYP2D6) for its metabolic transformation inside the host with the formation of hydroxylated primaquine metabolites. CYP2D6 exists in multiple alleles that cause varying degrees of primaquine metabolism and activities. Thus, G6PD deficiency, decreased metabolism, poor bioavailability, and higher cost leaves primaquine fraught with risk and uncertainty in clinical and health practice [7]. Since mid-nineteenth century, primaquine has been the most widely used drug for acting on the hypnozoite forms of *P. vivax* and *Plasmodium ovale*; however, its shorter half-life, lesser therapeutic index, long-term administration, and susceptibility to tolerance in *P. vivax* infections in many geographic domains (requiring increased doses) have prompted the search for a suitable alternative to produce radical cure. Thus, in an attempt to develop a longer-acting, more potent and less toxic drug for the radical cure and causal prophylaxis of malaria, Walter Reed Army Institute of Research and GlaxoSmithKline co-developed tafenoquine (previously known as WR-238605 or etaquine) (**6**), an 8-aminoquinoline which is originally a synthetic analog of primaquine in 1979 [8, 9]. Similarly, in the search for a newer, safer, and potent antimalarial, the Central Drug Research Institute (CDRI) selected CDRI 80/53 for further development as radical curative agent. This, later on, became bulaquine or ebulaquine (**7**), which acts as a potent antimalarial agent. Though an analog of primaquine, it is much safer as compared to the parent drug and causes only one-third as much as methemoglobinemia. This is also established as a radical curative and causal prophylactic against sporozoite-induced *Plasmodium cynomolgi* infection in rhesus monkeys and is also safe in subacute toxicity studies in rats and rhesus monkeys with no teratogenic action (Figure 11.2) [10].

11.1.2 Mode of Action

The understanding of the mechanism of action of the aminoquinolines mandates knowledge of the entire life cycle of the malaria parasites, which is rather complex.

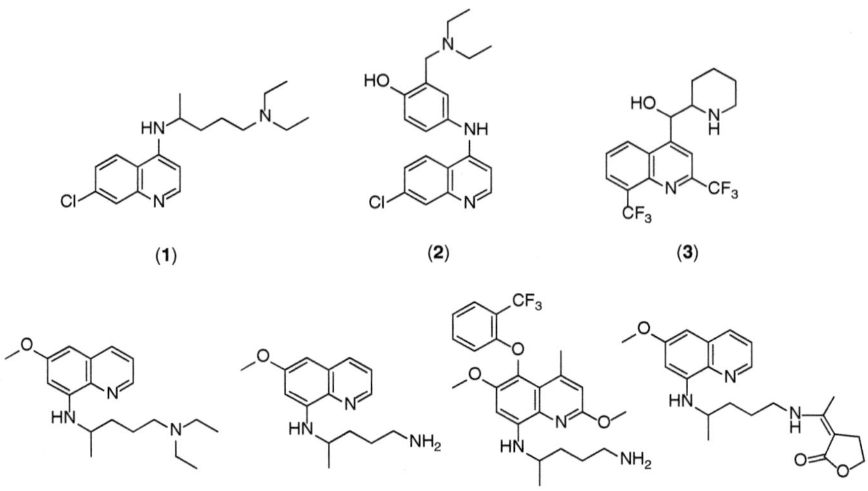

(1) (2) (3)

(4) (5) (6) (7)

Figure 11.2 Some well-established and classical 4- and 8-aminoquinoline antimalarial drugs.

The diversity of the symptoms of the disease is brought about by the erythrocytic stage of the parasite, which is harnessed by the human hosts.

The parasites digest more than 70% of the host cell hemoglobin present in the erythrocytes in order to synthesize amino acids, necessary to preserve osmotic stability, and make space for the parasite intracellularly. Hemozoin, formed as a product of hemoglobin degradation, is inevitable for the survival of the parasite inside host body. As a result, heme detoxification into hemozoin became the preliminary target of 4-aminoquinoline antimalarials [11]. It involves a very complex mechanism, followed by the release of ferriprotoporphyrin IX by *Plasmodium*-containing erythrocytes as the chloroquine receptor. After the drug binds to the ferriprotoporphyrin IX, this combination brings about the lysis of the parasitic as well as the erythrocytic membrane and intervenes the nucleoprotein synthesis in the parasites. The drug that enters into the acidic environment of the erythrocyte's lysosome gets protonated. This protonated drug then fails to leave the lysosome as it is repelled by the positively charged outlet pore, thus remaining bound to the host's hemoglobin preventing it from processing it properly [12]. Hence, the drugs of this class are mostly responsible for the inhibition of polymerization of heme and prevention of disposal of the polymers into the cytoplasm from the food vacuoles, thereby preventing hemozoin formation. This leads to free heme accumulation within the parasite, which is highly toxic to the latter [3]. However, the 4-aminoquinolines do not show any activity against the exo-erythrocytic stages of the malarial parasites and hence fails to prevent relapses of the malaria caused by *P. ovale* and *P. vivax*. Though the mechanism of development of resistance in the malarial parasites against the 4-aminoquinolines is not yet very well understood, researchers presume that resistance against chloroquine can be attributed to the increased level of drug efflux from the

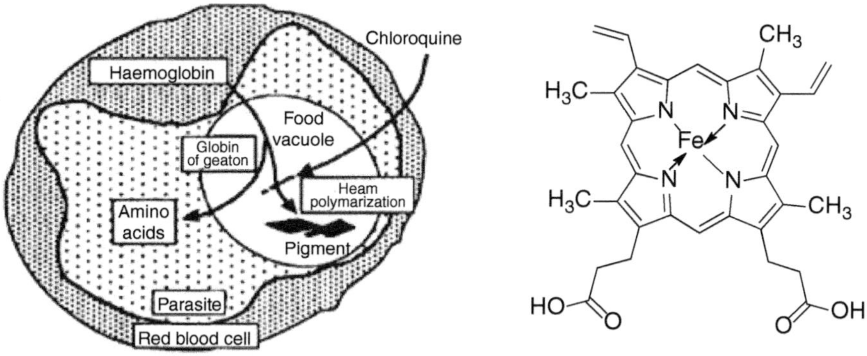

Figure 11.3 Mechanism of inhibition of hemozoin polymerization using chloroquine and ferriprotoporphyrin IX, the target of chloroquine.

chloroquine-resistant strains and reduced affinity of the drug for the heme, resulting in the lower uptake of the drug into the hemoglobin. Along with this, *Plasmodium falciparum* chloroquine-resistance transporter (*Pf*CRT) also adds to the development of resistance of the malarial parasite to chloroquine drug (Figure 11.3) [13].

Unlike the 4-aminoquinolines, 8-aminoquinolines have a narrow spectrum of antimalarial activity and are mainly used to target the exo-erythrocytic stages, such as immature gametocytic stages of the parasitic life cycle. In addition, the hepatic (both dormant and non-dormant) stages also fall prey to the 8-aminoquinolines. Primaquine helps to disorient the parasite's mitochondria, eventually by interference with the ubiquinone function as an electron carrier in the respiratory chain, resulting in the disruption of subsequent processes including maturation. The macro-gametocytes start showing a significant increase in the cristate mitochondria in the third morphological stage of *P. falciparum* gametocyte formation and these can be targeted only by primaquine. Selective accumulation of primaquine in the parasitic mitochondria leads to its swelling and ultimately affects the mitochondrial proliferation, thereby inhibiting further growth and development. Primaquine can act as a potential antimalarial agent by the production of highly reactive metabolites, especially the 4-amino-1-methylbutyl side chain that has been shown to generate superoxides that further generate oxidative potential intracellularly. Biotransformation of 8-aminoquinolines and their selective generation of oxidative stress in the parasitic cells is the probable mechanism for 8-aminoquinoline toxicity and efficacy. Tafenoquine has been reported to inhibit hematin polymerization, which may contribute to its blood-schizontocidal activity, although this effect has not been demonstrated for primaquine [8, 14].

11.1.3 SAR of Aminoquinolines

11.1.3.1 SAR of 8-Aminoquinolines

- The quinoline nucleus is of paramount importance as it is present in majority of 8-aminoquinoline antimalarials developed. However, rings like phenanthrene, anthracene, and naphthalene (**8**) also show significant schizonticidal activity and can replace quinoline. But, the tissue schizonticidal activity was reduced compared to primaquine when quinoline ring was substituted using acridine moiety.

- Substitution of the 8-aminoquinoline ring with other reduced quinoline ring analogs (**9, 10**) leads to decrease in the antimalarial activity.
- The presence of a 6-oxygen function is indispensable as is evident from all the work regarding SAR of 8-aminoquinolines done till date, where the 6-methoxy functionality of primaquine has been retained in most of the cases. Other groups like hydroxyl and 3-hydroxyethyl have also been used but they increased the toxicity profile apart from enhancing the antimalarial activity.
- Primaquine, when substituted using benzyloxy and certain substituted benzyloxy groups, acts as radical curatives but is lesser active and less toxic as compared to primaquine. Other analogs containing methoxy, amino, alkylamino, acetamido, chloro, alkyl, and vinyl radicals did not prove to be that efficient.
- Substitution at the third position of the quinoline ring generally leads to decrease in activity and toxicity associated with primaquine, e.g. phenyl.
- Substitution of the fourth position using smaller alkyl groups (for e.g. methyl and ethyl) and vinyl (**11, 12, 13**) substituents has been found to be very rewarding as they are equal or greater in activity and lesser toxic as compared to primaquine. These 4-alkyl or vinyl substituted primaquines mostly show radical curative properties.
- Introduction of oxygen functionality at the position 5 of the quinoline ring often leads to retention of activity along with lesser toxicity. When the fifth position of primaquine is substituted using functionalities like phenoxy, phenylthiol, or aniline (**14**), then highest level of tissue schizonticidal activity (as observed in case of tafenoquine) is observed in addition to reduced toxicity compared to primaquine (Figure 11.4).
- Substituents at the seventh position are not well tolerated and usually result in abolished activity of the quinoline ring as antimalarial.

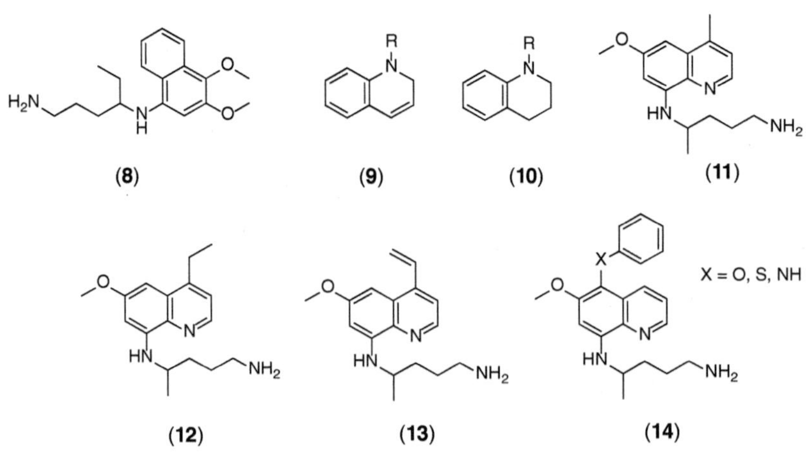

Figure 11.4 Various 8-aminoquinolines acting as antimalarial agents.

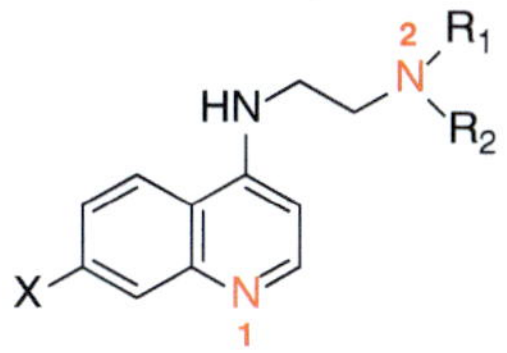

4-Aminoquinolines

X = –Cl, –Br, and –I
R_1, R_2 – alkyl, cycloalkyl, heterocycloalkyl

N_1 – 1st protonable nitrogen atom
N_2 – 2nd protonable nitrogen atom

Figure 11.5 Structural requirements in 4-aminoquinolines for antimalarial activities.

- Multiple substitutions, together at 2, 4, 5, and 6 positions, have been found to yield potent analogs.
- The chain length of the eighth position alkyl amino side chain has to be maintained between 2 and 6 carbon atoms, preferably ending with a terminal primary amino group. However, odd numbered methylene-containing side chains are found to exhibit better activity than even numbered side chains.
- Introduction of other heteroatoms into the basic side chain fails to enhance antimalarial profile [15].

11.1.3.2 SAR of 4-Aminoquinolines

The four basic structural requirements of a 4-aminoquinoline antimalarial, to be active against plasmodial strains, particularly chloroquine-resistant and chloroquine-sensitive *P. falciparum* strains, are as follows:

1. 4-Aminoquinoline moiety without alkyl substitution
2. A protonable nitrogen at the first position of the quinoline ring
3. A second protonable nitrogen at the terminal of the side chain attached to the 4-anilino nitrogen
4. A halogen atom at the seventh position, preferably chlorine, bromine, and iodine, but not fluorine (Figure 11.5) [16].

Along with these relatively stringent structural features, there is considerable room for variations in the aminoalkyl side chain and terminal amino groups for showing antiparasitic activity.

- The quinoline ring system itself is of great importance for the antimalarial efficacy. Other modifications of the quinoline ring generally lead to a loss of activity with the exceptions of chloroquine *N*-oxide (**15**) and 5-aza chloroquine (**16**), which are reported to have better activity than chloroquine in mouse model [17].
- A hydrophobic moiety in the seventh position is of prime importance, such as the chloro and other electron-withdrawing functional groups are required for the inhibition of both Fe(III) crystallization and parasite growth. Introduction of other substituents, such as methoxy, ethoxy, and methyl, to the quinoline ring lead to a decrease in efficacy [14].
- Introduction of a CF_3 group at the seventh position reduces antimalarial activity against chloroquine-susceptible and chloroquine-resistant *P. falciparum* strains. However, a 7-CF_3 group containing analogs exhibit excellent activity in conjugation with shortened carbon chains [17].

- The side chain containing 2–12 carbon atoms with a diverse range of terminal amino substituents, such as dimethylamino, diethylamino, dipropylamino, dibutylamino, pyrrolidinepiperidine, azepane, azocane, are active against chloroquine-sensitive *P. falciparum* strains. These structural features are very essential for the prevention of recognition and efflux by transporters present in the parasites. Shortening or lengthening the carbon chain ($\geq$3 or $\leq$10 carbon atoms) leads to loss of activity [12].
- 7-Iodo and 7-bromo aminoquinoline derivatives with diaminoalkane side chains, such as diethylaminoethyleneamino, diethylaminopropylamino, 2-methyl diethylaminoethylene amine, have proved to be equally active as the corresponding 7-chloro-4-aminoquinolines against both chloroquine-susceptible and -resistant *P. falciparum* strains [17].
- Short-chain chloroquine derivatives (**17**) are easily synthesizable from readily available starting materials, but they undergo rapid side chain dealkylation, which reduces their lipid solubility and thus is capable of increasing cross resistance with chloroquine [17].
- A hydrophilic group in the side chains leads to greater activity [16]. Presence of a hydroxyl group (**18, 19**) or an ether linkage in the intermediate side chain is well tolerated, resulting in significant increase in the therapeutic index [15].
- Introduction of quaternary carbon atom in the side chain (**20**) prevents biodegradation and thus increase half-life of the congener against resistant strains [18].
- Chloroquine resistance in parasites is mediated by P-glycoprotein exporter protein. In order to prevent active transport of chloroquine out of the cell, a bulky bisquinoline structure may be used to maintain antimalarial activity. Compounds of this class mainly constitute piperaquine, hydroxypiperaquine (**21**), dichloroquinazine (**22**), and 1,4-bis(7-chloro-4-quinolylamino)piperazine (**23**). In the bisquinoline series, maximum activity is observed with a connecting of two carbon atoms [17].
- Metal complexes have been in use to treat a platter of diseases, and fortunately, malaria has also not been left behind. Two novel chloroquine complexes of transition metals (Rh, Ru) (**24, 25**) have been synthesized and have been observed that the incorporation of these metal fragments conveniently enhances the efficacy of chloroquine without any significant incidences of acute toxicity. The Au–chloroquine complex (**26**) displayed high *in vitro* activity against chloroquine-resistant strains of *P. falciparum* and was considerably superior to the Ru and Rh complexes. When the carbon chain of chloroquine (CQ) was replaced by the hydrophobic ferrocenyl group (**27**), compound exhibited 22 times more potent antimalarial activity against schizonts than chloroquine *in vitro* against a drug-resistant *P. falciparum* strain (Figures 11.6 and 11.7a,b) [17].

The activity of the 4-aminoquinolines is mainly attributed to their unique affinity for the hematin complex, with their association constants being three times greater than the magnitude of that of simple quinoline rings and to the inhibition of hemozoin formation. In order to develop a potent antimalarials based on the 4-aminoquinoline moiety, the association constants of the congeners to be developed with the hematin have to be taken into consideration [18].

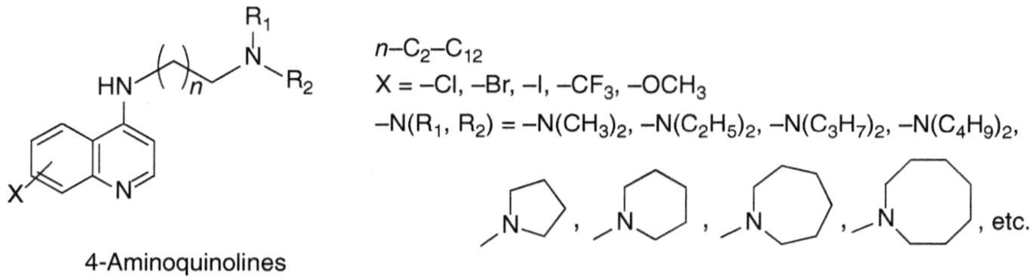

Figure 11.6 Structure–activity relationship of 4-aminoquinolines as antimalarials.

- Mere attachment of an alkyl side chain to the amino group of the 4-aminoquinolines has very little effects on the association constant.
- The Cl^- atom at the seventh position of 4-aminoquinoline, as in chloroquine, is the main hematin-binding nucleus and thus is extremely crucial, if not sufficient, for the antimalarial activity.
- The seventh position Cl^- atom is considered to be a critical feature for the inhibition of β-hematin formation and was confirmed by a complete loss of activity when a hydrogen atom replaced the seventh position chlorine atom.
- A basic nitrogen atom attached to the aminoalkyl side chain of the quinoline ring of the 4-aminoquinolines is essential in terms of the antiplasmodial activity. This helps the derivative to get entrapped into the acidic food vacuole of the parasite.
- The electronic nature of seventh position substituent has an important role to play in the maintenance of the pK_a (acid dissociation constant) of the terminal nitrogen atom present in the side chain. Strongly electron-withdrawing groups, such as CF_3 decreases the pK_a, while, electron-donating groups, such as NH_2 increases the value.
- The electronic nature seventh position substituent also plays a significant role in the maintaining the pK_a (acid dissociation constant of the quinolinium cation) of quinolinic nitrogen atom, required for the pH trapping of the compounds. Electron-donating groups such as NH_2, OCH_3, enhance the pK_a value, whereas strong electron-withdrawing groups such as NO_2 result in considerable decrease in the pK_a value [19].

11.2 Synthetic Approaches of 8-Aminoquinolines and 4-Aminoquinolines

11.2.1 Synthetic Approach of 8-Aminoquinolines

11.2.1.1 Synthetic Approach of Well-Established Drugs

The first obtained 8-aminoquinoline, pamaquine, exerts curative action against relapsing malaria (*P. vivax*) infections when administered in conjunction with quinine. However, the former suffers from a drawback of being excessively toxic, particularly to non-Caucasian races. It therefore became a dire necessity to synthesize a series of derivatives of 8-aminoquinoline, with increased

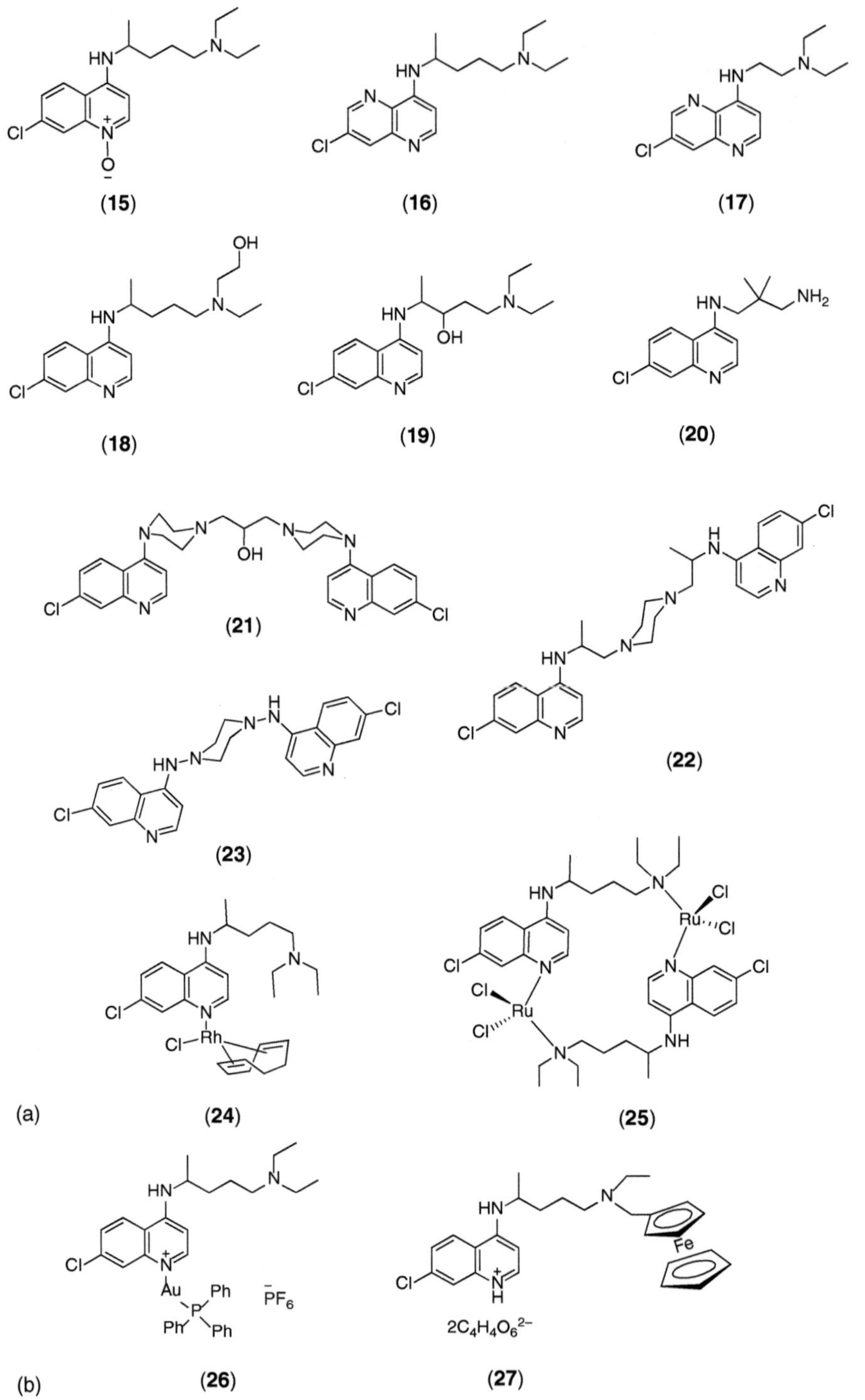

Figure 11.7 (a) Various chloroquine derivatives, including metal complexes, acting as active antimalarial compounds. (b) Transition metal complexes with chloroquine acting as active antimalarial compounds.

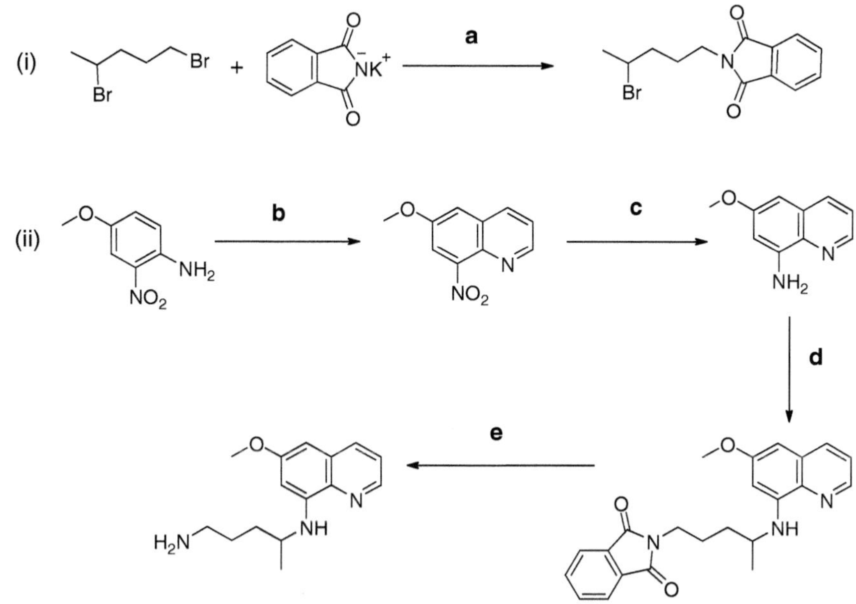

Scheme 11.1 Synthesis of primaquine; reagents and conditions: (a) acetone, reflux, 24 h; (b) glycerol, H_2SO_4 (concentrated), standard Skraup method; (c) $FeCl_3$, activated charcoal, $NH_2NH_2.H_2O$, MeOH, reflux, 60 °C, 12 h; (d) 4-bromo-1-phthalimidopentane, EtOH, reflux, 72 h or EtOH, phosphate buffer (pH 8), 75–80 °C, 79 h; (e) EtOH, $NH_2NH_2.H_2O$, reflux, 2 h.

antimalarial activity and decreased toxicity. As a result, primaquine came into existence. The synthesis of primaquine (Scheme 11.1) is achieved from the starting material 6-methoxy-8-nitroquinoline, which is afforded in a Skraup reaction from 4-methoxy-2-nitroaniline and glycerol in the presence of sulfuric acid. The nitro group in this compound is reduced to afford 6-methoxy-8-aminoquinoline. The amino group upon reaction with 4-bromo-1-phthalimidopentane gives 8-[(4-phthalimido-1-methylbutyl)amino]-6-methoxyquinoline, which upon hydrazinolysis, undergoes phthalimide deprotection, giving primaquine. The condensation reaction of 8-aminoquinoline with primary bromine group is preferred as compared to the secondary bromine in 1,4-dibromopentane because of its greater reactivity. 1,4-dibromopentane is refluxed with potassium phthalimide in acetone solution giving 1-phthalimido-4-bromopentane in good yields. Use of acetone as a solvent for this reaction is very crucial. When reaction was carried out in boiling ethanol, excessive dehydro-bromination took place, resulting in the formation of only polymeric materials. This novel method has been successfully optimized to manufacture primaquine on a large scale [20].

The major issue related to use of primaquine as suitable antimalarials is its toxicity and rapid metabolism followed by faster excretion. Literature search has revealed that this type of toxicity is imbibed by the chemical nature of the 8-amino side chain. Nuclear substituents also tend to have a significant impact upon relative toxicity. Elderfield developed several 8-[[(dialkylamino)alkyl]amino]-6-methoxyquinolines

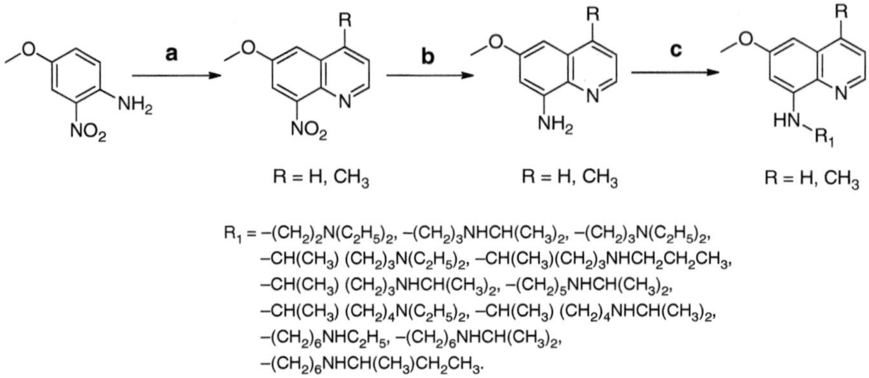

Scheme 11.2 Reagents and conditions: (a) glycerol (in case of 8-nitroquinoline) and 1,3,3-trimethoxybutane or methylvinylketone (in case of 8-nitrolepidine), H_2O, H_3PO_4, As_2O_5; (b) $SnCl_2$/HCl (for 8-aminoquinoline) and Fe/CH_3COOH (for 8-aminolepidine); (c) substituted or unsubstituted aminoalkyl halides, absolute alcohol, reflux, 60 °C.

and 8-[[(dialkylamino)alkyl]amino]-6-methoxy-4-methylquinolines that exhibited high antimalarial activity along with reduced toxicity relative to their unsubstituted analogs. It was found that the introduction of the 4-methyl group had increased the quinine equivalent by about 10-fold when tested against malarial strains in duck. In this method, 6-methoxy-8-nitroquinolines are prepared from 4-methoxy-2-nitroaniline by using modified Skraup method in presence of glycerol and then reduced to the corresponding amine using stannous chloride in hydrochloric acid or catalytically. 6-Methoxy-8-nitrolepidine, on the other hand, is synthesized from reaction between 4-methoxy-2-nitroaniline and 1,3,3-trimethoxybutane or methylvinylketone and then reduced to its amino congener more rapidly by iron and acetic acid rather than by catalytic hydrogenation. The side chains were then attached by coupling the 6-methoxy-8-aminoquinoline and 6-methoxy-8-aminolepidine with desired aminoalkylhalides using Rohrmann and Shonle method in which a mixture of starting materials was refluxed in absolute alcohol for 60 hours (Scheme 11.2) [21].

Carroll et al. synthesized 4-vinyl, 4-ethyl, and 4-[*p*-(arylthio)-ethyl]-8-aminoquinoline analogs. In order to achieve the synthesis of the desired target compounds, synthetic schemes for the preparation of 8-amino-6-methoxy-4-vinylquinoline (**I**), 8-amino-4-[(arylthio)-ethyl]-6-methoxyquinoline (**II**), and 8-amino-4-ethyl-6-methoxyquinoline (**III**) were devised (Scheme 11.3). The starting material, 6-methoxy-4-methyl-8-nitroquinoline was first subjected to Mannich reaction giving 4-[*p*-(dimethylamino)-ethyl]-6-methoxy-8-nitroquinoline hydrochloride, which upon neutralization, followed by treatment with methyl iodide and subsequent treatment with aqueous sodium hydroxide gave 6-methoxy-8-nitro-4-vinylquinoline. The reduction of the latter with stannous chloride and hydrochloric acid yielded compound **I**. Further condensation of the vinyl derivative with *p*-substituted thiophenols in DMF in presence of potassium carbonate gave the 8-amino-4-[(arylthio)-ethyl]-6-methoxyquinoline (**II**). For the synthesis of

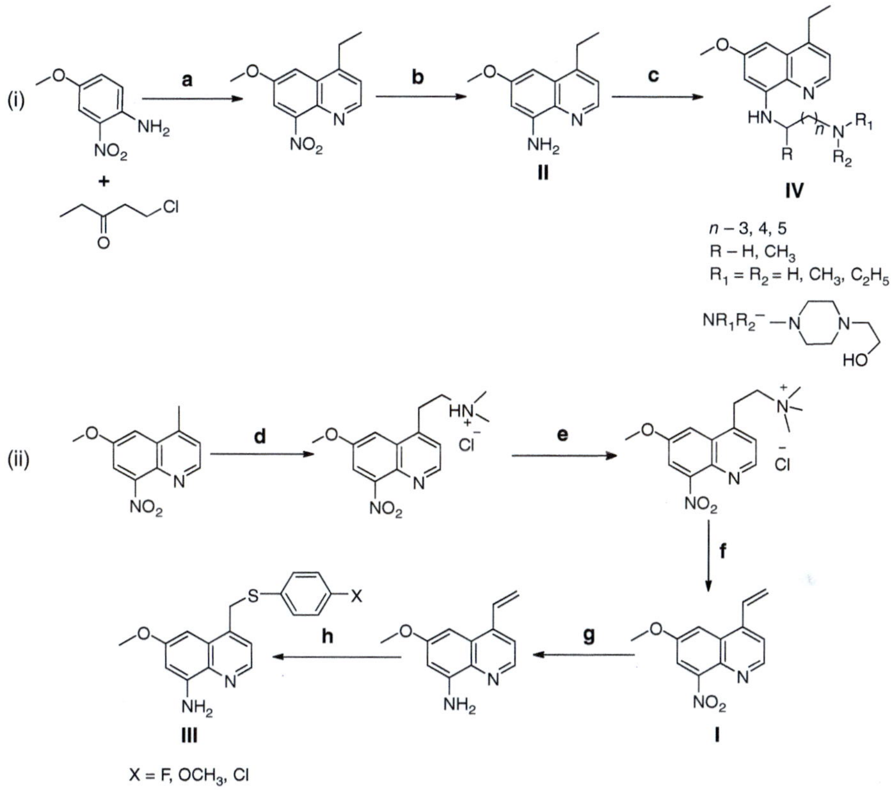

Scheme 11.3 Reagents and conditions: (a) H_2O, H_3PO_4, As_2O_5; (b)$SnCl_2$/HCl or H_2/Raney-Ni; (c) disubstituted or unsubstituted aminoalkyl chlorides, Et_3N; (d) $(CH_3)_2NH_2{}^+C1^-$, $(CH_2O)_n$, EtOH; (e) CH_3I, NaOH; (f) NaOH; (g) $SnCl_2$/HCl; (h) *p*-X-C_6H_4-SH, K_2CO_3, DMF.

8-amino-4-ethyl-6-methoxyquinoline (**III**), 4-methoxy-2-nitroaniline was converted to 4-ethyl-6-methoxy-8-nitroquinoline by a modified Skraup reaction and reduced with stannous chloride and hydrochloric acid or catalytically to give the desired amine. This amine can further be used as a precursor to develop various analogs (represented as compound **IV**) by attaching desired aminoalkyl side chains to the 8-amino group [22].

Carroll and coworkers further synthesized a series of 2,4-disubstituted 8-aminoquinoline analogs and evaluated against *P. berghei* in mice. Some of the analogs possessed significant activity almost equal to that of primaquine against *Plasmodium* strains. The synthetic scheme (Scheme 11.4) used to prepare target compounds involves condensation of 4-methoxy-2-nitroaniline with 3-penten-2-one under Skraup conditions to form 2,4-dimethyl-6-methoxy-8-nitroquinoline, that was subjected to Mannich condensation, followed by quaternization and then treatment with base yielded the 4-methyl-2-vinylquinoline (**I**). Catalytic reduction of the latter gave 8-amino-2-ethyl-6-methoxy-4-methylquinoline (**Ia**), whereas reduction with stannous chloride yielded 8-amino-6-methoxy-4-methyl-2-vinylquinoline (**Ib**).

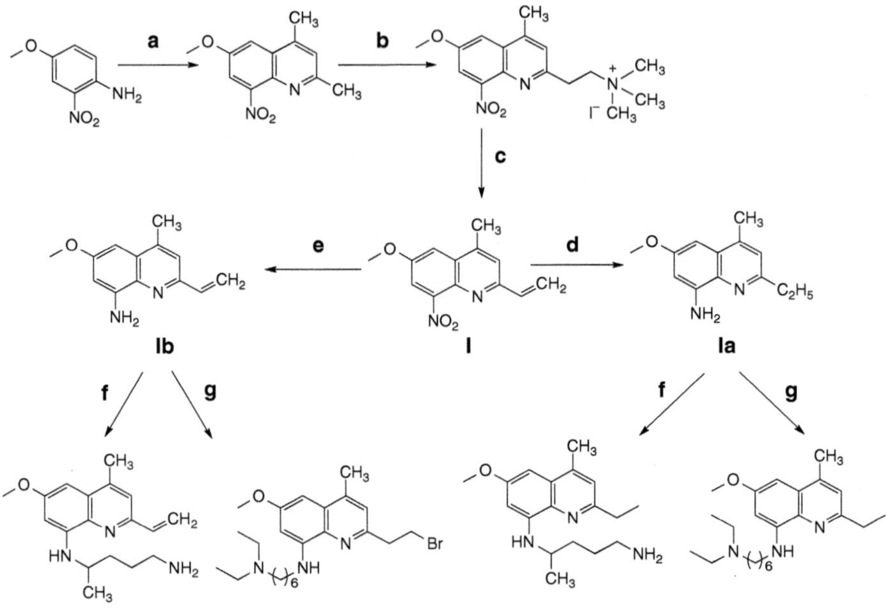

Scheme 11.4 Reagents and conditions: (a) 3-penten-2-one, As_2O_5, H_3PO_4; (b) CH_2O, $(CH_3)_2NH$, CH_3I; (c) NaOH; (d) H_2/Raney-Ni; (e) $SnCl_2$/HCl; (f) 4-amino-l-methylbutyl iodide, Et_3N, $NH_2NH_2.H_2O$; (g) diethylaminohexyl bromide.

Alkylation of the 8-amino group of **Ia** and **Ib** with 4-amino-1-methylbutyl and 6-diethylaminohexyl side chains yielded the expected products **IIa** and **IIIa** and **IIb** and **IIIb**, respectively [23].

Variable modifications of the antimalarial drug primaquine have been done so far, both at the quinoline ring and at the primary amino group with the desire to obtain antimalarial agents with improved bioavailability, prolonged activity, and reduced toxicity. Besides that, modifications in the terminal amino group have also been tried with the hope of preventing the metabolic pathway resulting in the formation of inactive and toxic carboxyprimaquine.

Given the utility of naturally occurring cinnamic acid as antimicrobial, antifungal, and antiviral, primaquine was conjugated with cinnamic acid derivatives to form hybrids of amide and acylsemicarbazide. The amides were prepared by the simple acylation of primaquine with cinnamic acid derivative chlorides (CADCl) or cinnamic acid derivative benzotriazolide (CADBt) (Scheme 11.5). The amides of primaquine and cinnamic acids with alkyl, halogen, or nitro substituents at different positions in the benzene moiety (*N*-cinnamoyl-primaquine conjugates, primacins) were afforded by coupling primaquine with the corresponding cinnamic acids in the presence of 2-(1*H*-benzotriazole-1-yl)-1,1,3,3-tetramethylaminium tetrafluoroborate (TBTU) and *N,N*-diisopropylethylamine (DIEA). Primacins have shown immense *in vitro* activity against malarial parasite *P. berghei*, compared to the parent drug [24].

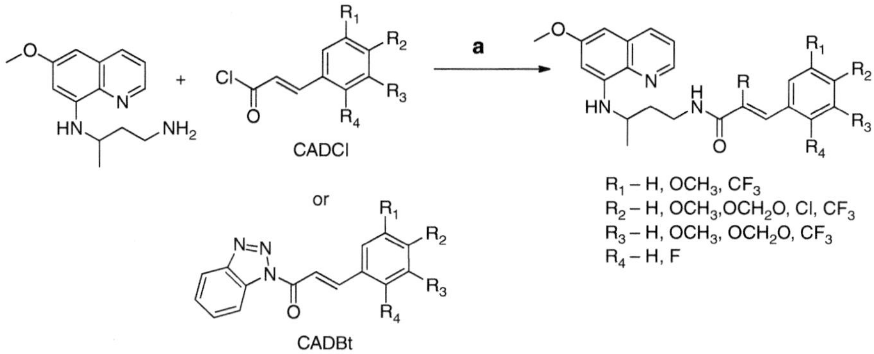

Scheme 11.5 Reagents and conditions: (a) Et_3N, TBTU, DIEA.

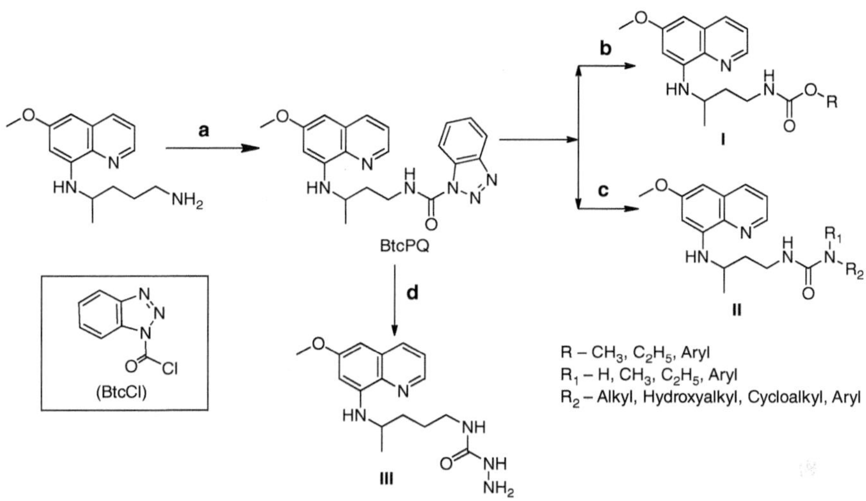

Scheme 11.6 Reagents and conditions: (a) benzotriazole carboxylic acid chloride (BtcCl), Et_3N; (b) Alkyl or Aryl alcohol, Et_3N; (c) primary or secondary amine or primaquine molecule, Et_3N; (d) $NH_2NH_2.H_2O$.

Moreover, acylation of primaquine with 1-benzotriazolecarboxylic acid chloride (BtcCl) produced a derivative (Btc-PQ) that served as the common precursor for the synthesis of carbamates (**I**) and ureas, respectively (Scheme 11.6). The antiplasmodial screening of these compounds revealed that *O*-alkylcarbamates potentially act as transmission-blocking antimalarial agents. In order to develop carbamates, alcoholysis of benzotriazolide was successfully done with methanol and ethanol, whereas the reaction failed with other alcohols. Later on, several *O*-alkyl and *O*-aryl primaquine-carbamates were synthesized as plausible prodrugs, which help to prevent oxidative deamination of primaquine to inactive carboxyprimaquine. Aminolysis of Btc-PQ was carried on under mild conditions, in the presence of triethylamine to prepare ureas (**II**), including twin derivatives, which contained two primaquine molecules, linked together with carbonyl group. Btc-PQ was reduced with hydrazine

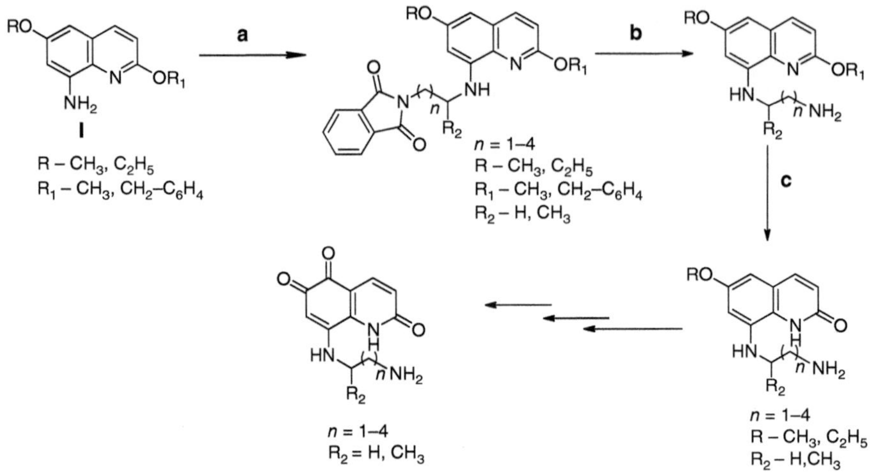

Scheme 11.7 Reagents and conditions: (a) sodium acetate, *N*-(bromoalkyl)phthalimide, 66% ethanol, reflux, 3 d; (b) ethanol/chloroform; (c) H_2/Pd/C.

hydrate to give rise to primaquine-semicarbazide (**III**), which serves as a useful intermediate for further reactions [24].

6-Methoxy-8-aminoquinolines get converted to quinoline-*o*-quinone internally within the human body, which lend support to Schonhofer's theory depicting that the *in vivo* action of the 8-aminoquinolines upon the erythrocytic or tissue stages of the *Plasmodium* strains is due to the quinonoid products to which these drugs are metabolized to by the host. Thus, quinoline–quinones serve as an essential lead for the search of better antimalarials. Talati et al. fabricated experiments to synthesize both quinoline–quinones and carbostyrils. However, the synthetic schemes aimed at synthesizing the synthesis-substituted 8-aminocarbostyril-5,6-quinones could not yield the target compounds but a series of 2-benzyloxy- or 2-hydroxy-6-alkoxy-8-(aminoalkyamino)quinolines were obtained, which served as the immediate precursor of the carbostyril-*o*-quinones (Scheme 11.7) [25].

Jain et al. have synthesized a class of 8-quinolinamine analogs exhibiting potent antimalarial activity against *P. falciparum* strains. The target compound was synthesized using the following synthetic scheme (Scheme 11.8), starting with 4,5-dimethoxy-2-nitroaniline, which upon undergoing direct ring-alkylation using a silver catalyzed radical oxidative decarboxylation of trimethylacetic acid by ammonium persulfate produced 4-alkyl-2-*tert*-butyl-5,6-dimethoxy-8-nitroquinoline. Selective demethylation of the 5-methoxy group with concentrated hydrochloric acid yielded 4-alkyl-2-*tert*-butyl-6-methoxy-8-nitro-5-quinolinols, which upon further reaction with phosphorous oxychloride produced 4-alkyl-2-*tert*-butyl-5-chloro-6-methoxy-8-nitroquinoline. These chloro derivatives then reacted with 3-(trifluoromethyl)phenol in the presence of potassium hydroxide to produce 4-alkyl-2-*tert*-butyl-6-methoxy-8-nitro-5-(3-trifluoromethylphenoxy)quinoline. The

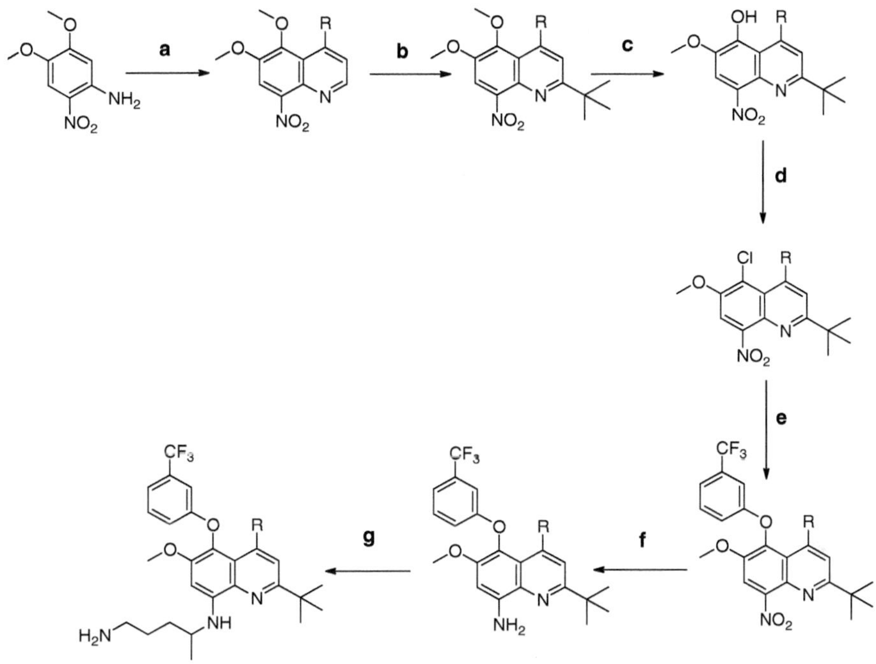

Scheme 11.8 Reagents and conditions: (a) glycerol, H_2SO_4, As_2O_5, 110 °C, 21 h; (b) $(CH_3)_3CCO_2H$, $AgNO_3$, $(NH_4)_2S_2O_8$, 10% H_2SO_4, CH_3CN, 70 °C, 15 min; (c) Conc.HCl, 95% EtOH 100 °C, 2 h; (d) $POCl_3$, 80 °C, 2 h; (e) 3-(trifluoromethyl)phenol, KOH, *p*-xylene, 12 h, 150 °C; (1) Raney-Ni/H_2, EtOH, 45 psi, 45 min; (g) Et_3N, 120 °C, 24 h; $NH_2NH_2.H_2O$; EtOH, reflux, 8 h.

latter was then converted to *N*-8-(4-amino-1-methylbutyl)-4-alkyl-2-*tert*-butyl-6-methoxy-5-(3-trifluoromethylphenoxy)-8-quinolinamines [26].

Vangapandu et al. designed and synthesized 5-alkoxy-4-ethyl-6-methoxy-8-nitroquinolines starting with 4-methoxy-5-alkoxy-2-nitroaniline and *o*-phosphoric acid in the presence of arsenic(V) oxide. The former was reduced with wet Raney-nickel catalyst in 95% ethyl alcohol at 45 psi to give 5-alkoxy-4-ethyl-6-methoxy-8-aminoquinolines, which upon further treatment with 2-(4-bromopentyl)-1, 3-isoindolinedione in the presence of triethylamine and subsequent hydrazinolysis with hydrazine hydrate in 95% ethyl alcohol under reflux conditions gave rise to 8-(1-amino-4-methyl)-5-alkoxy-4-ethyl-6-methoxy-8-aminoquinoline. This upon further treatment with several aryl carboxylic acids extended the side chain and gave other derivatives (Scheme 11.9). Some of these 8-quinolinamines have exhibited excellent *in vitro* and *in vivo* biological efficacy, even greater than the standard drug chloroquine against both drug-sensitive and drug-resistant malaria strains [27].

Han et al. developed a simple yet efficient protocol for the copper/bis(pinacolato) diboron-catalyzed C–H ethoxycarbonyldifluoromethylation of 8-aminoquinoline motifs using functionalized difluoromethyl bromides and iodides (Scheme 11.10), thereby leading to formation of desired products in moderate to good yields. This

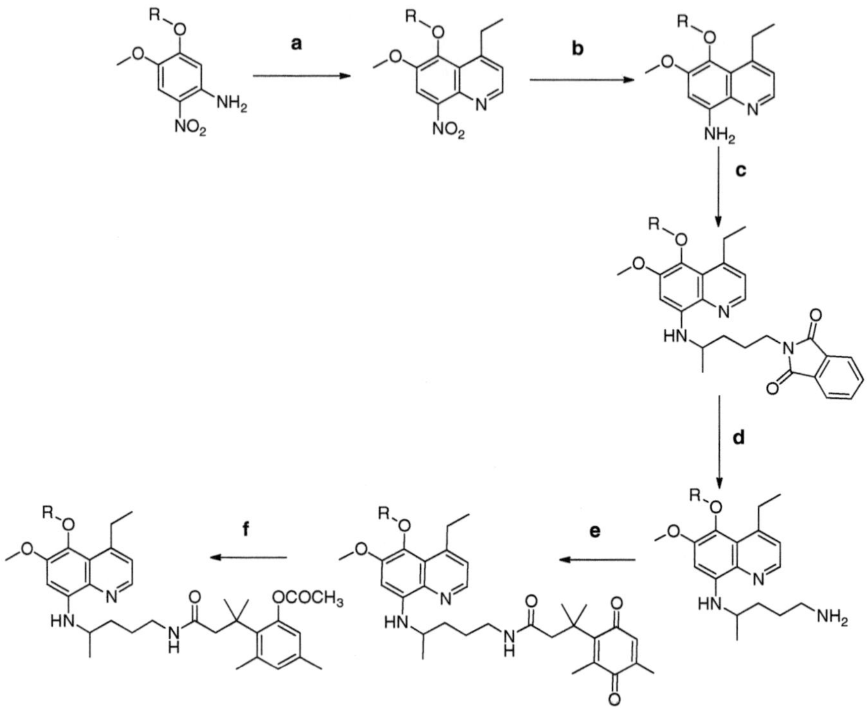

Scheme 11.9 Reagents and conditions: (a) 1-chloro-3-pentanone, 85% *o*-H_3PO_4, As_2O_5, 80 °C, 3 h; (b) Raney-Ni/H_2, EtOH, 45 psi, 45 min; (c) 2-(4-bromopentyl)-1,3-isoindolinedione, Et_3N, 120 °C, 24 h; (d) $NH_2NH_2.H_2O$, EtOH, Reflux, 8 h; (e) 3-(2,4-dimethyl-3,6-dioxo-1,4-cyclodienyl)-methylbutanoic acid, DCC, DMAP, DCM, 4 h; (f) 3-(2,4-dimethyl-6-methylcarbonyloxyphenyl)-3-methylbutanoic acid, DCC, DMAP, DCM, 4 h.

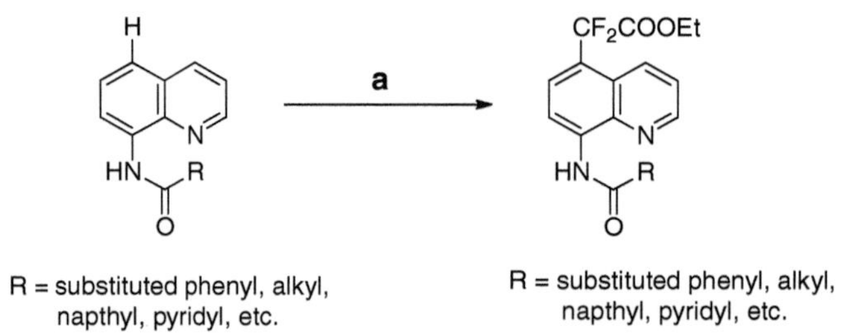

Scheme 11.10 Reagents and conditions: (a) $ICF_2COOEt/BrCF_2COOEt$, Cu(I), B_2Pin_2, 100 °C.

reaction can be conducted under mild conditions and exhibits good substrate tolerance [28].

Despite researchers have developed diverse ways of producing 8-aminoquinoline derivatives, the synthetic procedures so far developed are mainly dependent on traditional transition metal-catalyzed C–N coupling methods. Thus, Chen et al. developed an efficient method for the synthesis of 8-aminoquinoline derivatives through transition metal-free direct C–N coupling from fluoroquinolines and

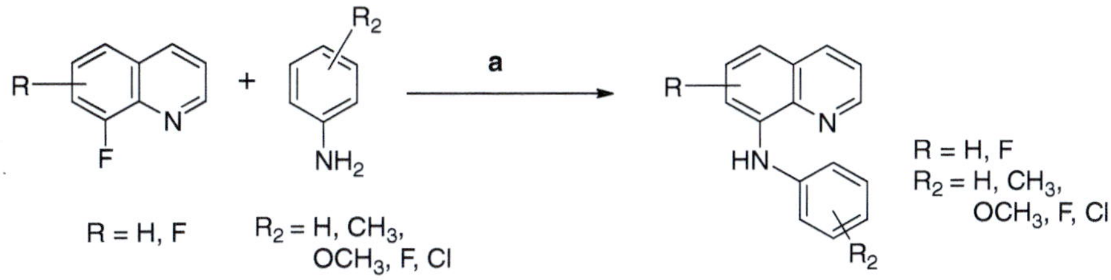

Scheme 11.11 Reagents and conditions: (a) lithium hydride (LiH), toluene, 110 °C.

arylamines (Scheme 11.11). It also showed significant chemo- and regio-selectivity for polyfluoroquinolines in which only C—F bond on 8-substituted position was cleaved. Thus, this method can be used as an inexpensive and efficient pathway to afford quinolin-8-amine derivatives in moderate to good yields [29].

11.2.1.2 Synthetic Approach of Recently Developed PQ Congeners

Although tafenoquine is a primaquine analog, it somewhat differs from its parent molecule in physicochemical properties, antimalarial potency, and toxicological and pharmacokinetic features. It has been explored that, tafenoquine is more active than primaquine in *in vitro* testing and *in vivo* preclinical animal models. The molecule has been tested in more than 2000 human subjects in clinical studies till date and has been found to exhibit equivalent activity (IC_{50} of 0.7–1.5 μM) to primaquine against culture-adapted chloroquine-sensitive strains, and considerably greater activity than primaquine against multidrug-resistant *P. falciparum* lines, with IC_{50} values ranging from 0.06 to 0.3 μM. It is conceivable that tafenoquine's enhanced blood schizontocidal potency compared with primaquine is because it exerts greater oxidative stress on multidrug-resistant parasitized erythrocytes [10]. The synthesis of tafenoquine has been achieved using the following synthetic scheme (Scheme 11.12), starting with chlorination of 6-methoxy-4-methylquinolin-2(1*H*)-one using sulfuryl chloride, followed by nitration of the eighth position with concentrated nitric acid. The resulting compound was then condensed with 3-(trifluoromethyl) phenol in presence of a base and then treated subsequently with phosphorus oxychloride and with sodium methoxide to afford a methoxy group at the second position. The eighth nitro group was reduced to amino by hydrazine and then treated with 4-iodo-1-pthalimidopentane in the presence of diisopropylamine and finally hydrazinolyzed to yield tafenoquine [30] (https://newdrugapprovals.org/tag/tafenoquine).

Bulaquine was picked up for further drug development because of its enhanced antirelapse efficacy in simian model (25 mg/day × five days), which is eightfolds more than primaquine (15 mg/day × five days) and its low levels of methemoglobin toxicity in comparison to standard drug primaquine. A mixture of primaquine base with freshly distilled 2-acetylbutyrolactone and few drops of a base like piperidine were stirred using magnetic stirrer at room temperature for an hour or so, to produce solidified bulaquine (Scheme 11.13). The product was then titrated in ether and filtered and crystallized from alcoholic solvent like propanol to get the pure bulaquine [31] (https://newdrugapprovals.org/2014/05/01/bulaquine).

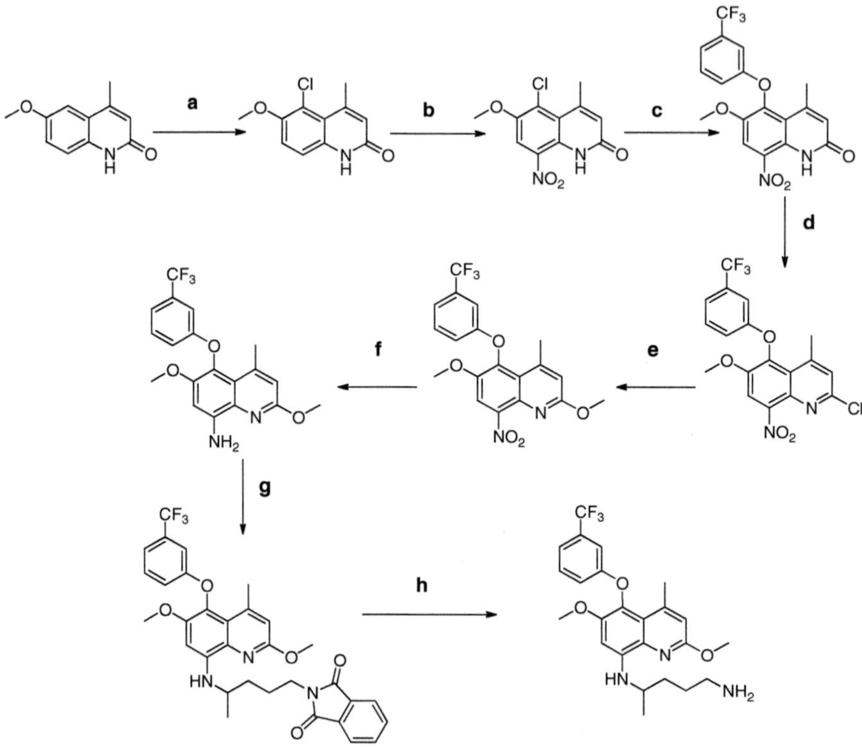

Scheme 11.12 Synthesis of tafenoquine; reagents and conditions: (a) SO_2C1_2; (b) HNO_3; (c) 3-(trifluoromethyl)phenol, KOH; (d) $POCl_3$; (e) NaOMe; (f) $NH_2NH_2.H_2O$, Pd/C; (g) 4-iodo-1-phthalimidopentane, diisopropylamine; (h) $NH_2NH_2.H_2O$.

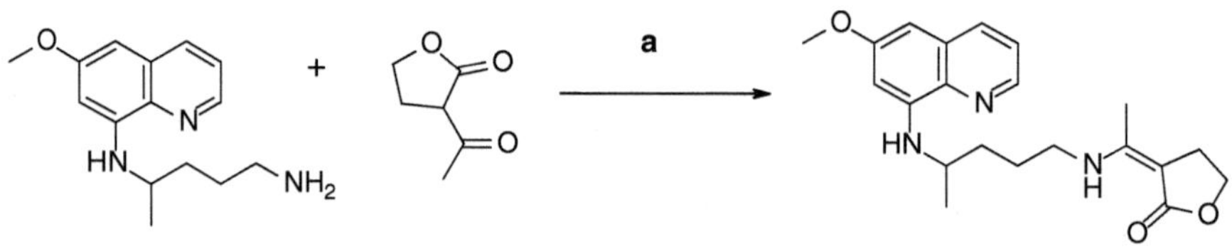

Scheme 11.13 Synthesis of bulaquine; reagents and conditions: (a) piperidine, stir, rt, 1 h.

11.2.2 Synthetic Approaches of 4-Aminoquinolines

11.2.2.1 Synthetic Approaches to Well-Established Drugs

In the past, 4-aminoquinolines have been synthesized using Hofmann or Curtius degradations from the corresponding quinoline-4-carboxylic acids. Moreover, easy accessibility of 4-chloroquinoline derivatives prompts the synthesis of 4-aminoquinolines by simple replacement of the fourth position chlorine using ammonia. However, this proves to be unwielding as the chlorine atom is somewhat inert in nature. Alternatively, a modified procedure of Andersag, Breitner, and Jung, which involves reduction of 4,7-dichloroquinoline in presence of phenol,

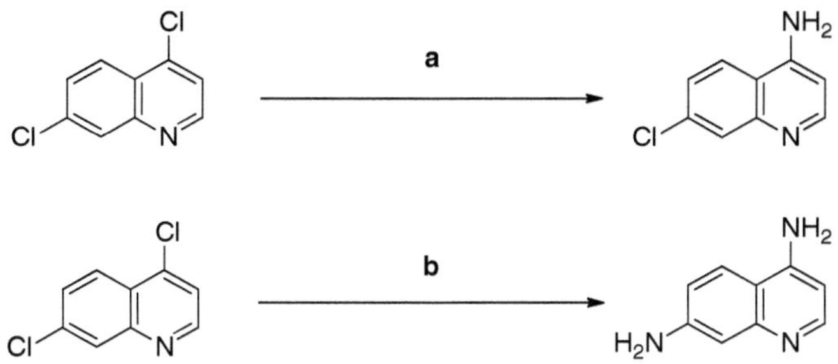

Scheme 11.14 (a) Dry NH_3, phenol, 170–175 °C, reflux, 6 h; (b) dimethylamine(anhyd), phenol, stir and heat, 200 °C, 24 h.

readily furnished 4-amino-7-chloroquinoline. When 4,7-dichloroquinoline was subjected to the reaction with dimethylamine in phenol at an elevated temperature and pressure resulted in replacement of both chlorine atoms with the formation of 4,7-bis-dimethylaminoquinoline (Scheme 11.14). 4-Amino-7-chloroquinoline has also been prepared by the general method of Backeberg by reduction of 7-chloroquinoline-4-phenylhydrazine [32].

The activity of 4-aminoquinolines is mainly based on hematin polymerization inhibition. There exists a positive correlation between inhibition of hematin polymerization and hematin binding affinity for chloroquine. Functionalization of the fourth position amino group with small alkyl side chains tends to increase the hematin binding. In this venture, 4-(ethylamino)-7-chloroquinoline was prepared by reaction of 4,7-dichloroquinoline with ethylamine (Scheme 11.15) [33].

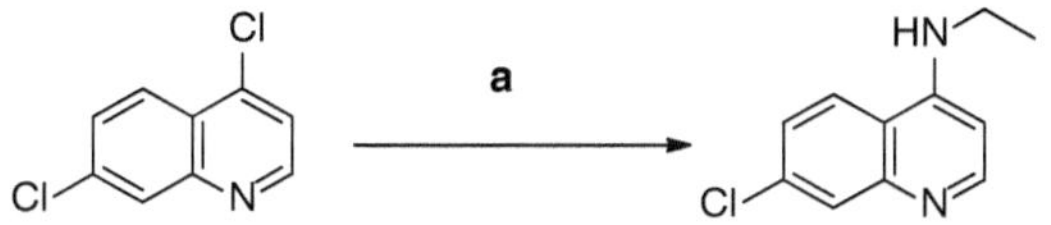

Scheme 11.15 Reagents and conditions: (a) diethylamine, stir and heat, 90–95 °C, 64 h.

Further attachment of basic nitrogen to the alkyl side chain is necessary for proper entrapment the molecule within the acidic vacuole. This led to the synthesis of chloroquine by Surrey and Hammer process consisting of the following steps: first, condensation of *m*-chloroaniline with ethyl oxaloacetate followed by pyrolytic cyclization, saponification, and thermal decarboxylation and then reaction with phosphorus oxychloride to give 4,7-dichloroquinoline, which ultimately reacts with 4-diethylamino-1-methylbutylamine to afford chloroquine (Scheme 11.16) [34]. Similarly, the 7-nitro analog of chloroquine was developed using the synthetic procedure, as described by Price and Roberts, involving the condensation of equimolar concentrations of 3-nitroroaniline with diethyl ethoxymethylene malonate yielded the corresponding arylaminomethylene ester which after cyclization, alkaline hydrolysis, and decarboxylation led to the formation of 4-hydroxy-7-chloroquinoline. Chlorination with phosphorus oxychloride produced 4,7-dichloroquinoline, which was treated with 2-amino-5-(diethylamino)pentane

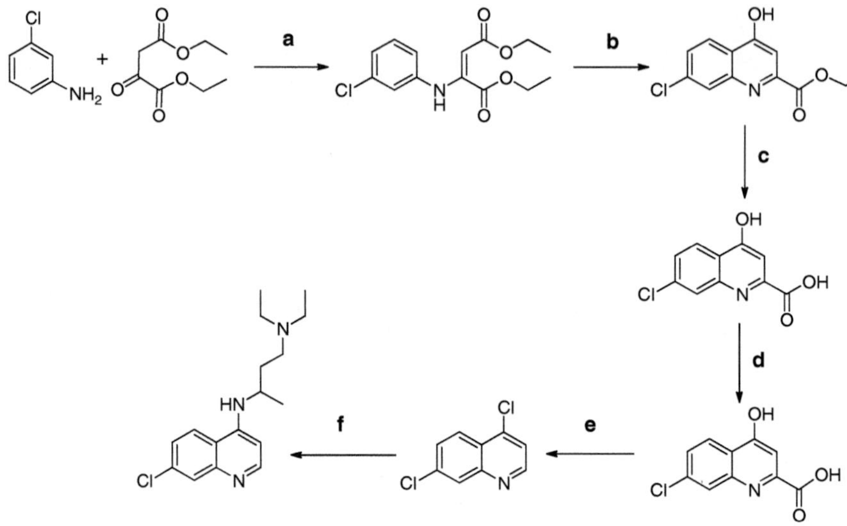

Scheme 11.16 Synthesis of chloroquine; reagents and conditions: (a) 100 °C; (b) 250 °C, mineral oil; (c) NaOH; (d) 250–270 °C, mineral oil; (e) $POCl_3$, (f) 4-diethylamino-1-methylbutylamine 165 °C, N_2.

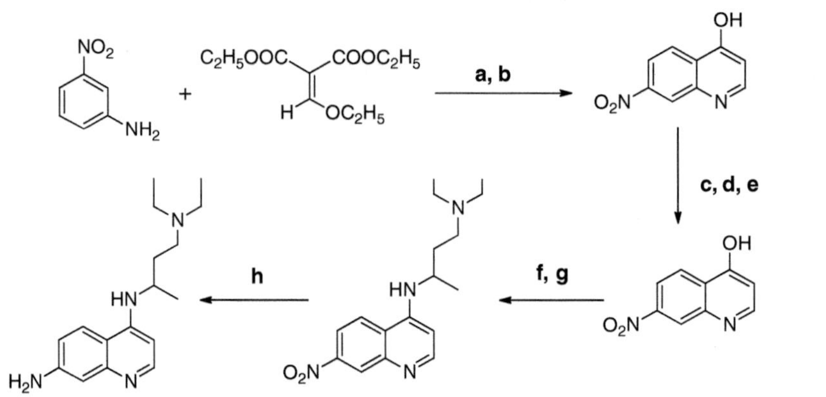

Scheme 11.17 Reagents and conditions: (a) 90 °C; (b) diphenyl ether, 255 °C; (c) 10% aq NaOH, HC1; (d) NH_4OH, $AgNO_3$; (e) diphenyl ether, 255 °C; (f) $POCl_3$, 110 °C; (g) 2-amino-5-(diethylamino) pentane, 120 °C; (h) H_2, Pd/C, 50 atm, EtOH, HCl (g).

to afford chloroquine. Catalytic hydrogenation of the seventh position nitro group further leads to the formation of 7-aminochloroquine (Scheme 11.17) [33].

Synthetic schemes involving aminolysis of the corresponding 4-halo, 4-alkoxy, or 4-aryloxyquinolines consist of harsh and hazardous conditions. To reduce the cost and to improve the yield of chloroquine, Gemma et al. developed a novel, low-cost, and versatile two-step strategy for the synthesis of diversely substituted chloroquine or mepacrine by the nucleophilic displacement of the halogen of 4-chloroquinolines by reaction with hydrazine in refluxing ethanol and reduction of the corresponding

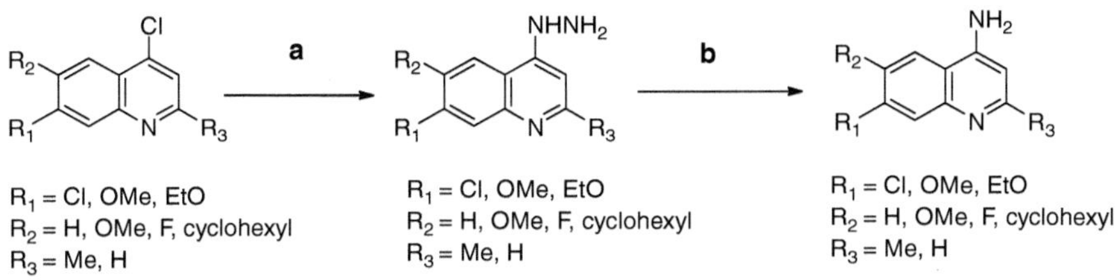

Scheme 11.18 Reagents and conditions: (a) $NH_2NH_2.H_2O$, MW, 150 W, 150 °C, 200 psi, 5 min; (b) $NiCl_2 \cdot 6H_2O$, $NiBH_4$, MeOH, stir, rt.

4-quinolinhydrazones by nickel borohydride in a microwave-assisted method to generate 4-aminoquinolines (Scheme 11.18) [35].

Madrid et al. have employed a modification of Price and Robert's method by replacing the ethoxymethylenemalonic ester with Meldrum's acid. The substituted anilines undergo an addition–elimination reaction with the methoxymethylene moiety (that is generated in situ in this reaction) to facilitate the ene–amine precursor for cyclization in the second step. Amine side chains are then attached to the fourth position of the chloroquinoline rings by nucleophilic substitution (Scheme 11.19) [17, 36].

For the past few decades, multicomponent reactions (MCRs) have also proved to be quite advantageous over conventional organic reactions due to their high convergence and requirement of minimum effort. Based on this alluring property of MCRs and the versatility of the antimalarial pharmacophores, Musonda et al. have recently used Ugi-4 component condensation (U-4CC) method involving an amine,

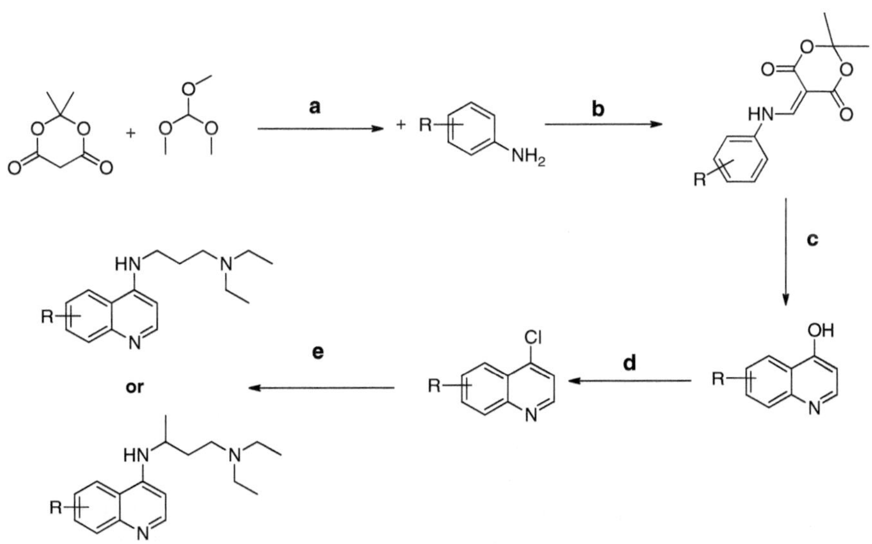

Scheme 11.19 Reagents and conditions: (a) reflux, 1 h; (b) DMF, reflux, 2 h; (c) diphenyl ether, 300 °C, 300 W, 5 min; (d) $POCl_3$, reflux, 3 h; (e) 3-diethylaminopropylamine or 2-amino-5-diethylaminopentane, 135–155 °C, 2 h.

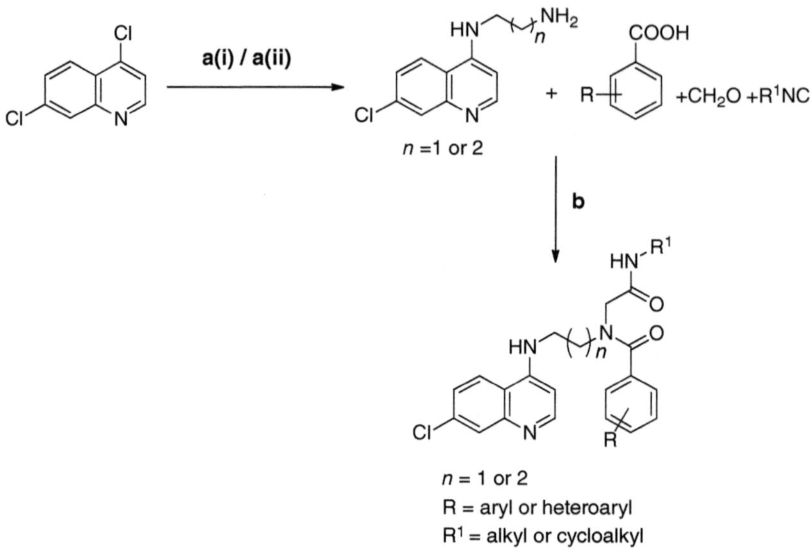

Scheme 11.20 Reagents and conditions: (a): (i) ethylene diamine, 80 °C, 1 h; or (ii) propanediamine, 135–140 °C, 3 h; (b) MeOH, rt, 36–48 h.

isocyanide, carboxylic acid, and an oxo compound, in order to produce novel compounds for screening against malaria parasites. The quinoline substructure was used as part of an amine input in the U-4CC reactions (Scheme 11.20), and the presence of a nitrogen atom in the carboxylic acid served as a second protonatable site, in order to aid the compound accumulation within the acidic parasite vacuole via pH trapping [17, 37].

Madrid achieved a new series of 4-aminoquinoline analogs with a shortened side chain and diverse functionalities on the alkylamine side chain by keeping both the 7-chloroquinoline nucleus and the shorter propylamine side chain, while substituting the distant basic group by using a variety of aldehydes, chosen on the basis of their chemical compatibility, structural diversity, and inclusion of drug-like features, to give a small library of 4-aminoquinolines. Upon the basis of the nature of the basic nitrogen substituent, that is, whether a small alkyl chain (propyl) or a bulky aromatic chain (benzyl), these aldehydes were selected. 4,7-Dichloroquinoline was allowed to react with diaminopropane to generate the amine, which upon two sequential reductive amination steps introduced two points of chemical diversity (Scheme 11.21) [17, 38].

4-Aminoquinolines have also been prepared by aromatic nucleophilic substitution of 4,7-dichloroquinoline. The guanidine derivatives and tetramethylguanidine derivatives were synthesized using simple steps. Mono Boc-protected 4-aminoquinoline has been synthesized by aromatic nucleophilic substitution of 4,7-dichloroquinoline with excess of a mono Boc-protected diaminoalkane (Scheme 11.22). These analogs had moderate *in vitro* antimalarial activity and were found to form a strong complex with hematin, thereby inhibiting the heme polymerization [17, 39].

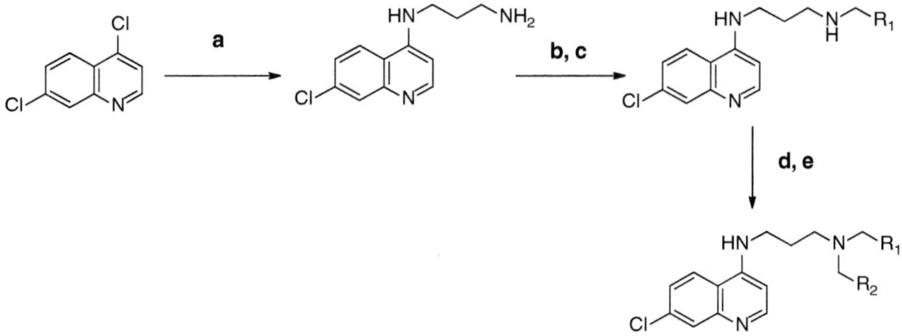

Scheme 11.21 (a) 1,3-Diaminopropane, MeOH, reflux, 2 h; (b) R_1CHO, MeOH, rt, 24 h; (c) $NaBH_4$, rt, 1 h; (d) R_2CHO, MeOH, rt, 24 h; (e) $NaBH_4$, rt, 1 h.

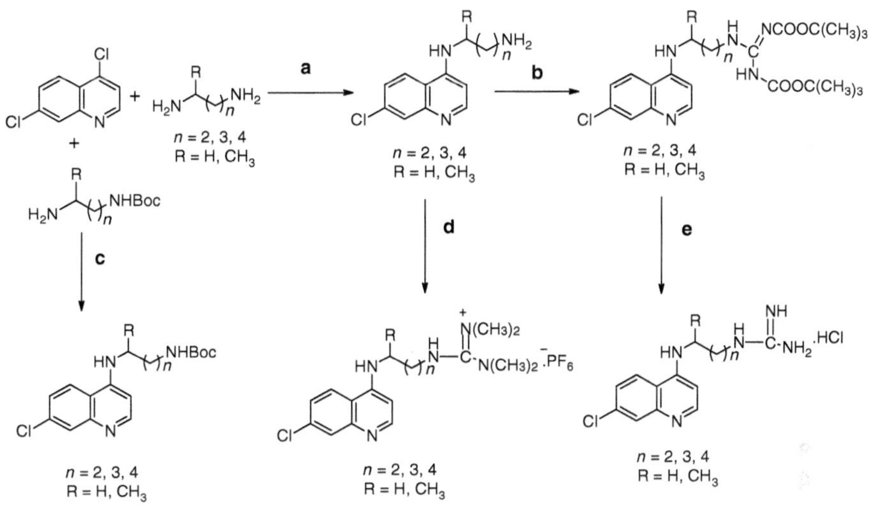

Scheme 11.22 Reagents and conditions: (a) 80 °C, 1 h, then 120–130 °C, 6–8 h; (b) 1,3-bis-(tert-butoxycarbonyl)-2-methyl-2-thiopseudourea, THF, 60 °C; (c) 80 °C, 1 h, then 120–130 °C, 6–8 h; (d) HBTU, dry CH_3CN, rt, 8 h; (e) 20% dioxane/HC1, rt, 1 h.

A promising approach in development of 4-aminoquinoline class of antimalarials is alteration of the CQ side chain. Current studies suggest that replacement of the basic tertiary nitrogen atom of CQ with other functionalities renders the molecules with improved metabolic stability and induces better resistance profiles. Substitution of bulky and/or hydrophobic substituents at lateral part of the side chain generates molecules that show promising activity against drug-resistant parasites. Kondaparla et al. reported the synthesis of a novel series of 4-aminoquinolines obtained by substitution of fixed set of bulky group substituent's such as ethyl, aryl, and benzyl piperazines at distal amino group of CQ while varying the side chain length. The synthesis of the compounds was achieved by aromatic nucleophilic substitution of varying hydroxyalkylamine with the desired quinoline scaffolds, such as 4,7-dichloroquinoline, 4-chloro-7-(trifluoromethyl)quinoline, that gave

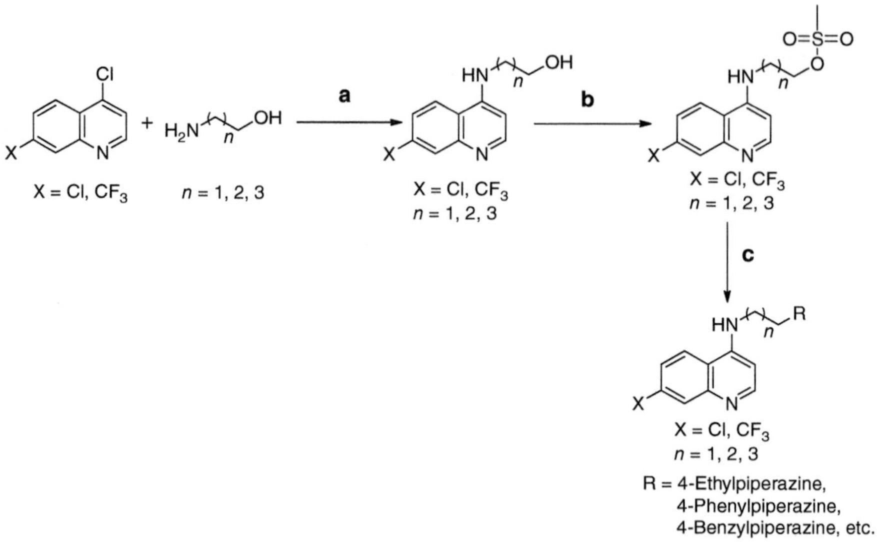

Scheme 11.23 Reagents and conditions: (a) TEA, 130 °C, inert atm, 12–14 h; (b) MsCl, TEA, 0 °C, inert atm, 6 h; (c) corresponding amine, Et_3N, CH_3CN, rt, 40 h, N_2 atm.

rise to 4-(hydroxyalkylamino)-7-substitutedquinolines in good yields. Further mesylation, followed by reaction of these mesylated intermediates with desired secondary amines (ethyl, aryl, and benzylpiperazines) led to formation of the final product (Scheme 11.23) [40].

In the desire to efficiently access the 4-aminoquinoline structural classes, several cascade reactions have been developed. 4-Aminoquinolines can be synthesized by reacting ynamides with nitrilium species, obtained from either arylating nitriles or dehydrating anilides. The former can also be obtained using Cu(I)-catalyzed cyclization of imidoylacetylenes and sulfonylazides. Apart from this, carbonylative Sonogashira reaction of 2-ethynylanilines with in situ amination at C_4 also generates the same. Palladium-catalyzed oxidative isocyanide insertion of *N*-aryl imines by double C–H activation also affords 4-aminoquinolines. Though generation of desired product can be easily achieved using the former methods, they include several drawbacks such as requirement of specialized starting materials, low yields, and involvement of toxic CO gas. Taking an insight from the associated disadvantages of the existing methods, Collet et al. developed a one-pot, two-step, and three-component synthetic route to substituted 4-aminoquinolines involving an imidoylative Sonogashira coupling followed by acid-mediated cyclization. This reaction is carried out using readily available starting materials and tolerates various substituents on the arene as well as the use of primary, secondary, and various functionalized isocyanides (Scheme 11.24) [41].

Considering the importance of the basic nature of side chain of the 4-aminoquinolines for their accumulation within acidic food vacuole of the parasite, Kumar et al. incorporated triazine in the side chain of 4-aminoquinoline pharmacophore to develop the new antimalarial agents. Triazine functionalized with

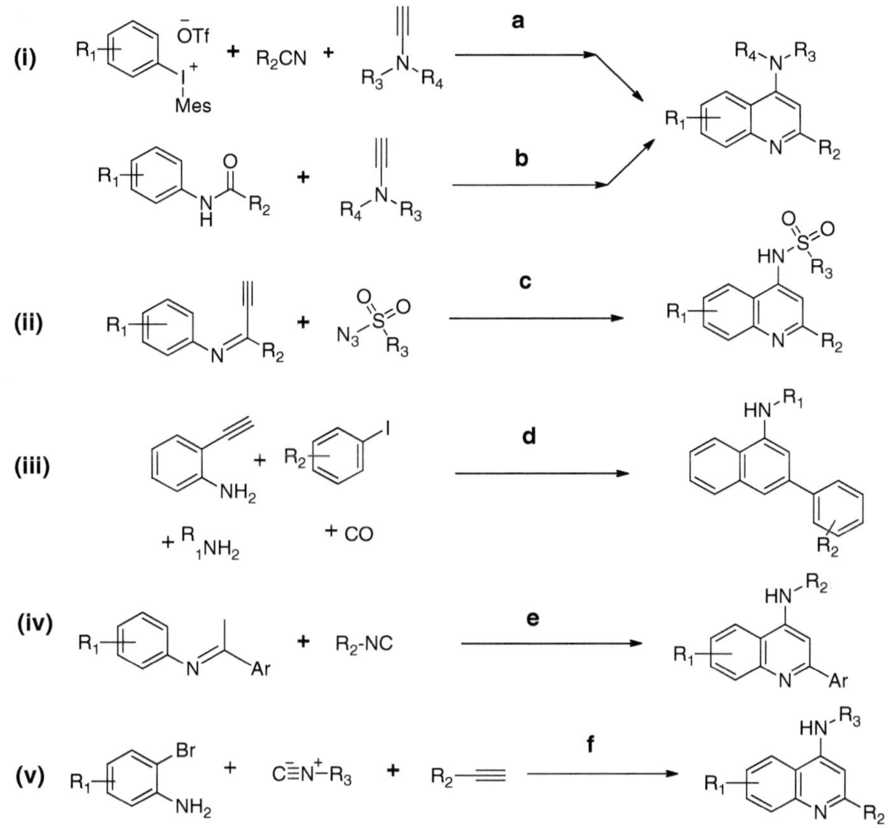

Scheme 11.24 Reagents and conditions: (a) CuTC (10 mol%); (b) Tf_2O, 2Cl-pyridine; (c) CuCl (10 mol%); (d) $Pd(OAc)_2$ (5 mol%), $P(o\text{-}Tol)_3$ (7 mol%); (e) $Pd(OAc)_2$ (10 mol%), PivOH (30 mol%), O_2 (1 bar), 4A MS, MePh, 100 °C, 20 h; (f) $Pd(OAc)_2$ (5 mol%), XantPhos (10 mol%), CuBr (15 mol%), Cs_2CO_3 (2 equiv), DMF, 90 °C, 15 h then 2 M HCl, rt, 15 min.

piperazine was linked to 4-aminoquinoline to form a new hybrid (Scheme 11.25), which exhibited antimalarial activity against both chloroquine-sensitive 3D7 and chloroquine-resistant N-67 strains of *P. falciparum* [42, 43]. After this, they went on to synthesize new side chain modified 4-aminoquinoline derivatives and quinoline–acridine hybrids and evaluated them against *P. falciparum* NF54 strain *in vitro* only to find some promising antimalarial analogs. The scheme for the synthesis of hybrid quinoline–acridine derivatives involves amination of 4,7-dichloroquinoline with piperazine, furnishing the 7-chloro-4-piperazin-1-yl-quinoline which then undergoes nucleophilic substitution with corresponding methanesulfonic acid 2-(6-chloro-2-methoxy-acridin-9-ylamino)ethyl ester and methanesulfonic acid 3-(6-chloro-2-methoxy-acridin-9-ylamino)propyl ester to yield the hybrid quinoline–acridine (6-chloro-2-methoxyacridin-9-yl)-{2-[4-(7-chloro-quinolin-4-yl)-piperazin-1-yl]-ethyl}-amine and (6-chloro-2-methoxy-acridin-9-yl)-{2-[4-(7-chloro-quinolin-4-yl)-piperazin-1-yl]-propyl}-amine, respectively (Scheme 11.26) [44]. Recently, Kumar et al. combined naphthalimides with 4-aminoquinolines, with

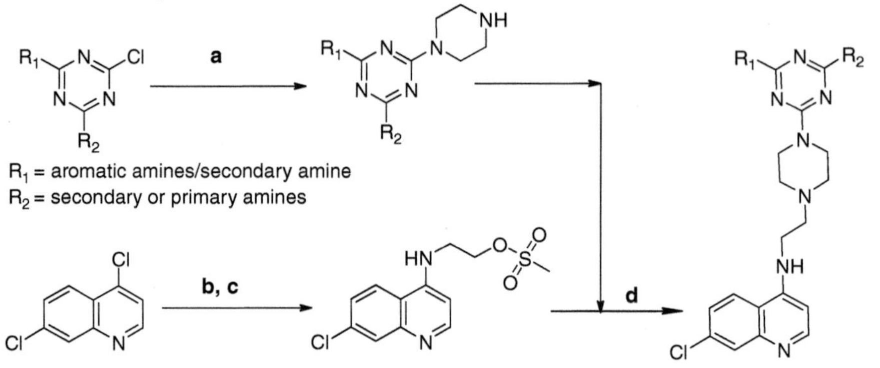

Scheme 11.25 Reagents and conditions: (a) piperazine, 0 °C, 2 h, THF; (b) $H_2N-CH_2-CH_2-OH$, *n*-BuOH, 90 °C, 8 h; (c) CH_3SO_2Cl, Pyridine, 0 °C, 3 h; (d) MW, 30s, NMP.

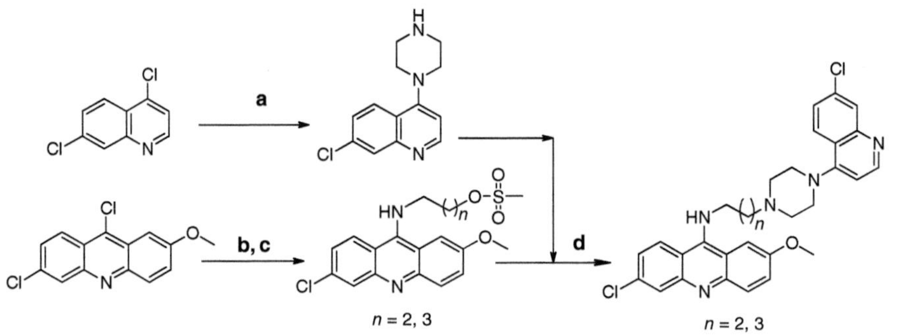

Scheme 11.26 Reagents and conditions: (a) piperazine, *n*-BuOH, 100 °C, 10 h; (b) 2-amino-ethanol or 3-amino-propan-1-ol, *n*-BuOH, 100 °C, 8 h; (c) methanesulfonyl chloride, dry THF, 0 °C, 3 h; (d) 7-chloro-4-piperazin-1-yl-quinoline, NMP, MW, 30 s.

varied spacer lengths, so as to develop potent antimalarials. Different secondary amines (piperidine, morpholine, and hydroxyethylpiperazine) have been incorporated at the C-4 position of the naphthalimide core, in order to enhance the basicity of the resulting scaffolds to promote concentration within the acidic vacuole of the parasite. The target scaffolds were afforded by reaction between 1,8-naphthalic anhydride and 4-diaminoquinolines (Scheme 11.27) [45].

A novel series of thiophene- and furan-based aminoquinoline derivatives were found to be potent inhibitors of β-hematin polymerization. Since, π–π stacking is the major driving force behind the hematin-chloroquine complex formation, introduction of an additional π-system to the 4-aminoquinoline scaffold (such as thiophene and furan) was thought to be helpful for inhibiting hemozoin polymerization from hematin. The synthesis of the desired end products was achieved by Suzuki–Miyaura reaction conditions, starting with thiophene and furan derivatives and respective arylboronic acids, followed by subsequent

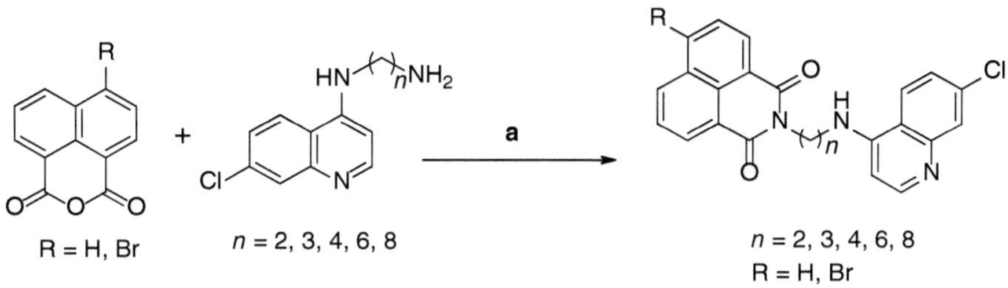

Scheme 11.27 Reagents and conditions: (a) NMP, 150 °C, 2 h.

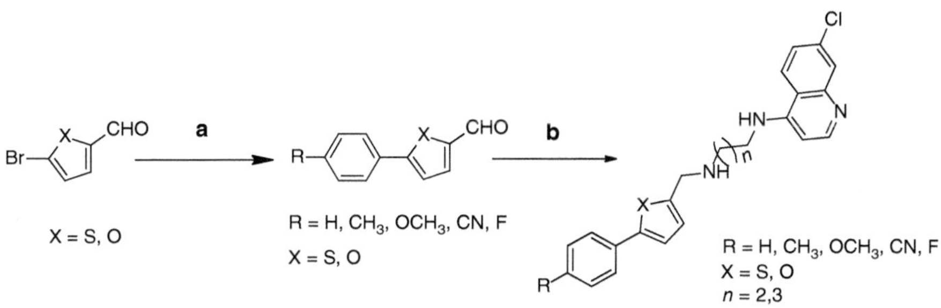

Scheme 11.28 Reagents and conditions: (a) $ArB(OH)_2$, $Pd(OAc)_2$, PPh_3, DME, Na_2CO_3 (aq), EtOH, 90 °C; (b) *N*-(7-chloroquinolin-4-yl)ethane-1,2-diamine or *N*-(7-chloroquinolin-4-yl)propan-1,3-diamine, CH_2Cl_2, MeOH, AcOH, $NaBH_4$, rt, 18 h.

reductive amination using *N*-(7-chloroquinolin-4-yl)ethane-1,2-diamine or *N*-(7-chloroquinolin-4-yl)propan-1,3-diamine (Scheme 11.28) [46].

A new class of tetrazole and 4-aminoquinolines was designed and synthesized based on the idea of circumventing metabolic *N*-dealkylation by incorporating bulkier substituents such as aromatic and tetrazole rings while varying the length of the alkyl side chain. The synthesis started with treating the key quinolinediamines with various aromatic aldehydes under MCR conditions in the presence of *tert*-butylisocyanide and trimethylsilane azide ($TMSN_3$) and subsequent cleavage of the *tert*-butyl group to afford the target compounds (Scheme 11.29) [47].

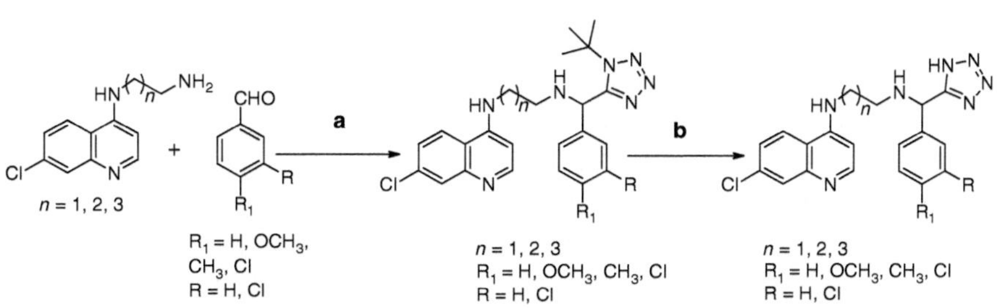

Scheme 11.29 Reagents and conditions: (a) *tert*-butyl isocyanide $TMSN_3$, MeOH, 40 °C, 24 h; (b) 32% HCl (aq), 120 °C, 4–8 h.

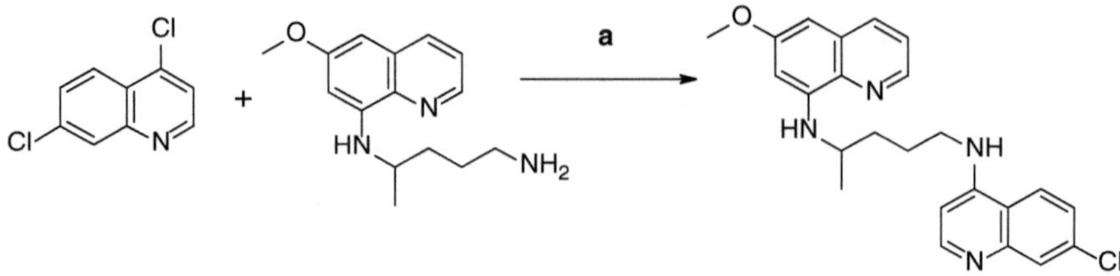

Primaquine–chloroquine hybrid

Scheme 11.30 Reagents and conditions: (a) K_2CO_3, Et_3N, NMP, N_2, 135 °C, 4 h.

11.2.2.2 Synthetic Approach of PQ–CQ Hybrid

Pal et al. synthesized primaquine–chloroquine twin drug and evaluated its heme binding property. The synthetic scheme (Scheme 11.30) proceeds with condensation of primaquine-biphosphate and 4,7-dichloroquinoline in presence of triethylamine and potassium carbonate in *N*-methyl-2-pyrrolidinone under inert atmosphere provided by nitrogen producing the primaquine–chloroquine hybrid in moderate yield. This hybrid could chelate free iron and reduce ferric ion thereby showing antioxidant abilities. It could also prevent hydroxyl free radical and heme-mediated protein degradation [43].

11.3 Conclusion and Future Perspectives

We have briefly described various synthetic approaches of 4-aminoquinolines and 8-aminoquinolines employed for the development of diverse antimalarial agents. The drug discovery programs conducted between the mid-1960s to the mid-1980s have failed to replace the antimalarial drugs, chloroquine and primaquine. 4-Aminoquinolines, specifically chloroquine, are known to bind to ferriprotoporphyrin IX and 8-aminoquinolines, namely primaquine, display marked gametocytocidal activity against all species of human malaria, including multiresistant *P. falciparum* strains and are also effective against all exo-erythrocytic forms of the parasite, thus providing a chemotherapeutic target for further rational design of drug analogs. A major progress in this research area has been done during the past two decades, resulting in the design and synthesis of viable candidates of 4-aminoquinoline and 8-aminoquinoline classes. Though, the occurrence of resistance threatens the antimalarial effectivity of the drugs in these classes, new analogs of the existing drugs, with nucleus modification or side chain alteration or novel conjugate formation with other heterocycles, have been deployed in conjunction of the existing first-line drugs. Such modifications help to extend life span of the drugs *in vivo* by bypassing metabolic pathways and also reduce toxicity associated with the established antimalarial molecules. The synthetic schemes that have been employed in the syntheses of these classes of drugs have evolved over the years, the very recent being transition metal-catalyzed reactions. Despite the disadvantages and drawbacks associated with 4-aminoquinolines and 8-aminoquinolines, they are still widely in use and serving as the major scaffold for further antimalarial drug design.

Gradual evolution of scientific research and ideas of scientists have moved the hybrid drug concept from the simple combination of two active moieties into a single chemical entity to a delivery/targeted system capable of selective activation inside the parasite. More recently, this concept was extended to compounds acting on different stages of the parasite life cycle. Besides, strategies for malaria elimination, hybrid compounds acting on the blood and liver stages of infections, by blocking the transmission of the parasite from the host to the mosquito vector, have also been developed. Despite the success of the hybrid drug approach in developing antimalarial agents, there are several constraints that are still needed to be addressed.

Acknowledgment

The authors are indebted to National Institute of Pharmaceutical Education and Research, N.I.P.E.R., S.A.S. Nagar (Mohali), Punjab, India, for all the support and inspiration.

References

1 Basu, S. and Sahi, P.K. (2017). Malaria an update. *Indian Journal of Pediatrics* 84: 521–528.

2 World Malaria Report (2019). World Health Organization. https://www.who.int/publications-detail/world-malaria-report-2019.

3 Kaur, K., Jain, M., Reddy, R.P. et al. (2010). Quinolines and structurally related heterocycles as antimalarials. *European Journal of Medicinal Chemistry* 45: 3245–3264.

4 Singh, A., Rani, A., Gut, J. et al. (2017). Piperazine linked 4-aminoquinoline-chalcone/ferrocenyl-chalcone conjugates: synthesis and anti-plasmodial evaluation. *Chemical Biology & Drug Design* 90: 590–595.

5 Tse, E.G., Korsik, M., and Todd, M.H. (2019). The past, present and future of antimalarial medicines. *Malaria Journal* 18: 93–114.

6 Basilico, N., Parapini, S., Sparatore, A. et al. (2017). In vivo and in vitro activities and ADME-Tox profile of a quinolizidine-modified 4-aminoquinoline: a potent anti-*P. falciparum* and anti-*P. vivax* blood-stage antimalarial. *Molecules* 22: 2102–2117.

7 Meltzer, E. and Schwartz, E. (2019). Utility of 8-aminoquinolines in malaria prophylaxis in travelers. *Current Infectious Disease Reports* 21: 43–49.

8 Crockett, M. and Kain, K.C. (2007). Tafenoquine: a promising new antimalarial agent. *Expert Opinion on Investigational Drugs* 16: 705–715.

9 Waters, N.C. and Edstein, M.D. (2012). 8-Aminoquinolines: primaquine and tafenoquine. In: *Treatment and Prevention of Malaria* (ed. H.M. Staines and S. Krishna), 69–94. Springer Basel AG.

10 Mehrotra, N., Lal, J., Puri, S.K. et al. (2007). In vitro and in vivo pharmacokinetic studies of bulaquine (analogue of primaquine), a novel antirelapse antimalarial, in rat, rabbit and monkey highlighting species similarities and differences. *Biopharmaceutics & Drug Disposition* 28: 209–227.

11 Hu, Y., Gao, C., Zhang, S. et al. (2017). Quinoline hybrids and their antiplasmodial and antimalarial activities. *European Journal of Medicinal Chemistry* 139: 22–47.

12 Block, J.H. (2011). Antimalarials. In: *Wilson and Gisvold's Textbook of Organic, Medical and Pharmaceutical Chemistry*, 12e (ed. J.M. Beale Jr., and J.H. Block), 242–257. CCH, A Wolters Kluwer Business.

13 Nqoro, X., Tobeka, N., and Aderibigbe, B.A. (2017). Quinoline-based hybrid compounds with antimalarial activity. *Molecules* 22: 2268–2290.

14 Vale, N., Moreira, R., Gomes, P. et al. (2009). Primaquine revisited six decades after its discovery. *European Journal of Medicinal Chemistry* 44: 937–953.

15 McChesney, J.D. (1981). Considerations about the structure–activity relationships of 8-aminoquinoline antimalarial drugs. *Bulletin of the World Health Organization* 59: 459–462.

16 Hocart, S.J., Liu, H., Deng, H. et al. (2011). 4-Aminoquinolines active against chloroquine-resistant *plasmodium falciparum*: basis of antiparasite activity and quantitative structure–activity relationship analyses. *Antimicrobial Agents and Chemotherapy* 55: 2233–2244.

17 O' Neill, P.M., Ward, S.A., Berry, N.G. et al. (2006). A medicinal chemistry perspective on 4-aminoquinoline antimalarial drugs. *Current Topics in Medicinal Chemistry* 6: 479–507.

18 O' Neill, P.M., Bray, P.G., Hawley, S.R. et al. (1998). 4-Aminoquinolines – past, present, and future: a chemical perspective. *Pharmacology & Therapeutics* 77: 29–58.

19 Kaschula, C.H., Egan, T.J., Hunter, R. et al. (2002). Structure–activity relationships in 4-aminoquinoline antiplasmodials. The role of the group at the 7-position. *Journal of Medicinal Chemistry* 45: 3531–3539.

20 Elderfield, R.C., Mertel, H.E., Mitch, R.T. et al. (1955). Synthesis of primaquineand certain of its analogs. *Journal of the American Chemical Society* 77: 4816–4819.

21 Campbell, K.N., Elderfield, R.C., Genslera, W.J. et al. (1947). Some derivatives of 6-methoxy-8-aminolepidine. *Journal of the American Chemical Society* 69: 1465–1467.

22 Carroll, F.I., Berrang, B., Linn, C.P. et al. (1979). Synthesis of some 4-substituted 8-amino-6-methoxyquinolines as potential antimalarials. *Journal of Medicinal Chemistry* 22: 694–699.

23 Carroll, F.I., Berrang, B.D., and Linn, C.P. (1980). Synthesis of 2,4-disubstituted 6-methoxy-8-aminoquinoline analogues as potential antiparasitics. *Journal of Medicinal Chemistry* 23: 581–584.

24 Zorc, B., Perkovic, I., Pavic, K. et al. (2019). Primaquine derivatives: modifications of the terminal amino group. *European Journal of Medicinal Chemistry* 182: 111640–111659.

25 Talati, S.M., Latham, M.R., Moore, E.G. et al. (1970). Synthesis of potential antimalarials: primaquine analogs. *Journal of Pharmaceutical Sciences* 59: 491–495.

26 Jain, R., Jain, S., Gupta, R.C. et al. (1994). Synthesis of amino acid derivatives of 8-[(4-amino-1-methylbutyl)amino]-6-4-substituted quinolines as potential antimalarial agents. *Indian Journal of Chemistry* 33: 251–254.

27 Vangapandu, S., Sachdeva, S., Jain, M. et al. (2003). 8-Quinolinamines and their prodrug conjugates as potent blood-schizontocidal antimalarial agents. *Bioorganic & Medicinal Chemistry* 11: 4557–4568.

28 Han, S., Liang, A., Ren, X. et al. (2017). Copper-catalyzed remote C–H ethoxycarbonyldifluoromethylation of 8-aminoquinolines with bis(pinacolato)diboron as reductant. *Tetrahedron Letters* 58: 4859–4863.

29 Chen, J., Huang, D., and Ding, Y. (2017). Transition-metal-free site-selective C—F bond activation for synthesis of 8-aminoquinolines. *Tetrahedron Letters* 58: 4240–4242.

30 Tafenoquine-New Drug Approvals (2020). https://newdrugapprovals.org/tag/tafenoquine (accessed on 27 April 2020).

31 Bulaquine-New Drug Approvals (2020). https://newdrugapprovals.org/2014/05/01/bulaquine (accessed on 27 April 2020).

32 Elderfield, R.C., Gensler, W.J., Birstein, O. et al. (1946). Synthesis of certain simple 4-aminoquinoline derivatives. *Journal of the American Chemical Society* 68: 1250–1251.

33 Vippagunta, S.R., Dorn, A., Matile, H. et al. (1999). Structural specificity of chloroquine-hematin binding related to inhibition of hematin polymerization and parasite growth. *Journal of Medicinal Chemistry* 42: 4630–4639.

34 Johnson, W.S. and Buell, B.G.A. (1952). New synthesis of chloroquine. *Journal of the American Chemical Society* 74: 4513–4516.

35 Gemma, S., Kukreja, G., Tripaldi, P. et al. (2008). Microwave-assisted synthesis of 4-quinolylhydrazines followed by nickel boride reduction: a convenient approach to 4-aminoquinolines and derivatives. *Tetrahedron Letters* 49: 2074–2077.

36 Madrid, P.B., Sherrill, J., Liou, A.P. et al. (2005). Synthesis of ring-substituted 4-aminoquinolines and evaluation of their antimalarial activities. *Bioorganic & Medicinal Chemistry Letters* 15: 1015–1018.

37 Musonda, C.C., Taylor, D., Lehman, J. et al. (2004). Application of multi-component reactions to antimalarial drug discovery. Part 1: parallel synthesis and antiplasmodial activity of new 4-aminoquinoline Ugi adducts. *Bioorganic & Medicinal Chemistry Letters* 14: 3901–3905.

38 Madrid, P.B., Wilson, N.T., DeRisi, J.L. et al. (2004). Parallel synthesis and antimalarial screening of a 4-aminoquinoline library. *Journal of Combinatorial Chemistry* 6: 437–442.

39 Solomon, V.R., Puri, S.K., Srivastava, K. et al. (2005). Design and synthesis of new antimalarial agents from 4-aminoquinoline. *Bioorganic & Medicinal Chemistry* 13: 2157–2165.

40 Kondaparla, S., Soni, A., Manhas, A. et al. (2017). Antimalarial activity of novel 4-aminoquinolines active against drug resistant strains. *Bioorganic Chemistry* 70: 74–85.

41 Collet, J.W., Ackermans, K., Lambregts, J. et al. (2018). Modular three-component synthesis of 4-aminoquinolines via an imidoylative sonogashira/cyclization cascade. *The Journal of Organic Chemistry* 83: 854–861.

42 Kumar, A., Srivastava, K., Kumar, S.R. et al. (2008). Synthesis and bioevaluation of hybrid 4-aminoquinoline triazines as a new class of antimalarial agents. *Bioorganic & Medicinal Chemistry Letters* 18: 6530–6533.

43 Pal, C., Sarkar, S., Mazumdar, S. et al. (2013). Synthesis and biological evaluation of primaquine–chloroquine twin drug: a novel heme-interacting molecule prevents free heme and hydroxyl radical-mediated protein degradation. *Medicinal Chemistry Communications* 4: 731–736.

44 Kumar, A., Srivastava, K., Kumar, S.R. et al. (2010). Synthesis of new 4-aminoquinolines and quinoline–acridine hybrids as antimalarial agents. *Bioorganic & Medicinal Chemistry Letters* 20: 7059–7063.

45 Shalini, Legac, J., Adeniyi, A.A. et al. (2020). Functionalized naphthalimide-4-aminoquinoline conjugates as promising antiplasmodials, with mechanistic insights. *ACS Medicinal Chemistry Letters* 11: 154–161.

46 Opsenica, I.M., Verbic, T.Z., Tot, M. et al. (2015). Investigation into novel thiophene- and furan-based 4-amino-7-chloroquinolines afforded antimalarials that cure mice. *Bioorganic & Medicinal Chemistry* 23: 2176–2186.

47 Tukulula, M., Njoroge, M., Abay, E.T. et al. (2013). Synthesis and in vitro and in vivo pharmacological evaluation of new 4-aminoquinoline-based compounds. *ACS Medicinal Chemistry Letters* 4: 1198–1202.

12

Antimalarial Activity of Novel Class of 1,3-Benzoxaborole Derivatives Containing 1,3,4-Oxadiazole Moiety

Vinayak Adimule[1], Adarsha Haramballi Jagadeesha Gowda[2], Santosh S. Nandi[3], and Debdas Bowmik[4]

[1]*Angadi Institute of Technology and Management (AITM), Department of Chemistry, Savagaon Road, Belagavi 591108, Karnataka, India*
[2]*National University of Ireland, Centre for Research in Medical Devices, Gaillimh, Galway H91TK33, Ireland*
[3]*KLE Dr. M. S. Sheshgiri College of Engineering and Technology, Chemistry section, Department of Engineering Science and Humanities, Udyambhag, Belagavi, Karnataka 590008, India*
[4]*High Energy Materials Research Laboratory, Defence Research and Development Organization, Ministry of Defence, Government of India, Sutarwadi, Pune 411021, India*

12.1 Introduction

Transmittable parasite involved in spreading Malaria cause several infections which continues to damage human health more than half the world's populations [1–4]. *Plasmodium falciparum* transmitted to humans by infected mosquitoes causing morbidity and mortality [5–8]. Combination therapies are well known to treat malaria caused by *P. falciparum*; however, many derivatives containing 1,3,4-oxadiazole and other heterocyclic compounds reported with higher efficacy values and more water solubility [9–10]. Most importantly, resistance to endoperoxide and resistance to *P. falciparum* have been wide spread for malarial treatment [11–13]. This situation brought renewed urgency for developing most resistance and easy, safe to use antimalarial compounds [14, 15]. Recently, novel derivatives of 2-substituted-1,3-bezoxazole reported by M.S.R. Murty et al. [16] as potential anticancer agents. Novel pyrazole containing compounds containing 1,2,4-triazoles has been synthesised by A.M. Vijesh et al. [17] and investigated for potential antimicrobial and analgesic agents. Regioselective design, synthesis and biological evaluation of novel class of benzoxazole derivatives have been reported by S. Ananya et al. [18] in the year 2015. Analogues of chloroquine and amodiaquine have been studied in detail by A.R. Parhizgar et al. [19] and tested for antimalarial properties. Novel class of 1-imino derivatives of 7-chloro-3-substituted-3,4-dihydro-1,9(2H,10H)-acridinediones antimalarial compounds designed and synthesised by J.K. Stephen et al. [20]. Structural design for

Drug Development for Malaria: Novel Approaches for Prevention and Treatment, First Edition.
Edited by Pravin Kendrekar.

benzoxazole novel class derivatives as potential cholesteryl ester transfer protein (CETP) inhibitors has been studied by S.K. Abdul Amin et al. [21] in the year 2019 and reported the detail activity against *P. falciparum* parasite. New generation of 4-aminoquinoline antimalarial compounds using predictive pharmacokinetic and toxicology models has been studied by R. Sunetra et al. [22] and reported the diversified modifications in the structure of the quinolone compounds. Novel, efficacious, antimalarial lead compounds containing *N*-aryl-2-aminobenzimidazole derivatives designed and synthesised by R. Sreekanth et al. [23] and investigated for their efficacy against *P. falciparum*. Based on the evidences author envisages, the boron containing benzoxaborole bearing 1,3,4-oxadiazole moiety finds promising candidate for effective treatment of malarial infection. The library of compounds containing 1,3-bezoxyborole-6-carboxylic acids has been synthesised in the present investigation and tested for *in vitro* efficacy [24–27] and solubility of the derivatives. Most importantly, the derivatives **13**, **14**, and **16** showed good potency against *P. falciparum* with IC_{50} of 10, 18, and 20 nM, respectively.

12.1.1 Materials and Methods

Synthetic materials, chemical reagents, solvents for reactions and column-chromatographic purifications purchased from Sigma–Aldrich, Alfa Assar, Spectrochem Pvt Ltd, S-D Fine Chemical Ltd, and any further purification carried out used as obtained. ^{1}H-NMR (proton nuclear magnetic resonance) and ^{13}C-NMR (carbon nuclear magnetic resonance) spectroscopy (dimethyl sulphoxide [DMSO]-d6 solvent) carried out to analyse the chemical shifts (expressed in ppm) of the intermediate compounds **6a–10a** and final compounds **12–16** using Bruker Avance Z-gradient and equipped for gradient shimming standard probe: 5 mm BBFO Z-gradient smart probe with automatic tune. High performance liquid chromatography (HPLC) from Shimadzu Nexera model with automatic diagnosis and solvent flow pilot (smart flow control) increases the flow rate which can be employed to assess the purity of the synthesised compounds. Liquid crystal mass spectroscopy (LCMS) was carried out for the synthesised compounds using Shimadzu LCMS-8060NX LC-MS/MS system with triple quadrupole and buffer A (H_2O containing 0.2% phosphoric acid) and buffer B (CH_3CN or methanol) used as mobile phases. The column was eluted with a gradient of 85–95% buffer A and 5–15% buffer B with auto-controlled mechanism set in the instrument from a time period of one minute with variation of 35% of buffer A and 5% of buffer B solution flow rate of 1 ml/min with a column temperature of 30 °C and UV detection. Silica gel (#100–200 mesh), all the *in vitro* studies on the *P. falciparum*, was carried out by procuring the cell lines from MTCC (Microbial Type Culture Collection, Chandigarh, India from the authorisation of the institutional approval) and used by culturing it in the culture medium as specified by the MTCC.

12.1.2 Synthesis

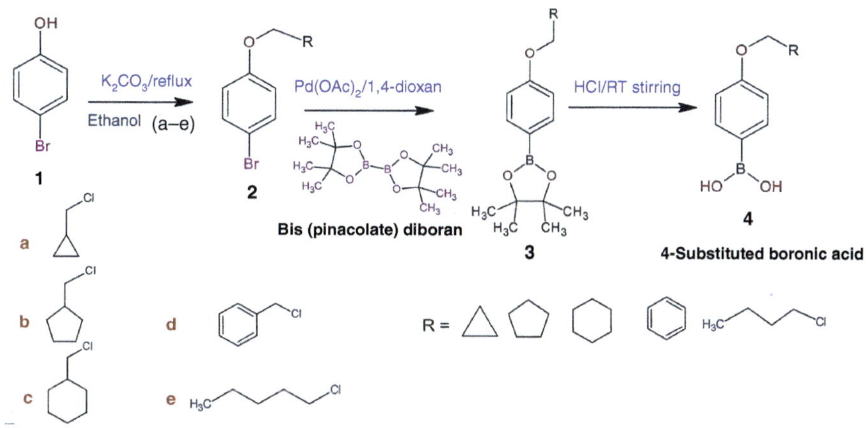

Figure 12.1 (Step I): Illustration of the synthesis of 4-ethoxy substituted phenyl boronic acid; reagents and conditions: (**2**) K_2CO_3 (2–3 M), absolute ethanol and reflux at 85 °C, (**a**–**e**) (1.1 M); (**3**) 1,4-dioxan, palladium acetate (0.5 equiv), bispinacolato diboron (1.2 M), K_2CO_3, reflux, RM at 80 °C; (**4**) concentrated hydrochloric acid in 1,4-dioxan, stirring at room temperature.

12.2 Experimental Procedure for *In Vitro* Studies on Antimalarial Activity

Strain W_2 and *P. falciparum* containing parasites were taken in a cultured medium added with human erythrocytes; RPMI-1640 added with 12% human serum (0.7% Albumax) maintained under oxygen, carbon dioxide and nitrogen atmosphere [28–30]. Serial dilutions of benzoxaborole containing 1,3,4-oxadiazoles from 100 μM to 50 nM solutions in 96 well plates (including 300 μl of media/well, 2% haematocrit, and 1% parasitaemia) and the parasites were made to synchronise into ring type by the treatment of 7% D-sorbitol. After completion of 48 hours incubations, unreacted and untreated cultures were fixed by adding 2% formaldehyde solution in water subsequently 5–7 μl of the test sample transferred to well plate containing 150–200 μl/well of staining solution. Fluorescence Spectrophotometer with the excitation of 485 nm and an emission of 525 nm was determined using flow cytometer, and the plots were drawn forward scatter against the emission values. Normalised values converted to percentage control activity and the IC_{50} values calculated by plotting graph using excel software. The values from the independent experiments and standard deviations with the errors were calculated [31–33].

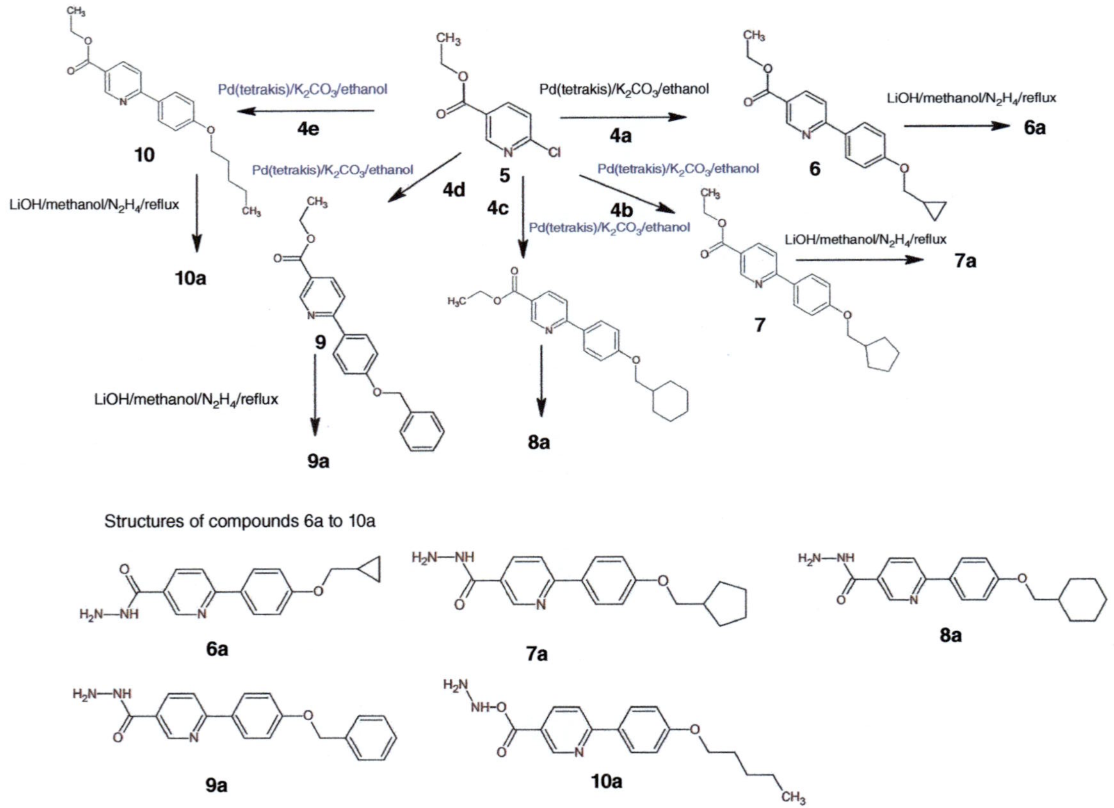

Figure 12.2 (Step II): Synthetic reaction scheme of compounds of **6a–10a**; reagents and conditions; (**6**) **4a**, tetrakis(triphenylphosphine) palladium(0), K_2CO_3, absolute ethanol, reflux for 10 hours; compound **6a**: $LiOH/H_2O/CH_3OH$ for 1 hour and N_2H_4, absolute ethanol, reflux for 3 hours: (**7**) **4b**, tetrakis (triphenylphosphine) palladium(0), K_2CO_3, absolute ethanol, reflux for 11 hours; compound **7a**: $LiOH/H_2O/CH_3OH$ for 1 hour and N_2H_4, absolute ethanol, reflux for 3 hours: (**8**) **4c**, tetrakis (triphenylphosphine) palladium(0), K_2CO_3, absolute ethanol, reflux for 15 hours; compound **8a**: $LiOH/H_2O/CH_3OH$ for 1 hour and N_2H_4, absolute ethanol, reflux for 3.5 hours: (**9**) **4d**, tetrakis(triphenylphosphine) palladium(0), K_2CO_3, absolute ethanol, reflux for 14 hours; compound **9a**: $LiOH/H_2O/CH_3OH$ for 1 hour and N_2H_4, absolute ethanol, reflux for 4.5 hours; (**10**) **4e**, tetrakis (triphenylphosphine) palladium(0), K_2CO_3, absolute ethanol, reflux for 18 hours; compound **10a**: $LiOH/H_2O/CH_3OH$ for 1 hour and N_2H_4, absolute ethanol, reflux for 3 hours.

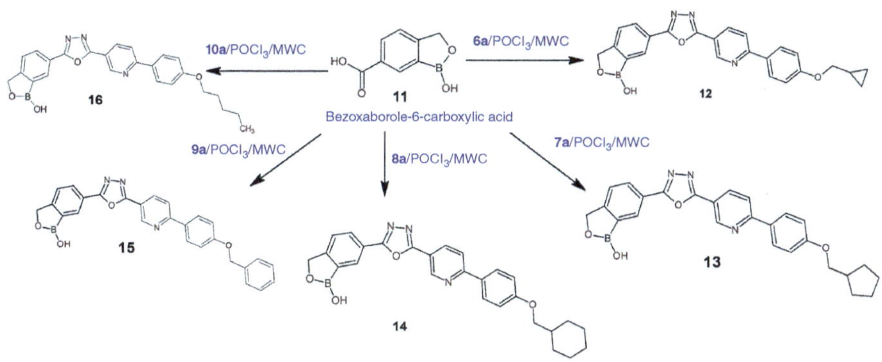

Figure 12.3 (Step III): Synthetic reaction scheme for final derivatives; reagents and conditions; (**12**) microwave cyclisation reaction (MWC), phosphoryl oxychloride, **6a**, for 3 minutes; (**13**) MWC, phosphoryl oxychloride, **7a**, for 3.5 minutes; (14) MWC, phosphoryl oxychloride, **8a**, for 5 minutes; (**15**) MWC, phosphoryl oxychloride, **9a**, for 4 minutes; (**16**) MWC, phosphoryl oxychloride, **10a**, for 3.8 minutes.

12.2.1 Experimentation

12.2.1.1 Analytical Results of the Intermediate Compounds (6a–10a)

^{1}H-NMR spectrum of 6-[4-(cyclopropyl methoxy)phenyll]pyridine-3-Carbo-hydrazide (**6a**): ^{1}H NMR: δ 0.23–0.37 (4H, 0.31 (dtd, J = 8.2, 7.6, 5.7 Hz), 0.30 (tdd, J = 8.3, 7.6, 5.7 Hz)), 0.87 (1H, ttt, J = 8.2, 7.6, 6.1 Hz), 4.46 (2H, d, J = 6.1 Hz), 7.10 (2H, ddd, J = 9.1, 1.6, 0.5 Hz), 7.78 (2H, ddd, J = 9.1, 1.6, 0.5 Hz), 8.15–8.25 (2H, 8.19 (dd, J = 7.8, 1.8 Hz), 8.24 (dd, J = 7.8, 0.61 Hz)), 9.04 (1H, dd, J = 1.77, 0.61 Hz); LCMS-$[M+H]^{+}$-284.1; Molecular formula: $C_6H_{17}N_3O_2$; HPLC purity = 97.8%; Yield = 510 mg; Colour: Off white solid.

^{13}C-NMR spectrum of 6-[4-(cyclopropyl methoxy)phenyl]pyridine-3-carbo-hydrazide (**6a**): δ (ppm): 116.6, 127.6, 157.5, 1378.7, 131.5, 11.6, 129.4, 129.4, 72.4, 152.49, 118.4, 167.67, 3.2.

^{1}H-NMR spectrum of 6-[4-(cyclopentyl methoxy)phenyl]pyridine-3-carbo-hydrazide (**7a**): ^{1}H NMR: δ 1.51–1.78 (8H, 1.67 (ddddd, J = 11.8, 9.4, 7.6, 6.7, 5.5 Hz), 1.58 (dddd, J = 9.1, 8.2, 7.7, 7.1 Hz), 1.62 (dddd, J = 9.1, 6.9, 4.2, 1.8 Hz), 1.69 (ddddd, J = 11.8, 7.1, 5.4, 1.7, 1.4 Hz)), 2.39 (1H, dddtd, J = 8.2, 7.6, 7.1, 5.1, 4.2 Hz), 4.51 (2H, d, J = 5.0 Hz), 7.08 (2H, ddd, J = 9.0, 1.7, 0.41 Hz), 7.74 (2H, ddd, J = 9.0, 1.5, 0.4 Hz), 8.15–8.25 (2H, 8.18 (dd, J = 7.7, 1.7 Hz), 8.22 (dd, J = 7.72, 0.62 Hz)), 9.04 (1H, dd, J = 1.7, 0.6 Hz); $[M+H]^{+}$-312.17; Molecular formula: $C_{18}H_{21}N_3O_2$; HPLC purity = 97.9%; Yield = 610 mg; Colour: Off white Solid.

^{13}C-NMR spectrum of 6-[4-(cyclopentyl methoxy)phenyl]pyridine-3-carbo-hydrazide (**7a**): δ (ppm): 130.5, 115.6, 115.6, 164.06, 137.7, 129.0, 129.06, 119.4, 27.7, 27.7, 148.9, 153.4, 70.0, 25.4, 37.7, 128.6, 167.6.

^{1}H-NMR spectrum of 6-[4-(cyclohexyl methoxy)phenyl]pyridine-3-carbo-hydrazide (**8a**): ^{1}H NMR: δ 1.25–1.56 (10H, 1.31 (dtt, J = 12.1, 10.3, 2.8 Hz), 1.46 (dtd, J = 12.6, 10.3, 2.8 Hz), 1.46 (dq, J = 12.6, 2.8 Hz), 1.40 (dtt, J = 12.8, 10.3, 2.8 Hz), 1.38 (dquint, J = 12.8, 2.8 Hz), 1.34 (dquint, J = 12.1, 2.8 Hz)), 1.75 (1H, ttt, J = 10.3, 5.1, 2.8 Hz), 4.48 (2H, d, J = 5.1 Hz), 7.09 (2H, ddd, J = 9.0, 1.6, 0.4 Hz),

7.74 (2H, ddd, J = 9.0, 1.5, 0.4 Hz), 8.15–8.25 (2H, 8.18 (dd, J = 7.7, 1.7 Hz), 8.22 (dd, J = 7.7, 0.6 Hz)), 9.03 (1H, dd, J = 1.7, 0.6 Hz); LCMS-$[M+H]^+$-326.18; Molecular formula: $C_{19}H_{23}N_3O_2$; HPLC purity = 98.6%; Yield = 850 mg; Colour: white solid.

^{13}C-NMR spectrum of 6-[4-(cyclohexyl methoxy)phenyl]pyridine-3-carbohydrazide (**8a**): δ (ppm): 153.4, 38.9, 115.6, 148.9, 137.7, 26.3, 128.6, 119.1, 129.0, 130.5, 164.06, 71.2, 28.3, 25.3, 25.30, 167.67.

^{1}H-NMR spectrum of 6-[4-(benzyloxy)phenyl]pyridine-3-carbohydrazide (**9a**): ^{1}H NMR; δ ppm: [5.34 (2H, s), 7.11 (2H, ddd, J = 9.0, 1.6, 0.4 Hz), 7.32–7.50 (5H, 7.35 tt, J = 7.5, 1.3 Hz), 7.41 (dddd, J = 7.8, 7.5, 1.6, 0.6 Hz), 7.47 (dddd, J = 7.8, 1.3, 1.0, 0.6 Hz), 7.74 (2H, ddd, J = 9.0, 1.5, 0.4 Hz), 8.15–8.25 (2H, 8.18 dd, J = 7.7, 1.7 Hz), 8.23 (dd, J = 7.7, 0.6 Hz), 9.03 (1H, dd, J = 1.7, 0.6 Hz)]; LCMS-$[M+H]^+$-320.13; Molecular formula: $C_{19}H_{17}N_3O_2$; purity (HPLC) = 99.8%; Yield = 800 mg; Colour; off white solid.

^{13}C-NMR of 6-[4-(benzyloxy)phenyl]pyridine-3-carbohydrazide (**9a**): δ (ppm): 130.5, 128.6, 160.4, 137.7, 128.5, 128.5, 119.4, 148.9, 129.06, 128.9, 153.4, 69.9, 127.8, 136.7, 167.6, 115.6.

^{1}H-NMR spectrum of (hydrazinyloxy){6-[4-(pentyloxy)phenyl]pyridine-3-yl} methanone (**10a**): ^{1}H NMR: δ 0.87 (3H, t, J = 7.0 Hz), 1.29 (2H, h, J = 7.0 Hz), 1.38 (2H, tt, J = 7.5, 7.0 Hz), 1.82 (2H, tt, J = 7.5, 7.1 Hz), 4.28 (2H, t, J = 7.1 Hz), 7.09 (2H, ddd, J = 9.0, 1.5, 0.4 Hz), 7.74 (2H, ddd, J = 9.0, 1.5, 0.4 Hz), 8.15–8.25 (2H, 8.18 (dd, J = 8.4, 1.7 Hz), 8.22 (dd, J = 8.4, 0.6 Hz)), 9.03 (1H, dd, J = 1.7, 0.6 Hz); LCMS-$[M+H]^+$-316.16; Molecular formula: $C_{17}H_{21}N_3O_3$; HPLC purity = 98.7%; Yield = 740 mg; Colour: Pale brown solid.

^{13}C-NMR of (hydrazinyloxy){6-[4-(pentyloxy)phenyl]pyridine-3-yl}methanone (**10a**): δ (ppm): 128.6, 115.6, 119.4, 148.9, 68.2, 137.7, 153.4, 22.397, 14.0, 129.0, 160.5, 28.725, 167.6, 130.5, and 28.2.

12.3 Analytical Results of Intermediate Compounds (12–16)

12.3.1 NMR and CMR Analysis

^{1}H-NMR spectrum of 1,3-benzoxazole-6-1,3,4-oxadiazole derivatives of 2-[4-(cyclopropylmethoxy)phenyl]pyridine (**12**): ^{1}H NMR: δ 0.22–0.38 (4H, 0.30 (dtd, J = 8.1, 7.5, 5.5 Hz), 0.30 (tdd, J = 8.1, 7.5, 5.5 Hz)), 0.85 (1H, ttt, J = 8.1, 7.5, 6.9 Hz), 4.36 (2H, d, J = 6.9 Hz), 5.04 (2H, d, J = 13.8 Hz), 7.24 (2H, ddd, J = 8.6, 1.3, 0.4 Hz), 7.55 (1H, dd, J = 8.3, 0.5 Hz), 7.71 (2H, ddd, J = 8.6, 1.7, 0.4 Hz), 8.11 (1H, dd, J = 8.3, 0.5 Hz), 8.32 (1H, dd, J = 8.3, 1.5 Hz), 8.45 (1H, dd, J = 8.3, 1.5 Hz), 8.69 (1H, dd, J = 1.5, 0.5 Hz), 9.33 (1H, dd, J = 1.5, 0.5 Hz); LCMS-$[M+H]^+$-424.14; Molecular formula: $C_{24}H_{20}BN_3O_4$; HPLC purity = 98.2%; Yield = 750 mg; Colour: white solid.

^{13}C-NMR spectrum of 1,3-benzoxazole-6-1,3,4-oxadiazole derivatives of 2-[4-(cyclopropyl methoxy)phenyl]pyridine (**12**): δ (ppm):130.6, 127.8, 119.4, 153.4, 123.48, 3.2, 3.21, 163.69, 129.0, 135.0, 10.6, 115.6, 158.5, 127.6, 65.5, 136.8, 131.3, 72.3, 148.9, 164.5, and 137.7.

^{1}H-NMR spectrum of 1,3-benzoxazole-6-1,3,4-oxadiazole derivatives of 2-[4-(cypentylmethoxy)phenyl]pyridine (**13**): ^{1}H NMR: δ 1.50–1.79 (8H, 1.68 (ddddd, *J* = 11.9, 9.4, 7.6, 6.8, 5.4 Hz), 1.58 (dddd, *J* = 9.2, 8.1, 7.6, 7.0 Hz), 1.61 (dddd, *J* = 9.2, 6.8, 4.1, 1.7 Hz), 1.69 (ddddd, *J* = 11.9, 7.0, 5.3, 1.7, 1.4 Hz)), 2.38 (1H, ddddt, *J* = 8.1, 7.6, 7.0, 4.1, 3.9 Hz), 4.45 (2H, d, *J* = 3.9 Hz), 5.04 (2H, d, *J* = 13.8 Hz), 7.19 (2H, ddd, *J* = 8.6, 1.3, 0.4 Hz), 7.62 (1H, dd, *J* = 8.3, 0.5 Hz), 7.71 (2H, ddd, *J* = 8.6, 1.7, 0.4 Hz), 8.11 (1H, dd, *J* = 8.3, 0.5 Hz), 8.32 (1H, dd, *J* = 8.3, 1.5 Hz), 8.45 (1H, dd, *J* = 8.3, 1.5 Hz), 8.69 (1H, dd, *J* = 1.5, 0.5 Hz), 9.33 (1H, dd, *J* = 1.5, 0.5 Hz); LCMS-$[M+H]^{+}$-452.17; Molecular formula: $C_{26}H_{24}BN_{3}O_{4}$; HPLC purity = 99.8%; Yield = 950 mg; Colour: brown solid.

^{13}C-NMR spectrum of 1,3-benzoxazole-6-1,3,4-oxadiazole derivatives of 2-[4-(cypentylmethoxy)phenyl]pyridine (**13**): δ (ppm): 70.0, 164.5, 163.6, 129.0, 129.0, 115.6, 137.7, 123.48333, 119.4, 130.6, 148.9, 27.78, 27.78, 25.44, 135.0, 164.06, 127.8, 125.5, 136.8, 65.5, 131.3, 153.4.127.694 05, 37.733 33.

^{1}H-NMR spectrum of 1,3-benzoxazole-6-1,3,4-oxadiazole derivatives of 2-[4-(cyclohexyl methoxy)phenyl]pyridine (**14**): ^{1}H NMR; *δ* ppm: [1.25–1.56 (10H, 1.31 dtt, *J* =12.1, 10.3, 2.8 Hz), 1.46 (dtd, *J* =12.6, 10.3, 2.8 Hz), 1.46 (dq, *J* =12.6, 2.8 Hz), 1.40 (dtt, *J* = 12.8, 10.3, 2.8 Hz), 1.38 (d quint, *J* = 12.8, 2.8 Hz), 1.34 (d quint, *J* =12.1, 2.8 Hz), 1.79 (1H, ttt, *J* =10.3, 4.8, 2.8 Hz), 4.46 (2H, d, *J* =4.8 Hz), 5.04 (2H, d, *J* =13.8 Hz), 7.19 (2H, ddd, *J* =8.6, 1.3, 0.4 Hz), 7.62 (1H, dd, *J* =8.3, 0.5 Hz), 7.71 (2H, ddd, *J* =8.6, 1.7, 0.4 Hz), 8.11 (1H, dd, *J* =8.3, 0.5 Hz), 8.32 (1H, dd, *J* =8.3, 1.5 Hz), 8.45 (1H, dd, *J* =8.3, 1.5 Hz), 8.69 (1H, dd, *J* =1.5, 0.5 Hz), 9.33 (1H, dd, *J* =1.5, 0.5 Hz)] ; LCMS-$[M+H]^{+}$-468.2; Molecular formula: $C_{27}H_{26}BN_{3}O_{4}$; purity (HPLC) = 98.5%; Yield = 890 mg; Colour; pale yellow solid.

^{13}C-NMR spectrum of 1,3-benzoxazole-6-1,3,4-oxadiazole derivatives of 2-[4-(cyclohexylmethoxy)phenyl]pyridine (**14**): δ (ppm): 164.5, 65.5, 71.2, 153.4, 137.7, 127.6, 148.9, 125.5, 127.8, 38.9, 130.6, 131.3, 119.4, 136.8, 163.6, 115.6, 135.0, 123.4, 129.0, 129.0, 164.06, 25.3, 28.3, 26.3.

^{1}H-NMR spectrum of 1,3-benzoxazole-6-1,3,4-oxadiazole derivatives of 2-[4-(benzyloxy)phenyl]pyridine (**15**): ^{1}H NMR: δ 5.04 (2H, d, *J* = 13.8 Hz), 5.50 (2H, s), 7.21 (2H, ddd, *J* = 8.6, 1.3, 0.4 Hz), 7.31–7.50 (5H, 7.34 (tt, *J* = 7.7, 1.3 Hz), 7.41 (dddd, *J* = 7.8, 7.7, 1.6, 0.6 Hz), 7.47 (dddd, *J* = 7.8, 1.3, 1.0, 0.6 Hz)), 7.55 (1H, dd, *J* = 8.3, 0.5 Hz), 7.71 (2H, ddd, *J* = 8.6, 1.7, 0.4 Hz), 8.11 (1H, dd, *J* = 8.3, 0.5 Hz), 8.32 (1H, dd, *J* = 8.3, 1.5 Hz), 8.45 (1H, dd, *J* = 8.3, 1.5 Hz), 8.69 (1H, dd, *J* = 1.5, 0.5 Hz), 9.33 (1H, dd, *J* = 1.5, 0.5 Hz); LCMS-$[M+H]^{+}$-462.16; Molecular formula: $C_{27}H_{20}BN_{3}O_{4}$; HPLC purity = 99.0%; Yield = 741 mg; Colour: white solid.

^{13}C-NMR spectrum of 1,3-benzoxazole-6-1,3,4-oxadiazole derivatives of 2-[4-(benzyloxy)phenyl]pyridine (**15**): δ (ppm): 163.6,123.4, 69.9, 148.9, 135.0, 127.852 27, 129.066 67, 115.6, 127.694 05, 119.4, 125.5, 128.9, 164.5, 128.5, 160.42, 127.8, 137.7, 65.5, 136.7, 131.3, 130.6, 153.4, 136.8.

^{1}H-NMR spectrum of 1,3-benzoxazole-6-1,3,4-oxadiazole derivatives of 2-[4-(pentyloxy)phenyl]pyridine (**16**): ^{1}H NMR; *δ* ppm: [0.87 (3H, t, *J* =7.0 Hz), 1.29 (2H, h, *J* =7.0 Hz), 1.38 (2H, tt, *J* =7.5, 7.0 Hz), 1.82 (2H, quint, *J* =7.5 Hz), 4.21 (2H, t, *J* =7.5 Hz), 5.04 (2H, d, *J* =13.8 Hz), 7.18 (2H, ddd, *J* =8.6, 1.3, 0.4 Hz), 7.62 (1H, dd, *J* =8.3, 0.5 Hz), 7.71 (2H, ddd, *J* =8.6, 1.7, 0.4 Hz), 8.11 (1H, dd, *J* =8.3,

0.5 Hz), 8.32 (1H, dd, J = 8.3, 1.5 Hz), 8.45 (1H, dd, J = 8.3, 1.5 Hz), 8.69 (1H, dd, J = 1.5, 0.5 Hz), 9.33 (1H, dd, J = 1.5, 0.5 Hz)]; LCMS-$[M+H]^+$-442.19; Molecular formula: $C_{25}H_{24}BN_3O_4$; purity (HPLC) = 98.1%; Yield = 765 mg; Colour; pale yellow solid].

^{13}C-NMR spectrum of 1,3-benzoxazole-6-1,3,4-oxadiazole derivatives of 2-[4-(pentyloxy)phenyl]pyridine (**16**): δ (ppm): 163.6, 123.4, 69.9, 148.9, 135.0, 127.8, 129.0, 115.6, 127.6, 119.4, 125.5, 128.9 (164.5, 128.5, 160.42, 127.8, 137.7, 65.5, 136.7, 131.3, 130.66831, 153.4, 136.8.).

12.4 Synthesis Procedures for 4-Ethoxy Phenyl Boronic Acid (General Procedure for Compounds 2, 3, and 4)

12.4.1 Synthesis of 1-Bromo-4-(Cyclopropyl Methyl) Benzene (Compound 2)

100 ml RB (round bottom) flask fitted with a reflux condenser, added 4-bromophenol (5 g, 0.028 M), K_2CO_3 solid (1.5 molar ratio), compounds (**a–e**) (1.1 molar ratio), (chloromethyl) cyclopropane (7.615g) and diluted reaction mixture (RM) with 60 ml of absolute ethanol, refluxed for 10–12 hours. RM cooled, solvent was evaporated, diluted with 50 ml of cold water and the product was extracted with ethyl acetate (50 ml × 3 times), washed with brine (10 ml), evaporated and obtained off white solid; Molecular formula: C_6H_5BrO; Yield = 5.8 g; molecular weight 172.10; TLC (ethyl acetate:hexane; 45 : 55); LCMS-$[M+H]^+$ 172.9; ^{1}H NMR: δ 0.21–0.36 (4H, 0.31 (dtd, J = 8.2, 7.6, 5.8 Hz), 0.31 (tdd, J = 8.2, 7.6, 5.8 Hz)), 0.83 (1H, ttt, J = 8.2, 7.6, 6.4 Hz), 3.89 (2H, d, J = 6.4 Hz), 6.68 (2H, ddd, J = 8.6, 2.8, 0.65 Hz), 7.11 (2H, ddd, J = 8.6, 1.7, 0.62 Hz).

Similar synthetic procedure was followed for the compounds **2b**, **2c**, **2d**, and **2e** derivatives and analytical data as given below.

12.4.1.1 1-Bromo-4-(Cyclopentyl Methoxy)Benzene (Compound 2b)

Molecular Name:bromo-4-(cyclopentyl methoxy) benzene; Molecular formula; $C_{12}H_{15}BrO$; Yield = 6.8 g; molecular weight 255; TLC (ethyl acetate:hexane; 50 : 50); LCMS-$[M+H]^+$ 256; ^{1}H NMR; δ ppm: [1.52-1.80 (8H, 1.67 (dd ddd, J = 12.0, 9.5, 7.6, 6.8, 5.4 Hz), 1.59 (dddd, J = 8.8, 8.1, 7.6, 7.0 Hz), 1.61 (dddd, J = 8.8, 6.8, 4.1, 1.7 Hz), 1.69 (ddddd, J = 11.9, 7.0, 5.3, 1.7, 1.4 Hz), 2.36 (1H, dddtd, J = 8.1, 7.6, 7.0, 5.7, 4.1 Hz), 3.99 (2H, d, J = 5.7 Hz), 7.02–7.13 (4H, 7.10 (ddd, J = 8.5, 1.6, 0.6 Hz), 7.06 (ddd, J = 8.5, 2.5, 0.6 Hz)].

12.4.1.2 1-Bromo-4-(Cyclohexyl Methoxy)Benzene (Compound 2c)

Molecular formula :$C_{13}H_{17}BrO$; Yield = 4.3 g; molecular weight; 269; TLC (ethyl acetate: hexane; 60 : 40); LCMS-$[M+H]^+$-270; ^{1}H NMR: δ ppm: [1.25–1.58 (10H, 1.32 (dtt, J = 12.2, 10.4, 2.8 Hz), 1.42 (dtt, J = 12.9, 10.4, 2.9 Hz), 1.52 (d, J = 12.6, 2.9 Hz), 1.52 (dtd, J = 12.7, 10.4, 2.9 Hz), 1.41 (dquint, J = 12.9, 2.9 Hz), 1.42 (dquint, J = 12.3, 2.95 Hz), 1.78 (1H, ttt, J = 10.4, 5.9, 2.9 Hz), 4.00 (2H, d, J = 6.0 Hz), 7.02–7.12 (4H, 7.11 (ddd, J = 8.6, 1.7, 0.7 Hz), 7.06 (ddd, J = 8.5, 2.5, 0.6 Hz)].

12.4.1.3 1-(Benzyloxy)-4-Bromobenzene (Compound 2d)

Molecular formula ;$C_{13}H_{11}BrO$; Yield = 5.3 g; molecular weight; 263; TLC (ethyl acetate:hexane; 60 : 40) LCMS-$[M+H]^+$-264.1; ^1H NMR: δ ppm; [5.13 (2H, s), 6.58 (2H, ddd, J =8.6, 2.8, 0.6 Hz), 7.12 (2H, ddd, J =8.6, 1.7, 0.65 Hz), 7.32–7.45 (5H, 7.40 (tt, J = 7.8, 1.35 Hz), 7.51 (dddd, J = 7.8, 7.61, 1.70, 0.55 Hz), 7.55 (dddd, J = 7.9, 1.4, 1.2, 0.6 Hz)].

12.4.1.4 1-Bromo-4-(Pentyloxy) Benzene (Compound 2e)

Molecular formula: $C_{11}H_{15}$ Br; yield = 5.5 g; Molecular weight: 243; TLC (ethyl acetate: hexane; 45 : 55) LCMS-$[M+H]^+$- 244.2; ^1H NMR: δ ppm: [0.86 (3H, t, J =7.1 Hz), 1.30 (2H, J =7.2 Hz), 1.37 (2H, tt, J =7.6, 7.2 Hz), 1.83 (2H, quint, J =7.5 Hz), 4.05 (2H, t, J =7.5 Hz), 7.02–7.11 (4H, 7.01 (ddd, J =8.6, 1.7, 0.7 Hz), 7.07 (ddd, J =8.6, 2.8, 0.7 Hz)].

12.4.1.5 Synthesis of 4-Methoxy Phenyl-Bispinacolato Adduct (3a)

^1H NMR: δ: 0.27–0.39 (4H, 0.32 (dtd, J = 8.4, 7.6, 5.7 Hz), 0.32 (tdd, J = 8.3, 7.7, 5.9 Hz)), 0.74–0.95 (13H, 0.86 (s), 0.85 (ttt, J = 8.1, 7.6, 6.7 Hz)), 1.02 (4H, d, J = 11.6 Hz), 4.08 (2H, d, J = 6.5 Hz), 6.82 (2H, ddd, J = 8.3, 1.3, 0.7 Hz), 7.31 (2H, ddd, J = 8.3, 1.2, 0.7 Hz).

12.4.1.6 Synthesis of 4-Methoxy Phenyl Boronic Acid

^1H NMR: δ : 0.23–0.36 (4H, 0.32 (dtd, J = 8.2, 7.6, 5.7 Hz), 0.35 (tdd, J = 8.2, 7.6, 5.7 Hz)), 0.85 (1H, ttt, J = 8.2, 7.6, 6.7 Hz), 4.15 (2H, d, J = 7.2 Hz), 7.09 (2H, ddd, J = 8.2, 1.5, 0.6 Hz), 7.35 (2H, ddd, J = 8.2, 1.3, 0.6 Hz).

12.4.1.7 General Procedure for the Synthesis of Derivatives (Compounds 6–10) (Step II)

1 l RB flask fitted with N_2 inlet ethyl 6-chloropyridine-3-carboxylate (1.5 g, 0.008 10 M ratio) was added under stirring in absolute ethanol. To the RM 4-methoxy cyclopropyl phenyl boronic acid (1.5 g, 0.008 10 M ratio), K_2CO_3 (2 g), Tetrakis (triphenylphosphine) palladium(0) (0.25 mg) were added and refluxed for five to eight hours (Suzuki coupling) [34–36], completion of the reaction monitored by TLC, solvent evaporated with rota evaporator, diluted with cold water, product was extracted with ethyl acetate (25 ml × 3 times), washed with 10 ml of brine, evaporated completely. The solid product was obtained after sonication of the gel with *n*-pentane and obtained as coupled products **6–10**.

12.4.1.8 General Procedure for the Synthesis of Derivatives (Compounds 6a–10a)

Products obtained in the previous steps **6–10** were taken in round bottom flask fitted with N_2, added with methanolic solution of LiOH and kept for stirring two to three hours. Product formation was monitored with the TLC techniques. After completion of the reaction, solvent evaporated, added ice cold water, neutralised excess of LiOH by adding drop-wise NH_4OH solution up to pH = 8–9, precipitate formed was filtered, washed with 10–20 ml of cold water and dried [37]. Dried powder was refluxed in ethanol and added with 2–4 ml of hydrazine hydrate monohydrate [38–40] for 10–12 hours. Completion of the reaction was monitored by TLC, solvent was completely removed by rota evaporation, diluted with ice cold water and kept under stirring for one hour. The precipitate of corresponding hydrazine hydrate washed with cold water, dried, and obtained as **6a–10a** compounds.

12.4.1.9 General Procedure for the Synthesis of Derivatives (Compounds 12–16)

The hydrazides **6a–10a** obtained in the previous step were taken in a round bottomed flask under nitrogen atmosphere in the presence of phosphoryl oxychloride (2–4 ml), benzoxaborole-6-carboxylic acid [41–42] (1.1 M ratio) in microwave. Microwave irradiation was done in an interval of two to five minutes, product formation and completeness of the reaction were continuously monitored by TLC, cyclised product was cooled, diluted with 20 ml of ice cold water and added drop-wise NH_4OH solution under stirring (pH = 9), precipitate formed was filtered, washed with cold water, and extracted in 20–25 ml of ethyl acetate. The crude product was subjected for column-chromatography purification {ethyl acetate (35–80 ml): hexane (65–20 ml)}. The eluted fractions were concentrated and obtained final cyclised products 12–16.

12.5 Results and Discussion

12.5.1 *In Vitro* Antiplasmodial Activity

Parasites *P. falciparum* and W_2 strains cultured in RPMI medium (Sigma–Aldrich, India) added with 0.5% Albumax I (Alfa Assar, India), hypoxanthine (Sigma–Aldrich, India), gentamicin (Sigma–Aldrich, India), and human erythrocytes [43]. The entire cultured medium subjected for incubation at 35 °C. *In vitro* activity of the cultured, grown parasites was performed ranging from elute concentration 100 μM to 50 nM and appropriate amount of inhibited drug was calculated with the emission and absorption fluorescence spectrum with the help of reference strain W_2 adopted and reference strain W_2 was susceptible to chloroquine and quinine molecules. The bezoxaborole containing 1,3,4-oxadiazole drug molecules and respective quantities of the DNA treated with the cultured parasites using human erythrocytes as control cultures. The well plates added with the SYBR Green I [44–46] and fluorescent absorptivity were measured. Further 100–150 μl of the homogenised culture was transferred to 96-well plate, added with 100 μl of the SYBR Green I lysis with buffer solution (SYBR Green, 20 mM Tris base pH 7.5, 5 mm EDTA, 0.008–0.009 w/v% saponin, 0.08–0.09 w/v% Triton X-100). DMSO or typically water was used as a negative control [47] and chloroquine or quinine was made as positive control molecules [48–49]; these were added to well plates during experimentation. However, well plates kept at same temperature and read on a fluorescence plate reader using excitation and emission wavelengths of 485 and 540 nm, respectively. Concentrations inhibiting 50% of the parasite's growth were then calculated from the obtained experimental results using a regression program available on line (Figures 12.4–12.7 and Tables 12.1–12.3) [50].

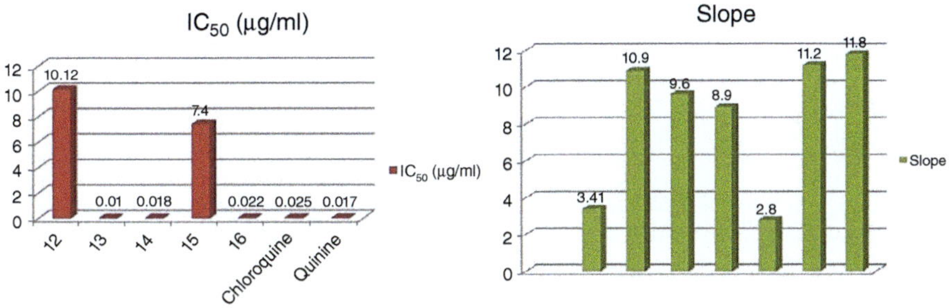

Figure 12.4 Bar diagram of the IC_{50} values for the compounds **13**, **14**, and **16** and their respective slope.

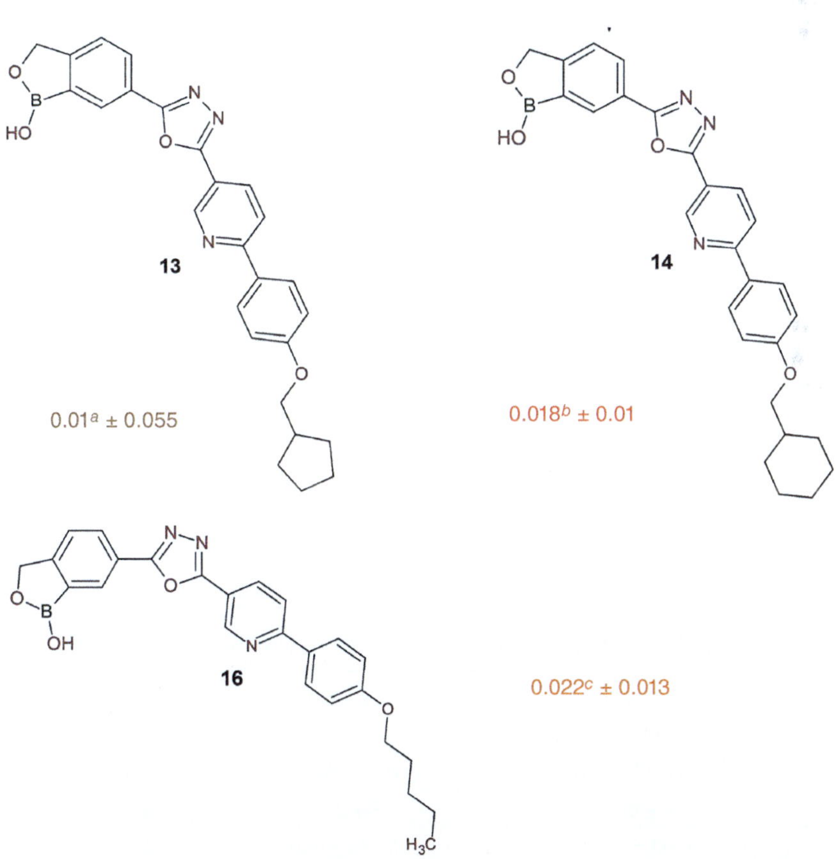

Figure 12.5 List of potent molecules having respective IC_{50} values against *P. falciparum*.

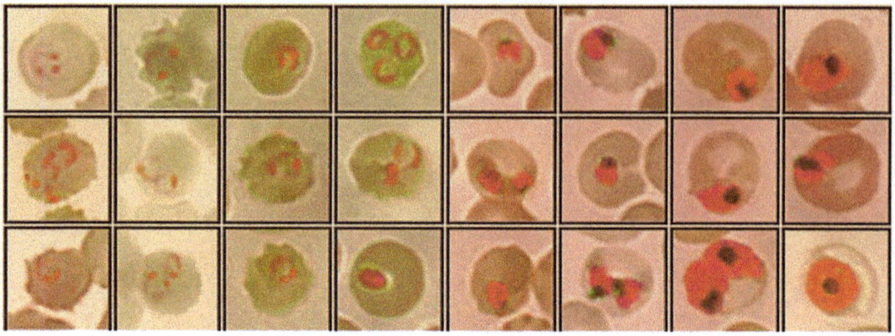

Figure 12.6 Pictures of *P. falciparum* inhibition against benzoxaborole 1,3,4-oxadiazole drug molecules with absorption and emission intensities of 485 and 590 nm, respectively.

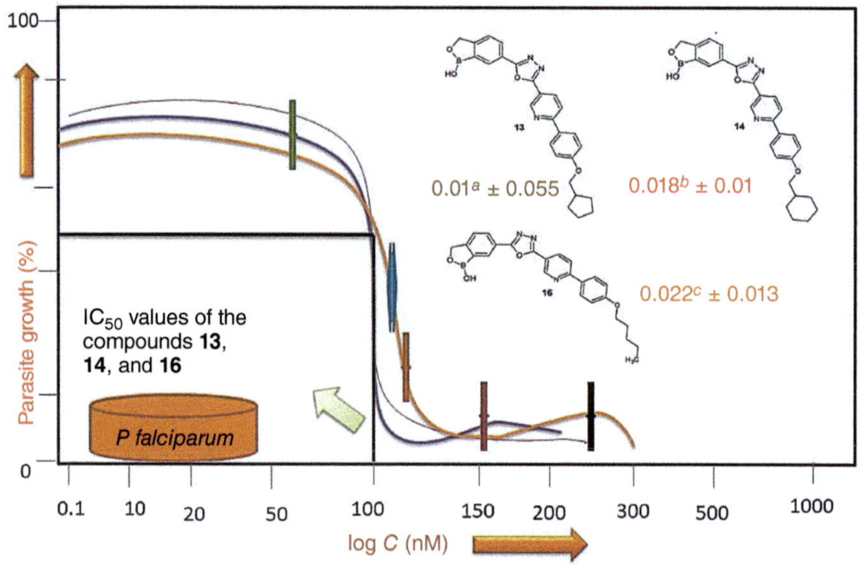

Figure 12.7 IC_{50} values for the curves against % growth of parasites and log of concentration for the potent drug molecules **13**, **14**, and **16**.

Table 12.1 IC_{50} values of the compounds **12–16** against *P. falciparum*.

Compounds	IC_{50} (Mean ± SD) (μg/ml)	Strains W_2 (μg/ml)	Slope
12	10.12 ± 0.011	11.2 ± 0.011	3.41
13	0.01[a)] ± 0.055	0.08 ± 0.055	10.9
14	0.018[b)] ± 0.01	0.25 ± 0.01	9.6
15	7.4 ± 0.2	7.8 ± 0.2	8.9
16	0.022[c)] ± 0.013	0.654 ± 0.013	2.8
Chloroquine	0.025 ± 0.01	0.55 ± 0.01	11.2
Quinine	0.017 ± 0.005	1.15 ± 0.005	11.8

a), b), c) Highest IC_{50} values.

Table 12.2 IC_{50} values of the compounds **6a–10a** against *P. falciparum*.

Compounds	IC_{50} (Mean ± SD) (μg/ml)	Strains W_2 (μg/ml)	Slope
6a	0.78 ± 0.013	2.28 ± 0.013	9.87
7a	0.25 ± 0.2	1.28 ± 0.2	5.47
8a	2.23 ± 0.3	3.47 ± 0.3	13.7
9a	6.6 ± 0.04	1.28 ± 0.04	11.9
10a	8.5 ±0.06	9.8 ± 0.06	4.95
Chloroquine	0.025 ± 0.01	0.55 ± 0.01	11.2
Quinine	0.017 ± 0.01	1.15 ± 0.02	11.8

Table 12.3 $C \log P$ values and solubility of the synthesised 1,3-bezoxazole 1,3,4-oxadiazole derivatives at 30 °C.

Compounds	$C \log P$	Solubility (μg/ml)	
		pH = 11	pH = 7
12	4.14	3.2 ± 0.06	5.57 ± 0.06
13	5.24	4.14 ± 0.012	6.25 ± 0.012
14	6.24	2.12 ± 0.7	8.75 ± 0.7
15	2.12	4.78 ± 0.05	9.87 ± 0.05[a)]
16	1.89	6.96 ± 0.09	4.81 ± 0.09
Chloroquine	6.98	8.7 ± 0.45	8.08 ± 0.45
Quinine	5.54	7.41 ± 0.48	7.19 ± 0.48

a) Highest solubility at pH = 7.

12.6 Conclusion

In the present research, a series of novel class of 1,3-benzoxazole derivatives containing 1,3,4-oxadiazole moiety were synthesised by microwave cyclisation of 1,3-bezoxazole-6-carboxylic acid (11) with intermediate compounds **6a–10a** under acidic conditions. All the compounds **6a–10a** and **12–16** were column purified and characterised by ^{1}H-NMR, ^{13}C-NMR, LCMS, and HPLC spectroscopic investigations. Intermediate and final compounds subjected for *in vitro* antimalarial studies using *P. falciparum* results showed remarkable properties. Compounds **13**, **14**, and **16** IC_{50} values are 10, 18, and 22 nM and $C \log P$ values are 5.24, 6.24, and 1.89, respectively. The aqueous solubility of the derivatives **13**, **14**, and **16** found to be 6.25 ± 0.012, 8.75 ± 0.7, and 4.81 ± 0.09 μg/ml, respectively. The presence of non-polar, penetrable and highly aqueous soluble side chains in the molecules **13**, **14**, and **16** and their $C \log P$ values made compounds possessing better IC_{50} values as compared with existing drug.

Authors Contributions

Dr Vinayak Adimule, Design, synthesis, characterisation of the 1,3-benzoxazole derivatives containing 1,3,4-oxadiazole compounds, preparation of the manuscript and Dr Debdas Bowmik, Design and interpretation of the spectral data of the synthesised compounds, partly by preparation of the manuscript. Mr Adarsha H.J. Gowda contributed for cell line activity against *P. falciparum* and partly by preparation of the manuscript. Dr Santosh S Nandi contributed in the preparation of the manuscript and formatting.

Acknowledgments

All the authors are thankful to MS Ramaiah Institute of Technology, Bangalore, CENSE, IISc, Bangalore for characterisation of the synthesised compounds, MTCC, for the cell line delivery and NUI, Ireland for the *in vitro* activity of the compounds.

Conflict of Interest

All authors declare that they do not have any conflict of interest.

References

1 Kevin, B.J. (2013). Evidence and implications of mortality associated with acute *Plasmodium vivax* malaria. *Clinical Microbiology Reviews* 26: 36–57. https://doi.org/10.1128/CMR.00074-12.
2 Juan, P.Q., Andre, M.S., Alberto, T. et al. (2011). Malaria-related anaemia: a Latin American perspective. *Memórias do Instituto Oswaldo Cruz* 106: 91–104. https://doi.org/10.1590/S0074-02762011000900012.
3 Jemma, D., Armin, P., Hans-Peter, B. et al. (2019). The *Plasmodium falciparum* Hsp70-x chaperone assists the heat stress response of the malaria parasite. *The FASEB Journal* 33: 14611–14624. https://doi.org/10.1096/fj.201901741R.
4 Susanta, K.G. and Manju, R. (2019). Malaria elimination in India—the way forward. *Journal of Vector Borne Diseases* 56: 32–40. https://doi.org/10.4103/0972-9062.257771.
5 D'Acremont, V., Christian, L., Blaise, G. et al. (2010). Reduction in the proportion of fevers associated with *Plasmodium falciparum* parasitaemia in Africa: a systematic review. *Malaria Journal* 9: 240. https://doi.org/10.1186/1475-2875-9-240.
6 Judith, A.O., Simon, I.H., Carlos, A.G. et al. (2004). The relationship between the *Plasmodium falciparum* parasite ratio in childhood and climate estimates of malaria transmission in Kenya. *Malaria Journal* 3: 17. https://doi.org/10.1186/1475-2875-3-17.

7 Yazoume, Y., Moshe, H., Valerie, L. et al. (2006). Housing conditions and *Plasmodium falciparum* infection: protective effect of iron-sheet roofed houses. *Malaria Journal* 5: 8. https://doi.org/10.1186/1475-2875-5-8.

8 O'Meara, W.P., Phillip, B., Tabitha, W.M. et al. (2008). Effect of a fall in malaria transmission on morbidity and mortality in Kilifi, Kenya. *The Lancet* 372: 1555–1562. https://doi.org/10.1016/S0140-6736(08)61655-4.

9 Hutt, M.P., Elslager, E.F., and Werbel, L.M. (1970). 2-Phenyl-5-(trichloromethyl)-1,3,4-oxadiazoles, a new class of antimalarial substances. *Journal of Heterocyclic Chemistry* 7: 511–518. https://doi.org/10.1002/jhet.5570070308.

10 Al-Wahaibi, L.H., Nandakumar, S.K., El-Emam, A.A. et al. (2019). Investigation of potential anti-malarial lead candidate 2-(4-fluorobenzylthio)-5-(5-bromothiophen-2-yl)-1,3,4-oxadiazole: Insights from crystal structure, DFT, QTAIM and hybrid QM/MM binding energy analysis. *Journal of Molecular Structure* 1175: 230–240. https://doi.org/10.1016/j.molstruc.2018.07.102.

11 Wang, X., Yan, J., Wang, M. et al. (2018). Synthesis and three-dimensional quantitative structure–activity relationship study of quinazoline derivatives containing a 1,3,4-oxadiazole moiety as efficient inhibitors against *Xanthomonas axonopodis pv. citri*. *Molecular Diversity* 22: 791–802. https://doi.org/10.1007/s11030-018-9837-0.

12 Bijan, P.D., Rebecca, A.W., David, W.B. et al. (1980). Synthesis and antitrypanosomal activity of some bis(4-guanylphenyl) five- and six-membered ring heterocycles. *Journal of Medicinal Chemistry* 23: 578–581. https://doi.org/10.1021/jm00179a022.

13 Horrocks, P., Pickard, M.R., Parekh, H.H. et al. (2013). Synthesis and biological evaluation of 3-(4-chlorophenyl)-4-substituted pyrazole derivatives. *Organic & Biomolecular Chemistry* 11: 4891–4898. https://doi.org/10.1039/c3ob27290g.

14 Shipra, B., Vijay, K., Simranjeet, S. et al. (2019). Synthesis, biological activities and docking studies of piperazine incorporated 1,3,4-oxadiazole derivatives. *Journal of Molecular Structure* 1191: 197–205. https://doi.org/10.1016/bj.molstruc.2019.04.106.

15 Parikh, P.H., Timaniya, J.B., Patel, M.J. et al. (2020, 2020). Design, synthesis, and characterization of novel substituted 1,2,4-oxadiazole and their biological broadcast. *Medicinal Chemistry Research* 29: 538–548. https://doi.org/10.1007/s00044-020-02505-8.

16 Murty, M.S.R., Ram, K.R., Rao, R.V. et al. (2011). Synthesis and preliminary evaluation of 2-substituted-1,3-benzoxazole and 3-[(3-substituted) propyl]-1,3-benzoxazol-2(3*H*)-one derivatives as potent anticancer agents. *Medicinal Chemistry Research* 20: 576–586. https://doi.org/10.1007/s00044-010-9353-y.

17 Vijesh, A.M., Arun, M.I., Prashanth, S. et al. (2013). New pyrazole derivatives containing 1,2,4-triazoles and benzoxazoles as potent antimicrobial and analgesic agents. *European Journal of Medicinal Chemistry* 62: 410–415. https://doi.org/10.1016/j.ejmech.2012.12.057.

18 Ananya, S., Leena, A., Nidhi, J. et al. (2015). One-pot sequential alkynylation and cycloaddition: regioselective construction and biological evaluation of novel benzoxazole–triazole derivatives. *ACS Combinatorial Science* 17: 39–48. https://doi.org/10.1021/co500135z.

19 Parhizgar, A.R. and Tahghighi, A. (2017). Introducing new antimalarial analogues of chloroquine and amodiaquine: a narrative review. *Iranian Journal of Medical Sciences* 42: 115–128. PMCID: PMC5366359.

20 Stephen, J.K., Margaret, J.D., Jocelyn, H. et al. (1992). Antimalarial drugs. 64. Synthesis and antimalarial properties of 1-imino derivatives of 7-chloro-3-substituted-3,4-dihydro-1,9(2*H*,10*H*)-acridinediones and related structures. *Journal of Medicinal Chemistry* 35: 3429–3447. https://doi.org/10.1021/jm00097a001.

21 Abdul Amin, S.K., Nilanjan, A., Shovanlal, G. et al. (2019). Reliable structural information for rational design of benzoxazole type potential cholesteryl ester transfer protein (CETP) inhibitors through multiple validated modelling techniques. *Journal of Biomolecular Structure and Dynamics* 37: 4528–4541. https://doi.org/10.1080/07391102.2018.1552895.

22 Sunetra, R., Peter, B.M., Paul, C. et al. (2010). Development of a new generation of 4-aminoquinoline antimalarial compounds using predictive pharmacokinetic and toxicology models. *Journal of Medicinal Chemistry* 53: 3685–3695. https://doi.org/10.1021/jm100057h.

23 Sreekanth, R., Shahul, H.P., Abhishek, S. et al. (2014). *N*-Aryl-2-aminobenzimidazoles: novel, efficacious, antimalarial lead compounds. *Journal of Medicinal Chemistry* 57: 6642–6652. https://doi.org/10.1021/jm500715u.

24 Clare, E.G., Marshall, M.H., Apurba, K.B. et al. (2011). In vitro efficacy of 7-benzylamino-1-isoquinolinamines against *Plasmodium falciparum* related to the efficacy of chalcones. *Bioorganic & Medicinal Chemistry Letters* 21: 786–789. https://doi.org/10.1016/j.bmcl.2010.11.099.

25 Carvalho, L.H., Brandao, M.G., Santos-Filho, D. et al. (1991). Antimalarial activity of crude extracts from Brazilian plants studied in vivo in *Plasmodium berghei*-infected mice and in vitro against *Plasmodium falciparum* in culture. *Brazilian Journal of Medical and Biological Research* 24: 1113–1123. https://pubmed.ncbi.nlm.nih.gov/1823001/.

26 Domarle, O., Blampain, G., Agnaniet, H. et al. (1998). In vitro antimalarial activity of a new organometallic analog, ferrocene–chloroquine. *Antimicrobial Agents and Chemotherapy* 42: 540–544. https://doi.org/10.1128/AAC.42.3.540.

27 Frederique, M., Mathias, M., Christine, L. et al. (2006). In vitro antimalarial activity of flavonoid derivatives dehydrosilybin and 8-(1;1)-DMA-kaempferide. *Acta Tropica* 97: 102–107. https://doi.org/10.1016/j.actatropica.2005.09.004.

28 Azas, N., Laurencin, N., Delmas, F. et al. (2002). Synergistic in vitro antimalarial activity of plant extracts used as traditional herbal remedies in Mali. *Parasitology Research* 88: 165–171. https://doi.org/10.1007/s004360100454.

29 Traore-Keita, K.F., Gasquet, M., Di Giorgio, C. et al. (2000). Antimalarial activity of four plants used in traditional medicine in Mali. *Phytotherphy Research* 14: 45–47. https://doi.org/10.1002/(SICI)1099-1573(200002)14.

30 Kuria, K.A.M., De Coster, S., Muriuki, G. et al. (2001). Antimalarial activity of *Ajugaremota Benth* (*Labiatae*) and *Caesalpinia volkensii Harms* (*Caesalpiniaceae*): in vitro confirmation of ethno pharmacological use. *Journal of Ethno pharmacology* 74: 141–148. https://doi.org/10.1016/S0378-8741(00)00367-6.

31 Sanon, S., Azas, N., Gasquet, M. et al. (2003). Antiplasmodial activity of alkaloid extracts from *Pavettacrassipes* (*K. Schum*) and *Acanthospermum hispidum* (*DC*), two plants used in traditional medicine in Burkina Faso. *Parasitology Research* 90: 314–317. https://doi.org/10.1007/s00436-003-0859-9.

32 Jacob, D., Johnson, R.A., Dennull, L.G. et al. (2007). Waters assessment and continued validation of the malaria SYBR Green I-based fluorescence assay for use in malaria drug screening. *Antimicrobial Agents and Chemotherapy* 51: 1926–1933. https://doi.org/10.1128/AAC.01607-06.

33 Sahu, R., Walker, L.A., Tekwani, B.L. et al. (2014). In vitro and in vivo antimalarial activity of tigecycline a glycylcycline antibiotic, in combination with chloroquine. *Malaria Journal* 13: 414. https://doi.org/10.1186/1475-2875-13-414.

34 Said, E., Nicole, C., Youssef, B. et al. (2003). An efficient synthesis of chalcones based on the Suzuki reaction. *Tetrahedron Letters* 44: 5359–5363. https://doi.org/10.1016/S0040-4039(03)01140-7.

35 Ning, L., Chun, L., Zilin, J. et al. (2011). Green synthesis of fluorinated biaryl derivatives via thermo regulated ligand/palladium-catalysed Suzuki reaction. *Journal of Organometallic Chemistry* 696: 2641–2647. https://doi.org/10.1016/j.jorganchem.2011.04.007.

36 Emilia, P., Nicolas, M., Patricia, M. et al. (2007). Suzuki–Miyaura cross-coupling reaction as the key step for the synthesis of some new 4′-aryl and alkyl substituted analogues of amodiaquine and amopyroquine. *Tetrahedron* 63: 12791–12810. https://doi.org/10.1016/j.tet.2007.08.115.

37 Braulio, I., Alba, M., Diana, B. et al. (2013). Synthesis of novel analogs of 2-pyrazoline obtained from [(7-chloroquinolin-4-yl) amino] chalcones and hydrazine as potential antitumor and antimalarial agents. *European Journal of Medicinal Chemistry* 67: 252–262. https://doi.org/10.1016/j.ejmech.2013.06.049.

38 Pieber, B., Glasnov, T., Kappe, C.O. et al. (2015). Continuous flow reduction of artemisinic acid utilizing multi-injection strategies-closing the gap towards a fully continuous synthesis of antimalarial drugs. *Chemistry of European Journal* 21: 4368–4376. https://doi.org/10.1002/chem.201406439.

39 Sandra, G., Gagan, K., Caterina, F. et al. (2006). Synthesis of *N*-1-arylidene-*N*-2-quinolyl- and *N*-2-acrydinylhydrazones as potent antimalarial agents active against CQ-resistant *P. falciparum* strains. *Bioorganic & Medicinal Chemistry Letters* 16: 5384–5388. https://doi.org/10.1016/j.bmcl.2006.07.060.

40 Kurasawa, Y., Yoshida, K., Yamazaki, N. et al. (2012). Quinolone analogues 11: synthesis of novel 4-quinolone-3-carbohydrazide derivatives with antimalarial activity. *Journal of Heterocyclic Chemistry* 49: 288–292. https://doi.org/10.1002/jhet.774.

41 Charles, Z.D., Yong-Kang, Z., Xianfeng, L. et al. (2010). Synthesis and biological evaluations of P4-benzoxaborole-substituted macrocyclic inhibitors of HCV NS3 protease. *Bioorganic & Medicinal Chemistry Letters* 20: 7317–7322. https://doi.org/10.1016/j.bmcl.2010.10.071.

42 Tsutomu, A., Yong-Kang, Z., Yvonne, R.F. et al. Identification of a 4-fluorobenzyl l-valinate amide benzoxaborole (AN11736) as a potential development candidate for the treatment of *Animal African Trypanosomiasis* (AAT). *Bioorganic & Medicinal Chemistry Letters* 28: 6–10. https://doi.org/10.1016/j.bmcl.2017.11.028.

43 Gumbo, M., Beteck, R.M., Mandizvo, T. et al. (2018). Cinnamoyl-oxaborole amides: synthesis and their in vitro biological activity. *Molecules* 23: 2038. https://doi.org/10.3390/molecules23082038.

44 Zulu, A.I., Oderinlo, O.O., Kruger, C. et al. (2020). Synthesis, structure and in vitro anti-trypanosomal activity of non-toxic arylpyrrole-based chalcone Derivatives. *Molecules* 25: 1668. https://doi.org/10.3390/molecules25071668.

45 Chunlin, Z., Wen, Z., Chunquan, S. et al. (2017). Chalcone: a privileged structure in medicinal chemistry. *Chemical Reviews* 117: 7762–7810. https://doi.org/10.1021/acs.chemrev.7b00020.

46 John, O. and Kelly, C. (2018). Recent updates in the discovery and development of novel antimalarial drug candidates. *RSC Medicinal Chemistry* 9: 437–453. https://doi.org/10.1039/C7MD00637C.

47 Duffey, M., Sanchez, C.P., Lanzer, M. et al. (2018). Profiling of the anti-malarial drug candidate SC83288 against artemisinins in *Plasmodium falciparum. Malaria Journal* 17: 121. https://doi.org/10.1186/s12936-018-2279-4.

48 Sabine, V.M., Tim, J., Kanyanga, C. et al. (2004). In vitro inhibition of β-haematin formation, DNA interactions, antiplasmodial activity and cytotoxicity of synthetic neocryptolepine derivatives. *Experimental Parasitology* 108: 163–168. https://doi.org/10.1016/j.exppara.2004.08.006.

49 Jenett-Siems, K., Mockenhaupt, F.P., Bienzle, U. et al. (1999). In vitro antiplasmodial activity of Central American medicinal plants. *Tropical Medicine & International Health* 4: 611–615. https://doi.org/10.1046/j.1365-3156.1999.00456.x.

50 Ravikumar, S., Ramanathan, G., Gnanadesigan, M. et al. (2012). In vitro antiplasmodial activity of spiro benzofuran compound from mangrove plant of Southern India. *Asian Pacific Journal of Tropical Medicine* 5: 358–361. https://doi.org/10.1016/S1995-7645(12)60059-5.

Part IV

A Vaccine Perspective

13

Recent Advances in Malaria Vaccine Development

Sailendra Kumar Mahanta

Department of Pharmacy, School of Health Sciences, The Assam Kaziranga University, Koraikhowa, NH-37, Jorhat, Assam 785 006, India

13.1 Introduction

As per WHO (World Health Organization, 2018) estimates, 228 million cases of malaria were recorded and 405 000 people lost their lives globally [1]. Malaria is a mosquito (female *Anopheles*) borne disease caused by a parasite of *Plasmodium* sp., and it transmits to humans through mosquito bites. Among the 100 species of *Plasmodium* known to humans, only the five species of *Plasmodium*, namely *Plasmodium falciparum* (*P. falciparum*), *Plasmodium malariae* (*P. malariae*), *Plasmodium vivax* (*P. vivax*), *Plasmodium ovale* (*P. ovale*), *Plasmodium knowlesi* (*P. knowlesi*) cause malaria. *P. falciparum* is known to cause maximum number of human deaths worldwide closely followed by *P. vivax*. Rest of the species cause only a small percentage of infections worldwide. The prevalence *of P. falciparum* is the highest in Africa (99.7%) followed by Eastern Mediterranean (71%), Western Pacific (65%), and South East Asia (50%) as per report of WHO. The prevalence *of P. vivax* (53%) is mainly predominant in South-East Asia, with India being the major contributor at 47% [1].

Rapid diagnostic test (RDT) kits are designed to detect the presence of *P. falciparum* exploiting the histidine-rich protein-2 (HRP2) present on the parasite surface. However, recently a lot of false-negative results are detected from the kits due to the absence of HRP2 on the surface of the parasite. The *P. falciparum* has evolved over the years, and certain regions of the world have already noticed the deletion of the genes *pfhrp2 and pfhrp3* in the parasite making it undetectable. So far 28 countries have reported the deletion of the gene *pfhrp2* from the parasite. Drug resistance has made it to the list of already existing challenges faced by mankind. Artemisinin resistance has cropped up in various parts of the world raising concerns considering the fact that it is the last line of drug-mediated defense we have against the parasite. *PfKelch13* mutation is identified recently as a marker for partial artemisinin resistance. Artemisinin-included combination therapies (ACTs) are increasingly popular among African countries such as

Drug Development for Malaria: Novel Approaches for Prevention and Treatment, First Edition.
Edited by Pravin Kendrekar.

artemether–lumefantrine (AL) combination, artesunate–amodiaquine (AS–AQ) combination, and dihydroartemisinin–piperaquine (DHA–PPQ) combination against *P. falciparum*. Chloroquine continues to be highly efficacious for *P. vivax* in most of the countries except Myanmar.

13.2 History of Malaria Vaccine Development

Almost six decades of research has been invested in the development of promising malaria vaccine. Preliminary work related to malaria vaccines dates back to 1942 where the administration of inactivated sporozoites to a domestic fowl demonstrated the development of immunity to subsequent exposure. The observed effect was attributed to the combination of cellular and humoral immune response [2]. Modern vaccine-related work gained momentum during the year 1960s when immunization studies were performed in mice administered with irradiated sporozoites and subsequent attempts to understand the mechanisms involved in the development of associated immunity [3–5]. Subsequent studies suggested that to achieve the highest level of protective immunity, one needs to be bitten by a large number of irradiated infective mosquitoes. In the early 1980s, circumsporozoite protein expressed on the surface of the sporozoites was identified raising hopes for development of a sporozoite vaccine. The gene sequencing and cloning of the sporozoite protein were carried out in search for the sporozoite vaccine. The period also saw a lot of progress in work for the development of a large number of blood stage vaccines (BSVs) due to the identification of several blood-stage antigens [6]. During the same period research also focused on the development of peptide-based vaccines such as SPf66 from Colombia and was evaluated in monkeys for development of immunity [7]. The experiment failed miserably. However, the only good news during the period came with the development of a new formulation from the circumsporozoite protein obtained from *P. falciparum* known as RTS, -S, in a novel adjuvant [8]. The formulated vaccine showed an excellent efficacy in sporozoite challenge tests [9]. The tests highlighted the detrimental role of cellular immunity in liver stage parasites in various animal models developed with the administration of irradiated sporozoites [10]. Spurred by the results there was a sudden surge in efforts to boost cellular immunity with focused research on plasmid DNA immunization. However, the first-generation DNA vaccines were less potent; hence, the focus shifted to boosting immunization techniques using viral vectors [11, 12]. RTS, -S vaccine has undergone rigorous tests and hogged the limelight in the year 2015 due to safety and efficacy clearance from the European Medicines Agency. The vaccine *RTS, -S*/AS01E (Mosquirix™) cleared the toughest scrutiny by WHO known as the Maturity Level 4 (ML4) [13]. Finally in the year 2019, *RTS, -S*/AS01E was used in a pilot implementation program for South African children, and the results were satisfying [14]. Clinical trial data during the last 20 years shows approximately 10 malaria vaccine trials each year (see Figure 13.1) [15].

Although trials related to *RTS, -S*/AS01E remained consistent throughout the period, trials related to whole sporozoite vaccines (WSVs) and transmission

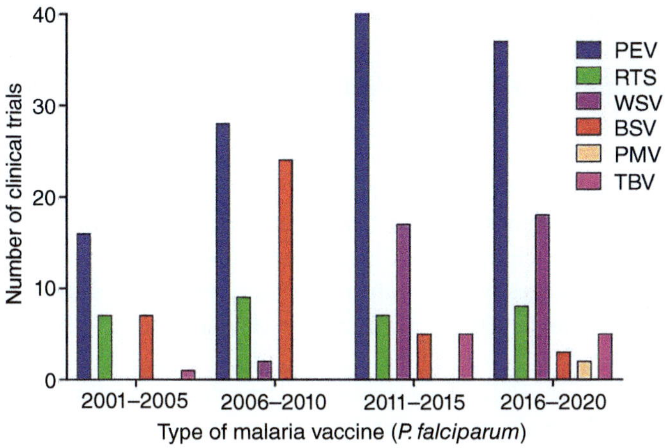

Figure 13.1 Clinical trials information for vaccines against *P. falciparum* at http://clinicaltrials.gov since 2000; PEV, pre-erythrocytic vaccines; *RTS*, *RTS* stands for the various components present in it i.e. "R" indicates the central repeat region of *P. falciparum* circumsporozoite protein (CSP), "T" indicates T-cell epitopes of the CSP; and the "S" indicated for Hepatitis B surface antigen (HBsAg). The above combination is fused in a single protein ("RTS"). WSV, whole sporozoite vaccine; BSV, blood stage vaccine; PMV, placental malaria vaccine; TBV, transmission blocking vaccines.

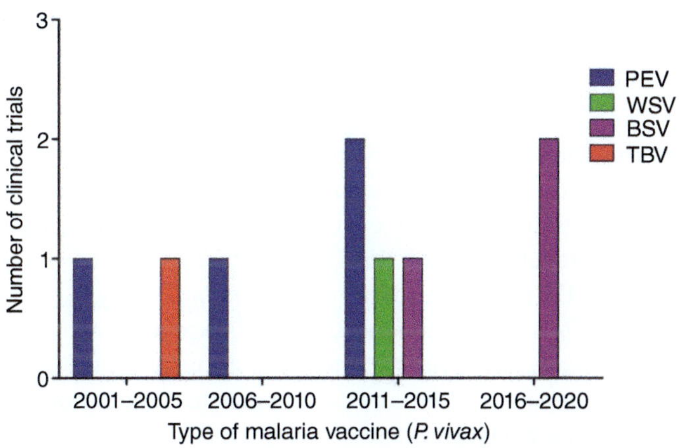

Figure 13.2 Clinical trials information for vaccines against *P. vivax* at http://clinicaltrials.gov since 2000.

blockade vaccines (TBVs) gained momentum during the period, while for BSVs decreased over the same time (see Figure 13.1) [15].

Moreover, only nine clinical trials for *P. vivax* were observed during the same period (see Figure 13.2) [15]. The reasons for such low numbers of clinical trials for the vaccine related to *P. vivax* may be due to the better efficacy of the existing drugs in most parts of the world.

13.3 Vaccine Design Targets and Approaches

In order to have a successful malaria vaccine, the life cycle of the malaria parasites need to be analyzed carefully and the stages where we can target the malaria parasite are identified. The life cycle of the malaria parasite is split between human beings and the female *Anopheles* mosquito. The genetic complexity of the parasite in addition to exposure of different antigens (proteins) to the human immune system makes it difficult to track with each infection. Since, the morphology of the parasite changes during the different stages of their entire life cycle, and the expression of antigens (proteins) changes frequently posing a serious challenge to its detection and initiating treatment.

Malarial parasites over the years have developed various mechanisms to evade the human immune system and remain undetected. The various stages of the life cycle of malaria parasite are discussed, and the approaches for vaccine design are shown in Figure 13.3.

Infection with malaria begins as soon as a person is bitten by a female *Anopheles* mosquito infected with the sporozoites of *Plasmodium* parasites. The sporozoites get injected in the blood stream with the bite and quickly move to the human liver. From the date of initiation of infection, the sporozoites multiply by asexual means in the liver without development of any visible symptoms over a period of 7–10 days. During this period the sporozoites mature into schizonts, or otherwise they remain in a dormant state known as Hypnozoites. During the last part of the stay of the schizonts in the liver, they form merozoites and are released into the blood. The merozoite stage of parasites is capable of starting asexual reproduction on their own. The symptoms associated with malaria are observed only in the presence of merozoites in the blood stream. After entering the blood stream, the merozoites make their way into erythrocytes and multiply rapidly. When the merozoite threshold load inside the RBC is exceeded, the RBC bursts and releases the merozoites into the blood stream. Inside the erythrocytes the merozoites attain a ring-like structure and are known as early trophozoite. In this stage, the merozoites derive nutrition from the erythrocytes to mature into a late trophozoite and subsequently the blood stage schizont. These are mature malaria parasites ready to be released into the blood once the threshold is attained. The cycle keeps on repeating itself, and the released merozoites from the erythrocytes keep on invading more erythrocytes.

Some of the late stage trophozoites develop into gametocytes and continue to stay in the blood. Subsequently, when a mosquito bites a human being carrying malaria parasite, it sucks the blood containing the gametocytes. These gametocytes further develop into mature gametes inside the mosquito and transform into oocytes that penetrate the gut wall lining of the mosquito and embed themselves on the gut wall lining as oocysts. Sporozoites continue to grow within the oocyst, and on attaining the threshold, the oocysts rupture and facilitate the movement of sporozoites into the gut cavity. The sporozoites finally reach the salivary glands of the mosquito from the gut. The infection continues as the mosquito having the malaria sporozoites bites a human being.

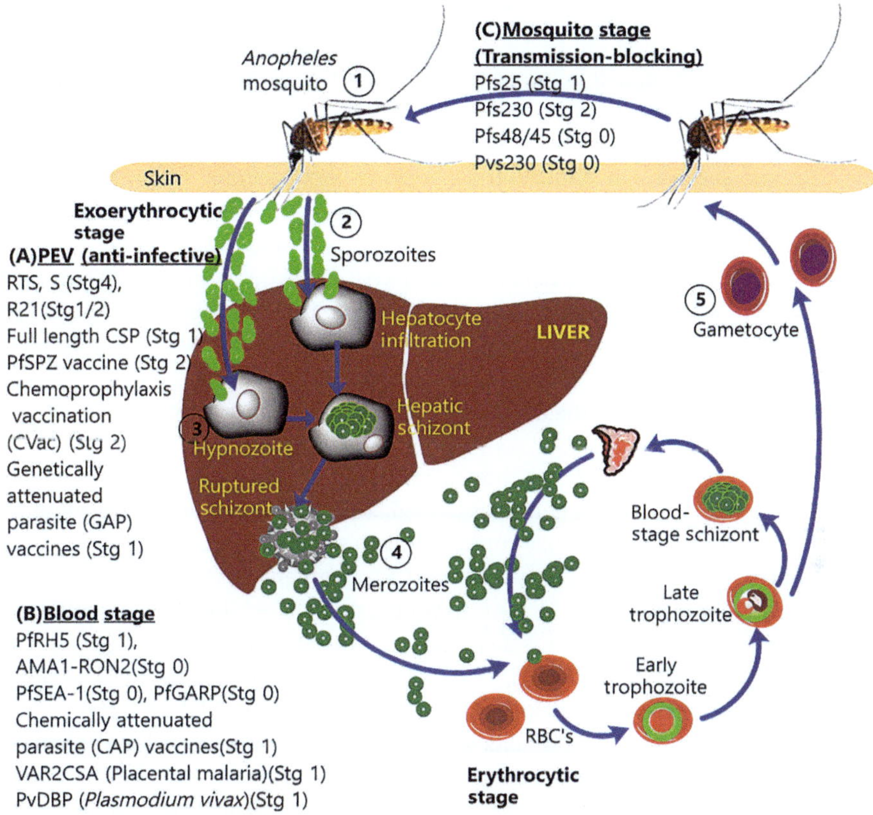

Figure 13.3 Life cycle of malaria, targets for vaccine design: 1. Vector (*Anopheles* mosquito); 2. The sporozoites (common target for most vaccines e.g. *RTS, -S*); 3. Hypnozoites and hepatic schizonts (vectored vaccines); 4. Erythrocytic stage: blood stage vaccines (merozoites are commonly targeted by protein present in adjuvant vaccine candidates); 5. Gametocytes and gamete formation within the mosquito; Malaria vaccine candidates from each category under clinical development (A) Pre-erythrocytic vaccines (PEV), (B) blood stage vaccines (BSV), (C) mosquito stage/transmission blocking vaccines, TBV [15]. The Stage (Stg) in brackets represents the Clinical Stage 0, 1, 2, 3, 4, respectively.

13.4 Types of Malaria Vaccine

13.4.1 Pre-erythrocytic Vaccines

Pre-erythrocytic vaccines (PEVs) specifically act on the antigens expressed on the surface of the sporozoites and liver stages (hypnozoites/liver schizonts) of *P. falciparum*. PEVs are designed to stimulate immune (T-cell mediated) responses that identify and destroy infected hepatocytes and sporozoites in the blood.

The efficacy of PEV dates back to 1970s wherein a human was exposed to irradiated WSVs through the bite of thousands of mosquitoes. The vaccine provided protection against homologous as well as heterogeneous *Plasmodium falciparum* sporozoites (PfSPZ). However, it did not protect from homologous blood stage merozoites and trophozoites. PEVs are also known as anti-infective vaccines (AIVs). *RTS, -S*/AS01E is the first PEV approved in the year 2019 for assessment of public safety through a pilot program in South Africa [16]. Depending on the immune response, duration of exposure, research focused on the development of vaccines that target the proteins expressed on the surface of sporozoite (Spz). Recent vaccines in clinical trials include Spz vaccines (attenuated), e.g. radiation-attenuated Spz, drug-attenuated Spz, and genetically attenuated Spz. Recombinant protein-based vaccines include *RTS, -S* and R21 and viral vector mediated vaccines such as Chad63 MVA ME-TRAP, CSVAC, ChAd63 METRAP, and MVA METRAP with the matrix-M adjuvant [17]. The list of selected malaria vaccine candidates from each category in preclinical or clinical trials is shown in Figure 13.3.

13.4.1.1 Vaccines Based on the RTS, -S, and CSP Encoded Sections of the Malaria Gene

The research finding that WSVs induce immunity in humans inspired genetic research on to it. The malaria gene was cloned, and this led to the identification of Circumsporozoite protein (CSP), a surface antigen of Sporozoites [18].

RTS, -S, (PEV), utilizes the *P. falciparum* CSP fragment with the central repeat gene section (abbreviated as "R"), the C terminus section (exhibiting T cell epitopes, abbreviated as "T"), and since it is fused with the hepatitis B surface antigen ("S"), it is abbreviated as "RTS." The *RTS, -S* PEV successfully reduced the clinical signs of severe malaria by approximately 36% (significant) in young children and approximately 26% (nonsignificant) in infants who have successfully received four doses of vaccine at 0, 1, 2, and 20 months, respectively. The discovery of *RTS, -S* PEV was a historical event in the area of malaria vaccines; however, the partial success in young children leaving behind the infants requires more clinical studies to perfect the PEV.

In order to enhance the immunogenicity of CSP-mediated vaccines, along similar lines a second-generation *RTS, -S* known as "R21" is being developed. R21 is administered with unfused Hepatitis virus surface antigen "S" and generates CSP-HbsAg fusion protein. R21 demonstrated mild immunogenic reactions in mice; however, the results showed that R21 protected the mice against exposure to transgenic sporozoites. Encouraged by the results obtained from the *in-vivo* studies, R21 has now moved into Phase I trial [19].

CSP shows high sequence specificity, and the validation came to the fore during the Phase 3 trial where the CSP showed increased protection against the parasite having a sequence matching [20]. The observation fueled an idea that proposed to modify the C terminal epitopes to target a variety of parasites. Moreover, the N-terminal section is not part of the *RTS, -S*; however, its role is detrimental to the interaction with the hepatocyte and mass entry of sporozoites [21]. Full-length CSP sequence-based vaccines are developed and undergoing clinical trials. CSP-based vaccines are modified at the epitopes based on the design of human monoclonal antibodies (mAbs) for increased recognition. The mAbs are obtained from humans exposed to PEVs or the malaria parasite [22–24]. Almost all the anti-CSP-mediated human mAbs interact with the central repeat section "R" followed by the N-terminal end and the least to the C-terminal end [22].

13.4.2 Whole Sporozoite Vaccines

Until 2010, the WSVs were not pursued in spite of demonstrated evidence in the year 1970 in support of its effectiveness in providing immunity against sporozoite challenge in humans. The perception of impracticality about the development of WSV changed after 2010 when Sanaria, a Biotechnology company, introduced a technology to harvest PfSPZ obtained from the saliva of mosquitoes exposed to *in-vitro* cultured malaria parasites [25]. Various attenuation strategies are employed for PfSPV, e.g. radiation attenuation (PfSPZ-R), chemical/drug attenuation (PfSPZ-CVac), genetic attenuation (PfSPZ-GA1) [26].

PfSPZ vaccine requires iv administration to provide immunity against sporozoites [15]. The efficacy of WSV is dose and regimen-dependent and the type of attenuated sporozoite under study [27, 28]. In individuals without malaria, PfSPZ-CVac attenuated using chloroquine provided long-lasting immunity (approximately two years) against homologous sporozoites and limited immunity against few vaccines [29, 30].

Irradiated sporozoites can enter the liver cells and mature within the cells, giving rise to damaged schizonts. The defective schizonts develop antigens having the potential to initiate a protective immune response with the activation of CD4 T cells, CD8 T cells, γδ T cells, and CSP protein Abs. However, defective schizonts fail to rupture and the merozoites do not make it to the blood stream and subsequently into the erythrocytes [31].

13.4.3 Blood Stage Vaccines (BSVs)

BSVs act on the asexual life cycle stage of the malaria parasite where it undergoes repetitive cycles of multiplication in erythrocytes causing the symptoms of malaria.

Each cycle duration in this repetitive phase varies across the malaria parasite species such as one and three days for *P. knowlesi* and *P. malariae*, respectively. The erythrocytic cycle is two days for *P. falciparum, P. vivax, and P. ovale*, respectively. At the completion of each erythrocytic cycle, merozoites are released into the blood and subsequently affect other erythrocytes. The cycle keeps repeating itself; however, a small fraction of erythrocytes evade the cyclic process and generate gametocytes that will subsequently infect mosquitoes.

The blood-stage parasite is the disease-causing stage in the life cycle of malaria. Moreover, IgG antibodies obtained from semi-immune individuals from Africa and Thailand were found to remove blood-stage parasites from such individuals [32]. Investigation into parasite preparations involving merozoites providing immunity dates back to 1977 where studies in monkeys demonstrated immunity against blood-stage malarial parasites [33].

The development of vaccines against the merozoites throws a lot of challenges since the merozoites within seconds infect a new erythrocyte after being released from one erythrocyte. Hence, circulating antibodies find it difficult to target the merozoites in blood. Moreover, antibody to merozoite ratio and antigen polymorphism are critical to the successful development of BSV. The antigens targeted for the development of BSV vaccines include MSP1, AMA1, EBA-175, and MSP3

[34]. In most of the cases, the high concentration of antibodies were maintained to achieve maximum immunity but failed to demonstrate efficacy against homologous parasites [35, 36]. GMZ2 (conserved domains of glutamate-rich protein, i.e. GLURP and merozoite surface protein-3 i.e. MSP3) is the only BSV vaccine to have demonstrated efficacy although low (14%), but statistically significant against naturally acquired infection [37]. Hence, the focus gradually shifted toward identification of novel antigen markers.

Plasmodium falciparum reticulocyte binding protein homolog 5 (PfRH5) interacts with erythrocytes by binding to basigin receptor present on the cell surface [38]. PfRH5 is a merozoite antigen having the ability to induce neutralizing antibody function. PfRH5-related preclinical investigations demonstrate enhanced immune-protection against blood-stage parasites, however, does not stimulate development vaccine induced antibodies. Moreover, a high concentration of the anti-PfRH5 IgG dose at 200 μg/ml is required to produce sustained immunity [39].

Apical membrane antigen 1 (AMA1) is another critical protein required for the growth of blood-stage malaria parasites. AMA1 interacts with the rhoptry neck protein (RON2), which is situated between the merozoite and erythrocyte interaction site. Upon binding with RON2, the antigenicity property of AMA1 increases tremendously [40]. *In-vivo* studies in monkeys demonstrate increased protection provided by AMA1-RON2 against heterologous blood-stage parasite challenges compared with AMA1 alone [41]. However, AMA1 shows extensive sequence polymorphism; hence more studies are required to validate its role in immunity.

Blood-stage parasite antigens translocate to the surface of the merozoite infested erythrocytes, thereby rendering them accessible for longer periods. Among the blood-stage parasite antigens, the *Plasmodium falciparum* erythrocyte membrane protein 1 (PfEMP1) interacts specifically with the malaria parasite antigens but could not develop enough research interest due to its high polymorphism, large size, and high content of cysteine residues [42].

Plasmodium falciparum glutamic-acid-rich protein (PfGARP) is a malaria parasite antigen (80 kDa) present on the membrane surface of erythrocytes that are infested with trophozoites. Antibodies targeting PfGARP kill erythrocytes containing trophozoites in culture by initiating apoptosis-like mechanisms in parasites. Preclinical studies in monkey show that vaccination with anti-PfGARP Abs provides partial protection against *P. falciparum* [43]. PfGARP-mediated vaccination can be co-administered with other vaccines for a more pronounced efficacy [44].

Plasmodium falciparum schizont egress antigen-1 (PfSEA-1), a malaria parasite antigen (244 kDa), is found to be expressed in erythrocytes infiltrated with malaria blood schizonts. The antibodies against PfSEA-1 decrease malaria parasite replication by preventing the rupture and release of schizonts into blood [45]. BSV lags significantly in comparison with its counterparts in vaccine development.

13.4.4 Placental Malaria Vaccines

In regions with a high prevalence of malaria, placental malaria (PM) is commonly observed where erythrocytes infested with *P. falciparum* accumulate in the placenta and trigger an inflammatory reaction affecting the placenta. Inflammatory PM is closely linked to anemia, pre-term low birth weight, and fetal death [46]. The placental accumulation of infected erythrocytes is facilitated due to the presence of antigen VAR2CSA on the membrane surface. VAR2CSA is a cysteine-rich transmembranous protein from the PfEMP1 family. It binds selectively to Chondroitin Sulfate A (CSA), which is located in between the villi of the placenta [47, 48].

Experimental evidence proves that parasites obtained from placenta routinely demonstrate expression of VAR2CSA [49]. Moreover, antibodies were found to inhibit infected erythrocytes binding to CSA and VAR2CSA. Women developing anti-adhesion antibodies due to VAR2CSA vaccination were found to be immune to effects of PM [50].

Based on the above preclinical results, recombinant VAR2CSA was developed that selectively binds to CSA at nanomolar concentrations [51]. Two vaccine candidates developed from VAR2CSA block the interaction of infected erythrocytes to CSA and avoid placental accumulation; however, the final results of the study are yet to come [52, 53]. The first vaccine PAMVAC (expressed in *Drosophila*) was tested in humans along with various human adjuvants. It was found safe, and it produced effective antibodies against homologous parasite challenges in humans [54]. The next PMV vaccine PRIMVAC is derived from VAR2CSA and prevents serious outcomes of *P. falciparum* during pregnancy. PRIMVAC was safe for human use, however, activated immune reactions, and stimulated development of antibodies against the VAR2CSA form expressed by transgenic NF54-CSA infested erythrocytes. Hence, an alternate schedule of immunization was proposed to address, the antigen concentration, and synergistic additions with the other VAR2CSA variants to improve the reactivity with other heterologous variants [55].

13.4.5 Transmission Blocking Vaccines (TBV)

TBV binds to surface antigens on gametocytes and facilitates antibodies that destroy malarial parasites in the blood meal of mosquitoes and disrupt the parasite cycle [56]. Antibodies against the surface antigens are developed in mice by exposing them to the sexual stage of the malaria parasite. The two gamete surface proteins Pfs230 and Pfs48/45 of *P. falciparum* are expressed by gametocytes during its presence in human blood [56] while Pfs25 and Pfs28 are zygote surface proteins (Zsp) that develop after sexual phase in the mosquitoes [57]. Pfs25 has garnered a lot of attention for clinical trials due to the effective serum transmission blocking activity as demonstrated in *in-vivo* preclinical studies. A lot of clinical trials are now focused on evaluating and replicating the lytic activity of Pfs230 against *P. falciparum* gametes as demonstrated in animal studies. However, Pfs25 and Pfs230 antigens demonstrated a low immunogenic profile [58].

Pfs25-EPA conjugate formulated with Alhydrogel® reportedly blocked the transmission of gametes of *P. falciparum* to female *Anopheles* mosquitoes [59]. Pfs48/45 is another gametocyte surface protein (GSP) expressed during the closing periods of gametocyte formation in erythrocytes. Pfs48/45 is a surface antigen expressed on both the male and female gametes, which interacts with Pfs230 to form a complex. Pfs48/45 and Pfs230 play a critical role in the maintenance of fertility associated with male gametes, hence, blocking it with antibodies seems to be a valid approach [60].

13.4.6 Vaccines for *P. vivax*

Plasmodium vivax has not received the kind of attention; it should have received in spite of having more number of hypnozoites leading to frequent relapse. Moreover, clinical trial information during the periods 2000–2020 shows only nine clinical trials, which is clearly not enough to reign in *P. vivax*. *P. vivax* vaccines undergoing trials in humans include *Plasmodium vivax* circumsporozoite protein (PvCSP) and Pvs25, of the pre-erythrocytic vaccine (PfCSP) and transmission blocking vaccines (Pfs25) [15]. *P. vivax* vaccine Pvs230D1-EPA is under development and may undergo Phase 1 trials in late 2021. Two BSV trials based on *P. vivax* have targeted the *P. vivax* Duffy-Binding Protein (PvDBP), which interacts with the Duffy Antigen Receptor present on red blood cells and is detrimental for the entry of merozoites [15, 61].

13.5 Conclusions

The progress in the number of malaria vaccine candidates in 2020 is significantly higher 20 years down the lane. The PEV, *RTS, -S*/AS01E is safe and has demonstrated its efficacy. *RTS, -S* has demonstrated considerable reduction in risk against clinical malaria. PEVs such as R21, PfSPZ (whole sporozoite vaccines), and CSP need to improve their efficacy profile. TBVs have made rapid strides into Phase 2 clinical trials during the last decade and proved to be synergistically efficacious in combination with PEVs against *P. falciparum*.

BSVs could not live upto its initial hype during the last 20 years targeting merozoite invasion proteins and have delivered disappointing results. Hence, novel immunogens and targets need to be identified. Active pursual of antigen discovery, structural insights into vaccine design is need of the hour to expand our malaria vaccine candidates.

References

1 World Health Organization (2018). *World Malaria Report 2018*. Geneva: World Health Organization.
2 Russell, P.F. and Mohan, B.N. (1942). The immunization of fowls against mosquito-borne *Plasmodium gallinaceum* by injections of serum and of inactivated homologous sporozoites. *The Journal of Experimental Medicine* 76 (5): 477–495.
3 Nussenzweig, R.S., Vanderberg, J., Most, H., and Orton, C. (1967). Protective immunity produced by the injection of X-irradiated sporozoites of *Plasmodium berghei*. *Nature* 216 (5111): 160–162.
4 Doolan, D.L. and Hoffman, S.L. (1997). Pre-erythrocytic stage immune effector mechanisms in *Plasmodium* spp. infections. *Philosophical Transactions of the Royal Society of London. Series B: Biological Sciences* 352 (1359): 1361–1367.
5 Clyde, D.F., McCarthy, V.C., Miller, R.M., and Woodward, W.E. (1975). Immunization of man against falciparum and vivax malaria by use of attenuated

sporozoites. *The American Journal of Tropical Medicine and Hygiene* 24 (3): 397–401.

6 Ballou, W.R., Sherwood, J., Neva, F. et al. (1987). Safety and efficacy of a recombinant DNA *Plasmodium falciparum* sporozoite vaccine. *The Lancet* 329 (8545): 1277–1281.

7 Patarroyo, M.E., Amador, R., Clavijo, P. et al. (1988). A synthetic vaccine protects humans against challenge with asexual blood stages of *Plasmodium falciparum* malaria. *Nature* 332 (6160): 158–161.

8 Stoute, J.A., Slaoui, M., Heppner, D.G. et al. (1997). A preliminary evaluation of a recombinant circumsporozoite protein vaccine against *Plasmodium falciparum* malaria. *New England Journal of Medicine* 336 (2): 86–91.

9 Bojang, K.A., Milligan, P.J., Pinder, M. et al. RTS,S Malaria Vaccine Trial Team(2001). Efficacy of RTS,S/AS02 malaria vaccine against *Plasmodium falciparum* infection in semi-immune adult men in the Gambia: a randomised trial. *Lancet* 358 (9297): 1927–1934.

10 Schofield, L., Villaquiran, J., Ferreira, A. et al. (1987). Gamma interferon, CD8+ T cells and antibodies required for immunity to malaria sporozoites. *Nature* 330 (6149): 664–666.

11 Wang, R., Doolan, D.L., Le, T.P. et al. (1998). Induction of antigen-specific cytotoxic T lymphocytes in humans by a malaria DNA vaccine. *Science* 282 (5388): 476–480.

12 McConkey, S.J., Reece, W.H.H., Moorthy, V.S. et al. (2003). Enhanced T-cell immunogenicity of plasmid DNA vaccines boosted by recombinant modified vaccinia virus Ankara in humans. *Nature Medicine* 9 (6): 729–735.

13 World Health Organization (2017). World Malaria Report 2017. Available at: http://www.who.int/malaria/publications/world-malaria-report-2017/report/en (accessed 20 October 2021).

14 Adepoju, P. (2019). RTS,S malaria vaccine pilots in three African countries. *The Lancet* 393 (10182): 1685.

15 Duffy, P.E. and Gorres, J.P. (2020). Malaria vaccines since 2000: progress, priorities, products. *npj Vaccines* 5 (1): 1–9.

16 Guerra Mendoza, Y., Garric, E., Leach, A. et al. (2019). Safety profile of the RTS,S/AS01 malaria vaccine in infants and children: additional data from a phase III randomized controlled trial in sub-Saharan Africa. *Human Vaccines & Immunotherapeutics* 15 (10): 2386–2398.

17 Molina-Franky, J., Cuy-Chaparro, L., Camargo, A. et al. (2020). *Plasmodium falciparum* pre-erythrocytic stage vaccine development. *Malaria Journal* 19 (1): 56.

18 Dame, J.B., Williams, J.L., McCutchan, T.F. et al. (1984). Structure of the gene encoding the immunodominant surface antigen on the sporozoite of the human malaria parasite *Plasmodium falciparum*. *Science* 225 (4662): 593–599.

19 Collins, K.A., Snaith, R., Cottingham, M.G. et al. (2017). Enhancing protective immunity to malaria with a highly immunogenic virus-like particle vaccine. *Scientific Reports* 7: 46621.

20 Neafsey, D.E., Juraska, M., Bedford, T. et al. (2015). Genetic diversity and protective efficacy of the RTS,S/AS01 malaria vaccine. *New England Journal of Medicine* 373 (21): 2025–2037.

21 Rathore, D., Sacci, J.B., de la Vega, P., and McCutchan, T.F. (2002). Binding and invasion of liver cells by *Plasmodium falciparum* sporozoites essential involvement of the amino terminus of circumsporozoite protein. *Journal of Biological Chemistry* 277 (9): 7092–7098.

22 Scally, S.W., Murugan, R., Bosch, A. et al. (2018). Rare PfCSP C-terminal antibodies induced by live sporozoite vaccination are ineffective against malaria infection. *Journal of Experimental Medicine* 215 (1): 63–75.

23 Cawlfield, A., Genito, C.J., Beck, Z. et al. (2019). Safety, toxicity and immunogenicity of a malaria vaccine based on the circumsporozoite protein (FMP013) with the adjuvant army liposome formulation containing QS21 (ALFQ). *Vaccine* 37 (29): 3793–3803.

24 Triller, G., Scally, S.W., Costa, G. et al. (2017). Natural parasite exposure induces protective human anti-malarial antibodies. *Immunity* 47 (6): 1197–209.e10.

25 Hoffman, S.L., Billingsley, P.F., James, E. et al. (2010). Development of a metabolically active, non-replicating sporozoite vaccine to prevent *Plasmodium falciparum* malaria. *Human Vaccines* 6 (1): 97–106.

26 Mueller, A.-K., Labaied, M., Kappe, S.H.I., and Matuschewski, K. (2005). Genetically modified *Plasmodium* parasites as a protective experimental malaria vaccine. *Nature* 433 (7022): 164–167.

27 Mordmuller, B., Surat, G.Z., Lagler, H. et al. (2017). Sterile protection against human malaria by chemoattenuated PfSPZ vaccine. *Nature* 542 (7642): 445–449.

28 Epstein, J.E., Paolino, K.M., Richie, T.L. et al. (2017). Protection against *Plasmodium falciparum* malaria by PfSPZ vaccine. *JCI Insight* 2 (1): 1–14.

29 Roestenberg, M., McCall, M., Hopman, J. et al. (2009). Protection against a malaria challenge by sporozoite inoculation. *New England Journal of Medicine* 361 (5): 468–477.

30 Roestenberg, M., Teirlinck, A.C., McCall, M.B.B. et al. (2011). Long-term protection against malaria after experimental sporozoite inoculation: an open-label follow-up study. *The Lancet* 377 (9779): 1770–1776.

31 Zaidi, I., Diallo, H., Conteh, S. et al. (2017). γδT cells are required for the induction of sterile immunity during irradiated sporozoite vaccinations. *The Journal of Immunology* 199 (11): 3781–3788.

32 Sabchareon, A., Burnouf, T., Ouattara, D. et al. (1991). Parasitologic and clinical human response to immunoglobulin administration in falciparum malaria. *The American Journal of Tropical Medicine and Hygiene* 45 (3): 297–308.

33 Siddiqui, W.A. (1977). An effective immunization of experimental monkeys against a human malaria parasite, *Plasmodium falciparum*. *Science* 197 (4301): 388–389.

34 Sirima, S.B., Cousens, S., and Druilhe, P. (2011). Protection against malaria by MSP3 candidate vaccine. *New England Journal of Medicine* 365 (11): 1062–1064.

35 Payne, R.O., Milne, K.H., Elias, S.C. et al. (2016). Demonstration of the blood-stage *Plasmodium falciparum* controlled human malaria infection model to assess efficacy of the *P. falciparum* apical membrane antigen 1 vaccine, FMP2.1/AS01. *The Journal of Infectious Diseases* 213 (11): 1743–1751.

36 Spring, M.D., Cummings, J.F., Ockenhouse, C.F. et al. (2009). Phase 1/2a study of the malaria vaccine candidate apical membrane antigen-1 (AMA-1) administered in adjuvant system AS01B or AS02A. *PLoS One* 4 (4): e5254.

37 Sirima, S.B., Mordmuller, B., Milligan, P. et al. (2016). A phase 2b randomized, controlled trial of the efficacy of the GMZ2 malaria vaccine in African children. *Vaccine* 34 (38): 4536–4542.

38 Crosnier, C., Bustamante, L.Y., Bartholdson, S.J. et al. (2011). Basigin is a receptor essential for erythrocyte invasion by *Plasmodium falciparum. Nature* 480 (7378): 534–537.

39 Douglas, A.D., Baldeviano, G.C., Lucas, C.M. et al. (2015). A PfRH5-based vaccine is efficacious against heterologous strain blood-stage *Plasmodium falciparum* infection in aotus monkeys. *Cell Host & Microbe* 17 (1): 130–139.

40 Srinivasan, P., Baldeviano, G.C., Miura, K. et al. (2017). A malaria vaccine protects *Aotus* monkeys against virulent *Plasmodium falciparum* infection. *npj Vaccines* 2 (1): 1–10.

41 Tonkin, M.L., Roques, M., Lamarque, M.H. et al. (2011). Host cell invasion by apicomplexan parasites: insights from the co-structure of AMA1 with a RON2 peptide. *Science* 333 (6041): 463–467.

42 Tessema, S.K., Nakajima, R., Jasinskas, A. et al. (2019). Protective immunity against severe malaria in children is associated with a limited repertoire of antibodies to conserved PfEMP1 variants. *Cell Host & Microbe* 26 (5): 579–90.e5.

43 Raj, D.K., Das Mohapatra, A., Jnawali, A. et al. (2020 Jun). Anti-PfGARP activates programmed cell death of parasites and reduces severe malaria. *Nature* 582 (7810): 104–108. PubMed PMID: 32427965. Epub 2020/05/20. eng.

44 Williams, A.R., Douglas, A.D., Miura, K. et al. (2012). Enhancing blockade of *Plasmodium falciparum* erythrocyte invasion: assessing combinations of antibodies against PfRH5 and other merozoite antigens. *PLoS Pathogens* 8 (11): e1002991. PubMed PMID: 23144611. Epub 2012/11/13. eng.

45 Raj, D.K., Nixon, C.P., Nixon, C.E. et al. (2014). Antibodies to PfSEA-1 block parasite egress from RBCs and protect against malaria infection. *Science* 344 (6186): 871–877. PubMed PMID: 24855263. Epub 2014/05/24. eng.

46 Desai, M., Ter Kuile, F.O., Nosten, F.O. et al. (2007). Epidemiology and burden of malaria in pregnancy. *The Lancet Infectious Diseases.* 7 (2): 93–104.

47 Fried, M. and Duffy, P.E. (1996). Adherence of *Plasmodium falciparum* to chondroitin sulfate A in the human placenta. *Science* 272 (5267): 1502–1504.

48 Salanti, A., Staalsoe, T., Lavstsen, T. et al. (2003). Selective upregulation of a single distinctly structured var gene in chondroitin sulphate A – adhering *Plasmodium falciparum* involved in pregnancy-associated malaria. *Molecular Microbiology* 49 (1): 179–191.

49 Resende, M., Nielsen, M.A., Dahlback, M. et al. (2008). Identification of glycosaminoglycan binding regions in the *Plasmodium falciparum* encoded placental sequestration ligand, VAR2CSA. *Malaria Journal* 7 (1): 1–11.

50 Tuikue Ndam, N.G., Fievet, N., Bertin, G. et al. (2004). Variable adhesion abilities and overlapping antigenic properties in placental *Plasmodium falciparum* isolates. *The Journal of Infectious Diseases* 190 (11): 2001–2009.

51 Clausen, T.M., Christoffersen, S., Dahlback, M. et al. (2012). Structural and functional insight into how the *Plasmodium falciparum* VAR2CSA protein mediates binding to chondroitin sulfate A in placental malaria. *Journal of Biological Chemistry* 287 (28): 23332–23345.

52 http://ClinicalTrials.gov (2018). NCT02647489: Safety and Immunogenicity of the Placental Malaria Vaccine Candidate PAMVAC Variously Adjuvanted (PAMVAC). University Hospital Tuebingen. http://ClinicalTrials.gov.

53 http://ClinicalTrials.gov (2019). NCT02658253: Trial to Evaluate the Safety and Immunogenicity of a Placental Malaria Vaccine Candidate (PRIMVAC) in Healthy Adults (PRIMALVAC). Institut National de la Santé Et de la Recherche Médicale, France. http://ClinicalTrials.gov.

54 Mordmuller, B., Sulyok, M., Egger-Adam, D. et al. (2019). First-in-human, randomized, double-blind clinical trial of differentially adjuvanted PAMVAC, a vaccine candidate to prevent pregnancy-associated malaria. *Clinical Infectious Diseases* 69 (9): 1509–1516. PubMed PMID: 30629148. Epub 2019/01/11. eng.

55 Sirima, S.B., Richert, L., Chêne, A. et al. (2020). PRIMVAC vaccine adjuvanted with Alhydrogel or GLA-SE to prevent placental malaria: a first-in-human, randomised, double-blind, placebo-controlled study. *The Lancet Infectious Diseases* 20 (5): 585–597.

56 Carter, R. and Chen, D.H. (1976). Malaria transmission blocked by immunisation with gametes of the malaria parasite. *Nature* 263 (5572): 57–60.

57 Grotendorst, C.A., Kumar, N., Carter, R., and Kaushal, D.C. (1984). A surface protein expressed during the transformation of zygotes of *Plasmodium gallinaceum* is a target of transmission-blocking antibodies. *Infection and Immunity* 45 (3): 775–777.

58 Read, D., Lensen, A.H.W., Begarnie, S. et al. (1994). Transmission-blocking antibodies against multiple, non-variant target epitopes of the *Plasmodium falciparum* gamete surface antigen Pfs230 are all complement-fixing. *Parasite Immunology* 16 (10): 511–519.

59 Talaat, K.R., Ellis, R.D., Hurd, J. et al. (2016). Safety and immunogenicity of Pfs25-EPA/Alhydrogel®, a transmission blocking vaccine against *Plasmodium falciparum*: an open label study in malaria naïve adults. *PLoS One* 11 (10): e0163144.

60 van Dijk, M.R., Janse, C.J., Thompson, J. et al. (2001). A central role for P48/45 in malaria parasite male gamete fertility. *Cell* 104 (1): 153–164.

61 Singh, K., Mukherjee, P., Shakri, A.R. et al. (2018). Malaria vaccine candidate based on Duffy-binding protein elicits strain transcending functional antibodies in a phase I trial. *npj Vaccines* 3 (1): 1–10.

14

Toll-Like Receptor-Based Adjuvants: A Gateway Toward Improved Malaria Vaccination

Deepika Kannan[1], Arshpreet Kaur[2], Deepak B. Salunke[2,3], and Shailja Singh[4]

[1] *Shiv Nadar University, Department of Life Science, NH91, Tehsil Dadri Gautam Buddha Nagar, Uttar Pradesh, 201314, India*
[2] *Panjab University, Department of Chemistry and Centre for Advanced Studies in Chemistry, Sector 14, Chandigarh, 160014, India*
[3] *Panjab University, National Interdisciplinary Centre of Vaccine, Immunotherapeutics and Antimicrobials, Sector 14, Chandigarh 160014, India*
[4] *Jawaharlal Nehru University, Special Centre for Molecular Medicine, New Mehrauli Road, Delhi 110067, India*

14.1 Introduction

Malaria, the world's deadliest parasitic disease, has been tolling the mortality rates for decades. Despite several promising progress to conquer the parasite, it is still responsible for the 25% annual death globally [1]. Since 2016, the global fight against malaria has stalled due to its complicated biological challenges. Resistance has been developed by parasites and mosquito vectors against first-line anti-malarial drugs and insecticides due to poor compliance of patients and socioeconomic barriers in drug distribution to endemic rural regions. These obstacles favor the drive toward malaria elimination through primary prevention, including the use of malaria vaccines [2].

There is an urgent need to develop highly efficacious, long-lasting, immunogenic vaccines against *Plasmodium*. Currently, RTS,S has been the only affluent subunit vaccine toward this goal that targets the pre-erythrocytic stage. The vaccine RTS,S/AS01 utilized the surface antigen *Plasmodium falciparum* circumsporozoite protein (*Pf*CSP) wherein 18 copies of the central repeat and the C-terminal domain of *Pf*CSP was fused with hepatitis B virus surface antigen (HBsAg). The formulation was further encapsulated within AS01 liposomal adjuvant to elicit a better immune response [3]. The partially successful malaria vaccine entered phase 3 clinical trial (from 2009 to 2014) where infants and children (5–17 months old) were immunized with four doses for four to five years. The vaccine efficiency prevented malaria cases by 39% and severe malaria cases by 29% in the defined age group (https://www.who.int/malaria/media/malaria-vaccine-implementation-qa/en). However, a decline in protection over a short period and the prolonged high antibody titer were major setbacks for the malarial vaccine. Nevertheless, the partial protection

Drug Development for Malaria: Novel Approaches for Prevention and Treatment, First Edition.
Edited by Pravin Kendrekar.

conferred by RTS,S/AS01 led to its advancement to phase 4 clinical trial in 2019, to further evaluate the safety context. The large-scale pilot program is introduced in three malaria-endemic sub-Saharan regions, Ghana, Kenya, and Malawi, including vaccination of nearly 360 000 children per year. The program contributed by malaria vaccine implementation programme (MVIP), associated with WHO and Expanded Programme on Immunizations (EPI), will focus on determining the efficacy of the vaccine in a large cohort of people and assess the associated side effects with its routine use, further enabling the wide-scale deployment of the only partially successful malaria vaccine to date [4]. To overcome the shortcomings, several strategies such as a change in the regimen, dosage of immunization, and structure-guided vaccine designing are also being studied to alter the immune responses toward RTS,S/AS01 [5, 6]. Such techniques may even assist in designing adjuvants or immunogens to elicit a stronger immune response that can last longer. A similar study by Oyen et al. focused on understanding the molecular and atomic specificity of the NANP raised monoclonal antibody (mAb) upon RTS,S/AS01 protection [6]. Authors observed the circumsporozoite protein (CSP)-specific mAb that recognizes two repeats NANP and NPNA, with the later eliciting a much better immune response. As a result, alteration in the amino acid sequence of these structures may further provide promising interaction, generating neutralizing antibodies and providing prolonged protection. Thus, mAb engineering may also seem like a probable intervention against malarial infection [6].

Unlike the pre-erythrocytic stage, one of the biggest challenges with the erythrocytic-stage malaria vaccine is the absence of major histocompatibility complex (MHC) molecule-mediated cellular immune responses. Hence, a strong dependency on humoral-mediated responses either through subunit vaccine or through naturally acquired immunity plays a vital role. Antibodies blocking the erythrocyte invasion or schizont egress proved effective. Over the decade, extensive efforts have been centered on merozoite and apical organelle-based antigens (MSPs, AMA1, EBA-175, *Pf*EMP1, etc). Substantial improvements in the identification of novel blood-stage candidates have been made utilizing several transcriptomic and proteomic approaches. However, antigenic diversity in *Plasmodium* blood-stage antigens is quite evident and does impede their use as a successful vaccine target [7]. Malaria Vaccine Development Branch had developed the AMA1-C1, a bivalent vaccine composed of aluminium hydroxide adjuvant with recombinant AMA1 of 3D7 and FVO strains. Although the phase 1 clinical trial showed moderate protection, no vaccination was observed in phase 2 clinical trial. The probable reason was the ability of the vaccine to provide only strain-specific immunity. Also, the invoked immunogenicity was insufficient demonstrating the need for strong adjuvants [8]. Another major blood-stage antigen is the *P. falciparum* reticulocyte-binding protein homolog 5 (*Pf*RH5), which interacts with basigin (CD147) on the erythrocyte surface during the invasion. *Pf*RH5 appears to have a 3.3-fold reduced density of polymorphism [9] with higher neutralization antibodies against parasites, evincing its ability against both homologous and heterologous strains of parasites [10–12]. With the requirement of an extended potency of a malarial blood-stage vaccine, the multi-protein complex blood-stage vaccine is also being studied. This includes *Pf*RH5, *Pf*Ripr, *Pf*CyPRA coupled with *Pf*RAP2, and *Pf*RhopH3. All these antigens are highly conserved and essential for blood-stage parasite survival and Ca^{2+}-dependent RBC invasion. The complex was analyzed for their ability to provide functional antibodies synergistically. The rationale behind such a complex multi-protein vaccine is temporal and gradient inhibition of parasite invasion steps by eliciting functional IgG. Thus, prolonged production of the protective antibody may result in increased avidity and potency against the disease. However, the results may be skeptical until the efficacy is monitored in malaria-endemic regions [13–15].

The third group of vaccines – transmission-blocking vaccines (TBVs) – focuses on herd immunity, with the principle of generating antibodies against parasite or mosquito midgut antigens. These antibodies are transported to the mosquito midgut during blood feed wherein the antibodies eliminate the parasite growth. Thus, two prime features for any TBV includes the ability to generate a strong humoral response in individuals and trigger an immune response in the vector annihilating immunocompetence. The survival of any pathogen within a vector requires an interacting ligand or attachment site in the vector. To establish an infection, parasite ookinete utilize several ligands on the midgut surface such as circumsporozoite- and thrombospondin-related anonymous proteins (CTRP), chitinase, von Willebrand Factor A domain-related protein (WARP), secreted ookinete adhesive protein (SOAP), two membrane attack ookinete proteins (MAOPs), cell traversal protein for ookinetes and sporozoites (CelTOS), several lectin adhesive-like proteins (LAPs), and ookinete surface antigens (*Pf*s25 and *Pf*s28). The first antigen to be used as a TBV was *Pf*s25. After yielding promising protective effect, the antigen was progressed for clinical trial phase 1a formulated with an adjuvant – Montanide ISA51. Several adjuvants such as EPA (exoprotein A of Pseudomonas aeruginosa), IMX313, and EPA/hydrogel were formulated with *Pf*s25 to elicit a safe, non-toxic immune response. With several of them dissipating high reactogenicity, the hydrogel-based vaccine was further continued for clinical testing [16]. Though a 50% reduction in the oocyst intensity was monitored, substantial antibody concentration was lacking. Huang et al. lately utilized adjuvantation of *Pfs*25 to nanoliposomes as a tool to enhance the antibody response [17]. A threefold high magnitude of antibody response was elicited, and mosquitoes fed with SNAP-treated mice blood rendered uninfected, without the parasite. The antibody response was prolonged till 250 days post immunization, proving it to be a promising approach. However, the question regarding the feasibility of such a particle-mediated vaccine in malaria-endemic fields still remains [17]. Several other TBVs such as *Pf*s45, *Pf*s48, *Pf*s230, and *Pf*s28 also depicted potent activity against *P. falciparum* gametes by inducing functional and transmission-blocking antibodies in animals. However, the majority of them are still under clinical trials with results awaited [18–20] (http://ClinicalTrials.gov ID NCT02942277; NCT03917654).

Regardless of several promising vaccine trials, the short-lived nature of immune responses, antigenic diversity, potential polymorphisms in the *Plasmodium* parasite, accumulated genetic drift, limited funding, and highly variable efficacy of vaccines have all contributed to the failure of all current approaches based on global malaria vaccination.

Bioengineering methods including antigen conjugation to toxin proteins, viral particles, viral vectors, and nanoparticles have been widely emerging to boost the humoral response. Moreover, vaccine adjuvantation has been historically used to maximize protective immunity, enhance, prolong, and modulate immune responses triggered by the recognition of vaccine antigens. However, clinically approved adjuvants such as alum, oil-in-water emulsions, saponin, and ISCOMs tested against malarial vaccines have all demonstrated suboptimal protection. These limitations associated with vaccine conjugation have triggered the use of synthetic adjuvants targeting the major groups of pattern recognition receptors (PRRs), toll-like receptors (TLRs), nod-like receptors (NLRs), and C-type lectin receptors (CLRs).

14.2 Host Immunological Responses in Malaria Conferring Protection

Immunity to malaria is very heterogeneous and depends on various aspects like host immune system, age, exposure to a parasite strain, frequency of infection, amount of protective antibody produced by the host, and several geographical factors. Immunological response may also vary based on the severity of infection in terms of uncomplicated malaria, severe malarial anemia, and cerebral malaria. Pathogenesis of malaria is chiefly attributed to pro-inflammatory cytokine release, cytoadherence, and sequestration of infected erythrocytes to endothelial cells and finally the elimination of altered or infected erythrocytes by splenic macrophages. Thus, both humoral- and cell-mediated immunities play a vital role in malarial pathogenesis.

14.2.1 Innate Immunity

Both CD4+ and CD8+ T cells provide innate immunity during malaria infection. During symptomatic malaria, monocytes, splenic macrophages, and dendritic cells (DCs) predominantly contribute to the cytokine outburst in the bloodstream. Experimental studies showed that parasite ligands during infection trigger DC maturation, further presenting malarial antigens, thereby stimulating interaction with receptors on naive CD4+ and CD8+ T cells. Activated T cells secrete cytokines or release pore-forming enzymes such as perforins, serine esterase, and granzymes that lyse the infected parasites [21, 22]. Additionally, activated T cells also secrete several cytokines or lymphokines that further activate the complement system in the host inhibiting the parasite penetration or maturation within the hepatocytes [23, 24] (Figure 14.1).

The following section summarizes the role of each of these immune effectors in the defense against *Plasmodium* parasite.

Macrophages: Macrophages are members of the innate immunity in malaria infection that mainly sense altered structures of infected erythrocytes, phagocytose these cells, and present the peptides on their surface to activate T cells and

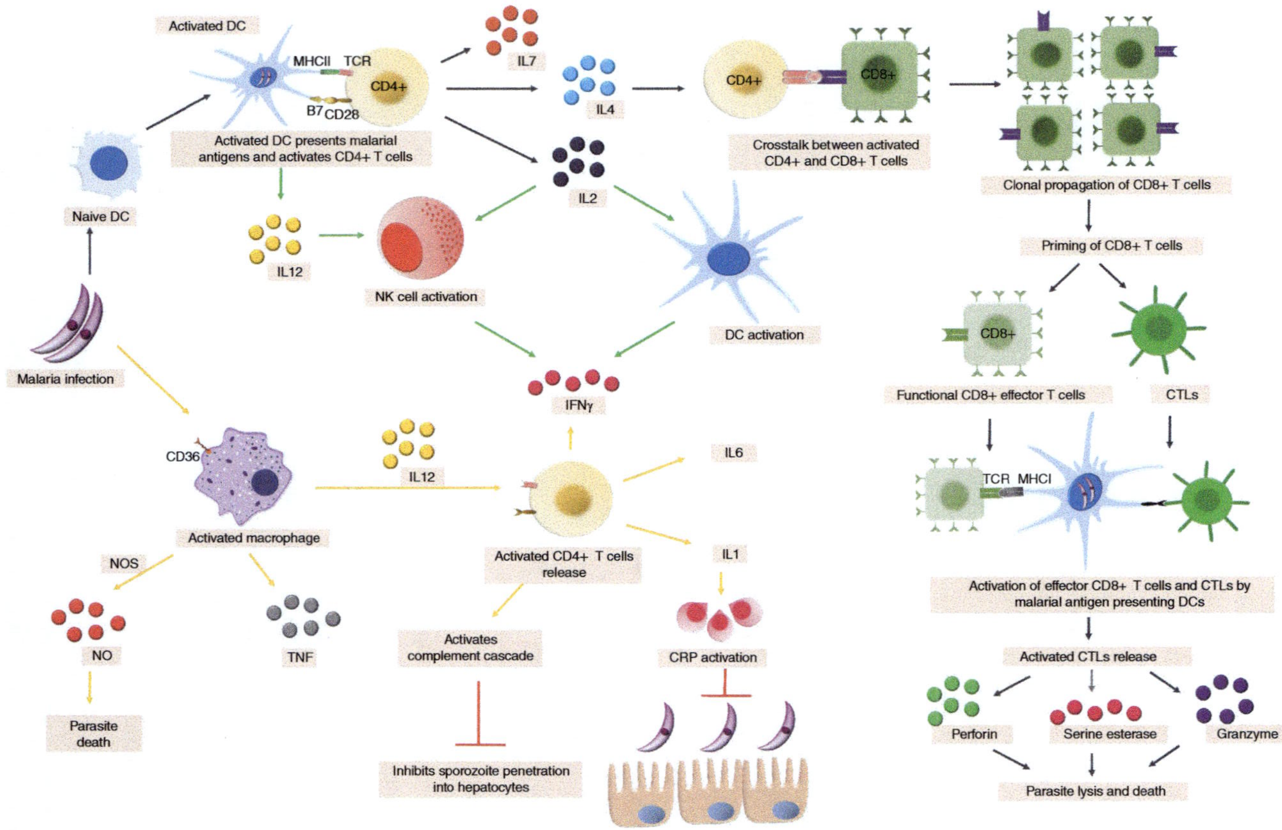

Figure 14.1 Innate immune response during malaria. Dendritic cells (DCs) play a vital role toward malarial immunity. Mature DC presents malarial antigens, stimulating interaction with receptors on naive CD4+ T cells. Activated CD4+ T cells secrete cytokines such as IL-4, IL-2, and IL-7, further mediating crosstalk between activated CD4+ T cells and CD8+ T cells. These interactions facilitate the clonal expansion of CD8+ T cells via STAT-6 IL-4-dependent mechanism. However, the interaction may not specifically be dependent on IL-4 alone. Priming of CD8+ T cells in the presence of CD4+ T cells at the initial stage of infection results in effector or memory CD8+ T cell formation. Functional CD8+ T cells and CD8+ cytotoxic T lymphocytes (CTLs) express a high level of adhesion molecule CD44. These molecules enable interaction between the effector CTLs and class-I MHC antigen-expressing infected hepatocytes. Activation of CTLs release pore-forming enzymes such as perforins, serine esterase, and granzymes that lyse the infected parasites. Additionally, activated T cells also secrete several cytokines or lymphokines such as IL-1, IL-6, IFN-γ, and TNF. These cytokines inhibit the exo-erythrocytic form of parasite by inducing the synthesis of nitric oxide (NO) via NO synthase and synthesis of acute-phase proteins such as C-reactive protein (CRP). NO synthesis and the presence of IFN-γ initiate the phagocytosis of parasites by activated macrophages. However, upregulated CRP molecules during malaria infection binds to the phosphorylcholine on parasite membrane and prevents sporozoite penetration.

B cells. Upon engulfing the infected erythrocytes, macrophages secrete several pro-inflammatory cytokines such as IL12, IFN-γ, and TNF-α by enhancing TLR expression on their surface [25]. TNF-α and IFN-γ play a central role in severe malaria infection by priming the host cells to produce nitric oxide (NO) by NO synthase. Induction of NO exerts a dual role in protection against blood-stage infection by acting as a self-regulatory molecule, enabling Th1 cell proliferation and pro-inflammatory cytokine release while regulating their overproduction by blocking the secretion of IL-2 and IFN-γ from Th1 response [26].

NK Cells: NK cells are cytotoxic lymphocyte that forms the first line of defense along with neutrophils and phagocytes against malaria infection. During increased parasite load, activated NK cells secrete increasing amounts of IFN-γ, which in turn induce macrophage activation and secretion of pro-inflammatory cytokines (IL-8) [27]. While in liver tissue, natural killer T cells (NK1.1+ TCRab) confer innate immunity. These cells provide defense by recognizing CD1 molecules expressed on the surface of infected hepatocytes, thereby secreting IL-4 or IFN-γ inhibiting the liver-stage parasite replication [28].

Dendritic Cells (DCs): DCs are known for their role in bridging between the innate and acquired immunity. During early *Plasmodium* infection, DCs detect and engulf infected erythrocytes that are circulating in the blood or spleen. These cells process and present the *Plasmodium* antigens from rupturing erythrocytes on their surface mediating an interaction to activate the CD4+ Th1 cells. Activated Th1 cells express certain co-stimulatory molecules and release a pool of cytokines such as IL-2, IL-4, IL-12, and IFN-γ. These cytokines further activate various effector T cells and B cells, initiating their clonal propagation and IgG class switching. IL-4 promotes IgM to IgG1 and IgM to IgE class switching, while IFN-γ and IL-12 induce class switching to IgG2a and IgG3 contributing to antibody-mediated responses during the early blood-stage infection. IL-12 in the blood further mediates the protection by NO synthesis [29, 30].

Presentation of malarial antigens also stimulates expression of class II MHC molecules that induces the expression of CD40, CD86, and CD80 and production of IL-12 and IFN-γ. IFN-γ and DC maturations enhance the antigen presentation, triggering the clonal expansion of naive CD4+ T cells. Expression of CD40 ligand on CD4+ T cells and its interaction with CD40 upregulates IL-12, facilitating Th1 differentiation. As a result, differentiated Th1 cells and activated macrophages further induce adaptive immune responses [31].

14.2.2 Adaptive Immunity

Immunity to malaria is modulated by a wave of innate followed by acquired immune responses. Being the symptomatic stage (devoid of MHC class I or II molecule), adaptive immunity is dominant in the blood stage of malaria. Several immune cells and factors are involved in conferring adaptive immunity. The following section describes the role of different adaptive immunity regulators during the erythrocytic stage.

B Cells: During acute infection, activation of several myeloid and lymphoid cells releases several cytokines promoting CD4+ T cell activation and Th1 differentiation. These T cells stimulate B cells, humoral responses, and phagocytosis, resulting in a reduction of parasite load. During blood stages, increased parasitemia levels results in ingestion of parasitized erythrocytes by macrophages and DCs. Toxic hemozoin from infected erythrocytes paralyzes these phagocytic cells inducing the production of IL-10 and TGF-β. IL-10 is a growth factor for B cells and induces B-cell differentiation into plasma cells eliciting a humoral response. The elicited humoral response varies depending on the antigenic diversity of several surface proteins expressed on the schizonts or merozoites. Antibodies against these proteins bind to the phagocytes and mediate parasite clearance by opsonization via Ab-dependent cellular inhibition. Some of the invasion inhibiting antibodies may bind to the surface of infected erythrocytes, preventing sequestration and promoting their elimination by the spleen. However, the absence of B cells succumbs malaria-infected individuals to severe pathogenesis. Mice models deficient of B cells were unable to clear the parasite load while the transfer of B cells to these deficient mice restored their ability of parasite clearance with Th1/Th2 response [32]. Langhorne et al. [33] obtained similar findings where B-cell knockout mice (μMT mice) sustained their T cell responses. However, these mice were unable to eliminate the parasite load. These studies strongly support the requirement of B cell in malaria pathogenesis and switching off the immune response from Th1 to Th2 during humoral immunity.

Th1/Th2 Response: Several studies including erythrocytic-stage *Plasmodium chabaudi* infection have provided evidence for CD4+ Th1-based activation of several effector mediator cells such as macrophages further triggering CD4+ Th2-based activation of B-cell responses for complete clearance of the parasite load [34–37]. Epidemiological investigation of individuals in endemic areas and several mice studies have been observed during acute or primary infection when the parasitemia is ascending, Th1 response-based IgG2a provides initial protection. As the disease progresses toward the chronic or secondary infection, switching of Th1 to Th2 response initiates a predominant IgG1 and IgG3 production, providing a greater level of protection [38–40].

Antibody Isotype: The humoral response generated against blood-stage malaria is also dependent on the Ab isotype. Predominantly, IgE, IgG, and IgM antibodies play a crucial role in malarial pathogenesis. Experimental data from *Plasmodium*-infected mice and humans showed elevated IgE titer in the blood in the case of severe and cerebral malaria. Complicated malaria patients exhibited a significantly higher concentration of IgE than uncomplicated patients [41, 42]. IgG, on the other hand, is known to be involved in the passive transfer of immunity against malaria. The most predominant serum antibody, IgG, is generated along with memory B cells against both the pre-erythrocytic and erythrocytic stage antigens. Protection against *Plasmodium* is attributed by several subclasses of IgG antibody. *Plasmodium* infection in humans living in endemic areas attributed IgG1 and IgG3 as the potent antibody conferring protection. These cytophilic Ab are found against several blood-stage antigens such as RESA, MSP1, and MSP2; however, the extent of protection is also determined by the age and several genetic factors in the host. Previous studies by Vukovic et al. and Majarian et al. showed mice challenged with *Plasmodium yoelii* and immunized with MSP119 generated anti-MSP119 IgG3 Ab that, when transferred passively to naive recipients, enabled the elimination of *P. yoelii* infection, protecting the mice [43, 44].

T-Follicular Helper Cells (Tfh): Tfh cells are the subsets of CD4+ helper T cells that in the germinal centers of secondary lymphoid organs promote B-cell formation and differentiation into long-lived plasma cells. The role of different Tfh cell subsets in malaria immunity is currently being explored. Studies have shown that the superior $CXCR3^-$Tfh cell subset providing better B cell helps not trigger malaria [45]. However, recent studies in malaria-exposed children demonstrated the involvement of Th1-polarized $PD1^+CXCR5^+CXCR3^+$Tfh cells in B-cell functioning during acute infection.

T-Regulatory Cells (Tregs): The other subset of CD4+ T cells, i.e. the regulatory T cells (CD4 + FOXP3+), provides an immunosuppressive response by secreting cytokines such as IL-10 and TGF-β. These cells in malaria immunity have proved detrimental associating with increased parasite progression and supporting disease severity [46]. Tregs have been associated with the suppression of T-cell responses and modulation of immune responses by the production of cytokines followed by the creation of an immunosuppressive environment. These conditions provide a niche to boost the parasite survival and establishment of chronic infections. As a result, immune responses may downregulate by the expansion of Tregs during vaccine administration [47]. Such findings provide new approaches where the trigger of $CXCR3^-$Tfh cell subset and limited expression of Tregs may enhance vaccine efficacy.

14.3 Crosstalk of PRRs in Host Immune System with Malarial Antigens

Malaria pathogenesis is associated with three physiological events: (i) infected or altered red blood cell clearance, (ii) cyto-adhesion of infected erythrocytes to endothelial cells, and (iii) cytokine storm. Evidence support encountering of *Plasmodium* parasites or iRBCs by antigen-presenting cells (APCs) initiating a cascade of innate and subsequent adaptive immune responses within the host [48]. Individuals priorly exposed to parasite infections elicit adaptive immune responses contributing to partial protective immunity. These antibodies generated against specific antigens by effector cells during previous exposure result in reduced risk of infection. However, this may vary upon infection to different *Plasmodium* strains [49].

The trigger of an immune response against parasite largely depends on the interaction between the PRRs on host cells and pathogen-associated molecular patterns (PAMPs) on *Plasmodium*. During *Plasmodium* infection, TLRs (TLR-1, 2, 4, 7, and 9) and NLRs (NALP3) are the major PRRs that recognize the PAMPs and initiate a series of signaling cascade, triggering host innate responses (Figure 14.2).

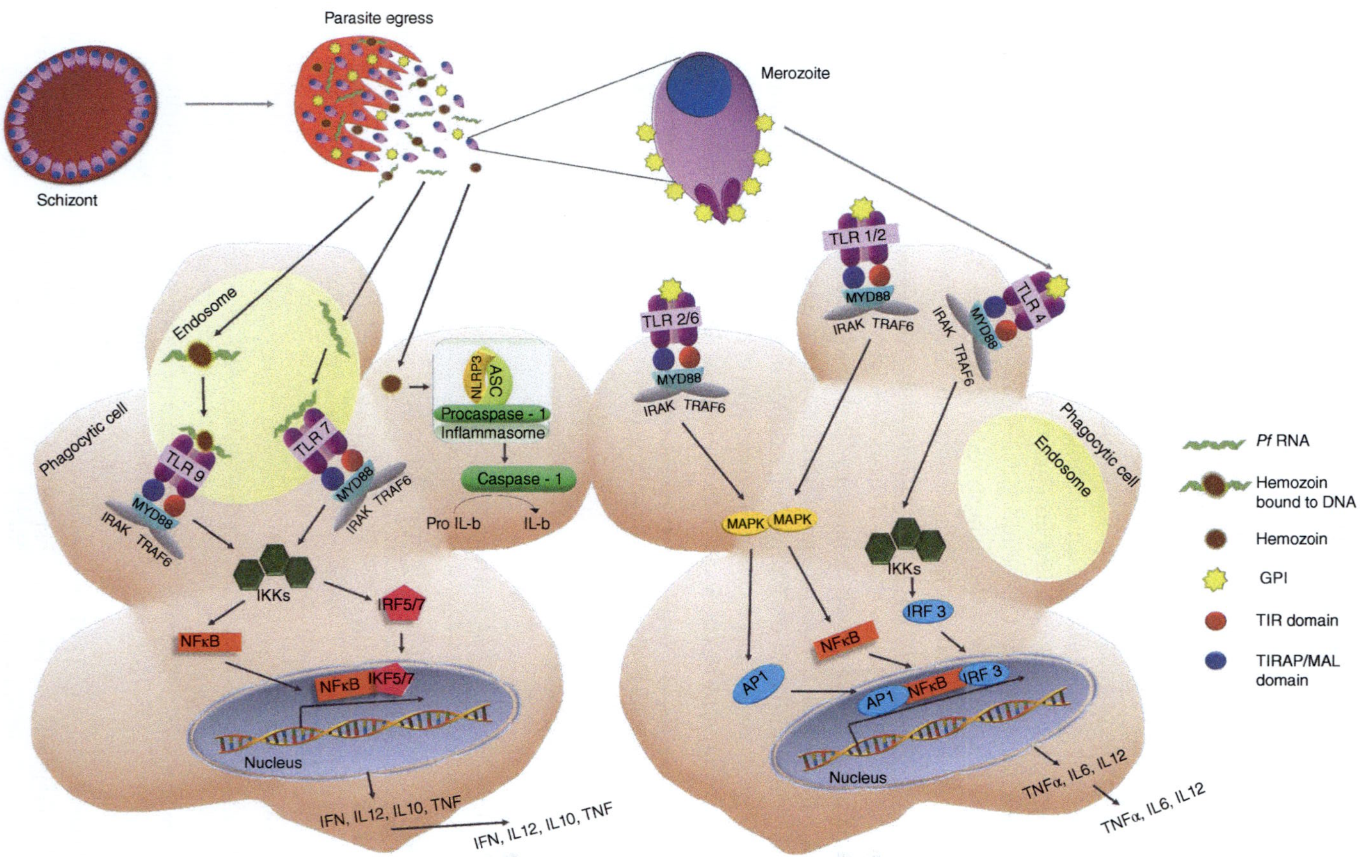

Figure 14.2 Illustration of the TLR signaling pathway in malarial pathogenesis. Different TLRs involved in malaria pathogen recognition and evoked an immune response.

Secretion of several inflammatory cytokines, chemokines, and type-1 IFN additionally induces maturation of plasmacytoid dendritic cells (pDCs) and activation of macrophages, triggering the adaptive responses and killing the parasites. The critical role of TLRs in protection against *Plasmodium* was observed when mice deficient for adaptor molecules MyD88 were susceptible for *Plasmodium berghei* infection due to impaired activation of Th1 cells and decreased production of Th1 cytokines [50, 51]. These findings that suggest in malaria the interplay between the PRRs and their ligands is essential in the activation of immune responses. Parasitized RBCs provide several ligand molecules that can interact with several TLRs and NLRs to evoke immunogenicity. Interaction of TLR9 with parasite pigment hemozoin and DNA induces activation of pDCs producing pro-inflammatory cytokines [52, 53]. Several anchors (glycosyl phosphatidyl inositol [GPI]) expressed on parasite membrane proteins interact with TLR1–2 and TLR2–4 complexes, activating the human DCs, macrophages, and B cells through MyD88 signaling [54, 55]. Although the interaction of other PRRs than TLRs is not much studied in malaria, recently, hemozoin was reported to activate the Nalp3 inflammasome complex. Mice models of cerebral malaria exhibited phagocytosis of hemozoin crystals, leading the activation of Nalp3 inflammasomes that induced IL-1β production and neutrophil recruitment [56, 57]. Though the scope of malaria immunity remains to be further unraveled, identification of new PAMPs and insights into their immune mechanism may rapidly progress malaria vaccination. A handful of known malarial PAMPs inducing beneficial immune responses are GPI, plasmodial RNA, and hemozoin (Table 14.1).

14.3.1 Glycosyl Phosphatidylinositols (GPI)

This abundant glycolipid is surface-expressed primarily to anchor several cellular proteins to the plasma membrane. As a plausible parasite component relative to

Table 14.1 Interaction of malarial ligands with their receptors and their immune response.

Ligand	PRR	Immune response
Triacyl lipopeptide	TLR1/2	MyD88-dependent NF-κB activation and production of cytokines such as TNFα, IL-6, IL-12, IFNγ, and nitric oxide
Diacyl lipopeptide	TLR2/6	MyD88-dependent NF-κB activation and production of cytokines and chemokines
Malarial GPI	TLR4	MyD88-dependent NF-κB activation and production of IFN-β and IFN inducible genes
Plasmodial RNA	TLR7	MyD88-dependent NF-κB activation and production of pro-inflammatory cytokines such as IFN-1 and TNF, stimulating a Th1 response
Hemozoin-*Pf*DNA complex	TLR9	MyD88-dependent NF-κB activation and production of cytokines such as TNFα and IL-1β and chemokines such as MIP-1a, MIP-1b, and MCP-1
Hemozoin	NLRP3	NalP3 inflammasome complex-mediated caspase-1-based secretion of IL-1β

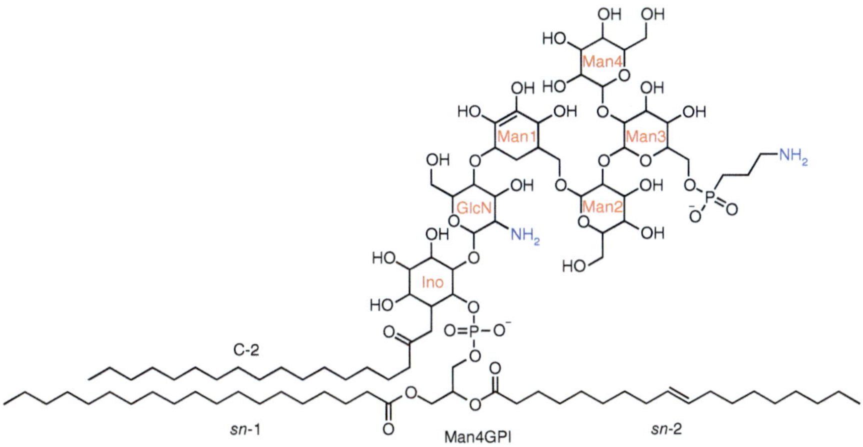

Figure 14.3 Structure of *P. falciparum* Man4-GPI ligand. The *P. falciparum* GPIs have four mannose sugar residues (Man), one glucosamine (GlcN), and one inositol (Ino). The three fatty acid substituents are at the C-2, *sn-1*, and *sn-2* positions. Mannoses are numbered as Man1, Man2, Man3, and Man4 according to their position.

pathogenesis, GPI of *Plasmodium* varies structurally relative to the diacylated glycerol moiety and fatty acid acylation, especially the presence of palmitate and myristate on C-2 of inositol and the presence of phosphoethanolamine (PE) on the first mannose residue [58]. These structural differences may contribute to the induction of pro-inflammatory responses by the innate immune system.

Literature very well states TLR2 as the probable PRR recognizing the *Plasmodium* GPIs. Structural insights by *in silico* studies have revealed that Man4 of GPI binds to the convex region of the TLR2/1 heterodimer [59]. Man4-GPI (Figure 14.3) has three lipid chains: (i) the acyl chain at the *sn*-1 position, (ii) inositol predominate chain, and (iii) fatty acid chain at the *sn*-2 position. Of these, the acyl chain and the inositol moiety get buried in the TLR2 pocket, while fatty acid region buries into the TLR1 pocket, exposing the head group of Man4-GPI out of the dimer pockets. While GPI regions were elucidated, residues Phe325, Asp327, and Asn294 of TLR2 and Gly313 and Gly316 of TLR1 participated in the interaction.

Being potent immune stimulators, *Plasmodium* GPI (preferentially the Man4 ligands) initially gets recognized by TLR-2/1 heterodimer or TLR4 (lesser extent) on monocytes and macrophages. Simultaneous interaction of these ligands with CD36 receptors on these cells and TLR dimerization trigger MyD88-dependent activation of MAPKs and NF-κB pathways. Dimerization of the TLR domains undergoes certain conformational changes with adaptor molecules (MyD88, TIRAP) inducing the IRAKs-TRAF6 signaling cascade. Post ubiquitinoylation and phosphorylation of the $I_{\kappa}B\alpha$ kinase complex (IKK) induces phosphorylation of downstream kinases such as ERK1/ERK2, p38, and JNK, promoting pro-inflammatory cytokine releases such as TNFα, IL-6, IL-12, IFN-γ, and nitric oxide from immune cells. Induction in the expression of adhesion molecules (ICAM-1, VCAM-1) on endothelial cells further contributes to the pathology [54, 60].

14.3.2 Plasmodial RNA

Parasite nucleic acids can act as potent stimulators to trigger the immune responses. *Plasmodium* RNA serves as a potent TLR7 agonist capable of eliciting a strong immune response against multiple *Plasmodium* species [61]. TLR7 is known to be involved in recognition of malaria, triggering early innate responses in several experimental studies. TLR7-mediated secretion of pro-inflammatory cytokines is strongly detectable during the early stage of infection [62, 63]. Cerebral malaria mouse models have depicted predominant secretion of these pro-inflammatory cytokines, several chemokines, and leukocytes relative to the pathogenesis [64, 65].

Contribution of TLR7 in malaria pathogenesis was studied *in vivo* in TLR7-deficient experimental cerebral malaria mice models for the development of hyper-parasitemia. TLR7−/− mice demonstrated better protection with an improved survival rate than the wild type. The deficient mice reported initial protection from cerebral malaria by suppressing the production of pro-inflammatory cytokines. Wild-type mice exhibited very high cytokine profiling of several pro-inflammatory cytokines such as IFN-1 and TNF, stimulating a type-1 immune response compared with type 2 [66]. The trigger to produce pro-inflammatory cytokine rush and activation of TLR7 downstream signaling is attributed to the early detection of *Plasmodium* RNA by TLR7. Supplementation of purified *P. falciparum* RNA to mice stimulated the TLR7 cascade while the response was abolished in TLR7−/− mice. *In vitro* bone marrow cells from mice models upon infection with parasitized RBCs also reported the susceptibility of wild-type cells toward infection while TLR7 deficient were less susceptible. Reports indicate the defect in the production of TNF and IFN-γ during the early stage of infection while the level of TNF and IFN-γ increases by the time infection peaks [62]. This suggests the involvement of TLR7 during early innate immune response mediated by *Plasmodium* RNA while protection against the malarial pathogenesis may involve several other MyD88-dependent and MyD88-independent PRRs.

14.3.3 Hemozoin (Hz)

Hemozoin is a detoxified waste product of hemoglobin degradation within the food vacuole of infected RBCs. It comprises hematin dimers linked by iron–carboxylate linkages and hydrogen bonds to form triclinic crystals. Structurally the crystals are arranged in two faces: (i) free propionic acid groups being very polar and hydrophilic in nature and (ii) hydrophobic flat porphyrin plane of the hematin dimers, lipophilic in nature [67]. Primarily upon schizont rupture, Hz is released and pools within circulating myeloid cells (macrophages and monocytes). Hz-induced immune signals by these phagocytes is contributed by internalization and lipid raft integrity.

Though the property of Hz to activate the immune cells is highly debatable [53, 68], Parroche et al. [53] reported that Hz coated with plasmodial DNA had an immunomodulatory activity while Hz alone failed. Inflammatory responses by Hz internalized within the endosomes of myeloid cells are MyD88 dependent. Potential receptors that mediate MyD88 dependent Hz-induced signaling pathways are TLR9 and NLRP3. TLR9 mediates immune responses against Hz by the specific interaction of cysteine residues within the extracellular domain of TLR. MyD88-dependent signaling cascade thus signals upregulation of IL-1β mRNA. Consequently, this releases a pool of cytokines such as TNFα and IL-1β and chemokines such as macrophage inflammatory protein-1a (MIP-1a), MIP-1β, and monocyte chemoattractant protein-1 (MCP-1) [69]. Prolonged internalization of Hz leads dysregulated cytokine production and impaired phagocytic ability. These variations cause the release of factors such as MIF erythropoietic inhibitor and adhesion molecules (CD11/CD18). Alterations in the plasma level of MIF cause suppression of erythropoiesis and development of severe malarial anemia. Recent studies have also reported TLR-independent MyD88-dependent activation of the NLRP3 inflammasome by malarial Hz. Opsonization of Hz by myeloid cells provides infection associated signals that activate the ASC/caspase-1 complex. Activated complex further carries synthesis and caspase-1-mediated cleavage of ProIL-1β into mature IL-1β. Excessive secretion of IL-1β causes deleterious effects further increasing malaria-related pathology. Mice models deficient of IL-1β and NLRP3 demonstrated better survival than wild-type mice [70].

14.4 Synthetic TLR Adjuvants: An Approach to Enhance Vaccine Immunogenicity

With the prerequisite need for a malaria vaccine, the potency of target peptides and associated low immunogenicity and efficacy are the pivotal points to be addressed. Plasmodial TLR agonists mentioned above, although can elicit an immune response, fail to establish a potent anti-parasitic effect. Natural TLR agonists from other organisms get associated with an increased risk of pathogenesis, contamination, and an adverse immune reaction such as allergies and complication. Thereby, to enhance the induction of vaccine-specific responses, these antigenic agonists need to be harnessed better. Adjuvants such as alum, Montanides, and Freund's adjuvant in the past have been employed for malarial vaccines; however, these had several downsides (explained in Table 14.2). To overcome these drawbacks in this review, we have focused on the use of a new class of synthetic TLR agonists as adjuvants against malarial pathogenesis (briefed in Table 14.3).

Synthetic TLRs (such as poly I/C, synthetic MPLA, imiquimod) are structural analogs of different natural ligands, mimicking in terms of their interactions with host PRRs, invoking enhanced immunogenicity.

14.4.1 TLR2

TLR2 expresses on the outer membrane of the myeloid cells with its co-receptors TLR1 and TLR6. The first true agonist of TLR2, identified as a mycoplasmal lipopeptide, *S*-[2,3-bis-(palmitoyloxy)-(2*R*)-propyl]-*R*-cysteinyl-GNNDESNISFKEK termed as macrophage-activating lipopeptide MALP-2 (Figure 14.4), was exemplified by the *S*-[2,3-bis(palmitoyloxy)-(2*RS*)-propyl]-R-cysteinyl-S-serine (PAM_2CS) chemotype [82, 83].

Table 14.2 Adjuvants in malarial vaccines and their pitfalls.

Adjuvants	Disadvantages
Complete Freund's adjuvant (CFA)	Causes adverse reactions in humans by attracting macrophages and other immune cells to the site of injection, causing granulomas and lesions
Alum	Inability to induce Th1/CTL-type responses required for intracellular pathogens
MF59	Stimulates immune cells resulting in lymphocyte, cytokine, and chemokine secretion but lower Th1-type immunity.
Montanides	Adverse local reaction, instability of antigens
Saponins (QS-21)	Severe allergic reactions
Immunostimulating complexes (ISCOMs)	Expensive, highly unstable, and difficult manufacturing

Among the several TLR2 agonists, only the lipopeptide-based ligands (PAM_3CSK_4 and PAM_2CSK_4) have been widely explored in malaria vaccines either as part of vaccine formulations or through conjugation with parasitic antigen/epitope [84–86]. Studies in clinical trials proved that the coupling of PAM_3Cys with tri-epitope-branched peptide of circumsporozoite (CS) elicited a higher immune response in *P. falciparum* sporozoite-immunized volunteers. PAM_3Cys is a lipopeptide TLR2 agonist that triggers an innate immune response; branched T1BT* includes T1 (a T cell epitope of CS conserved among all *Plasmodium* species), T* (a T cell epitope universally recognized by class II MHCs) triggering cellular immunity, and B (a B cell epitope region of CS) triggering protection by producing neutralizing antibody. Volunteers immunized with PAM3Cys-T1BT*-adjuvanted CS peptide vaccine produced sporozoite-specific neutralizing antibody, a pool of CD4+ T cell population including CTLs and effector T cells [87]. The efficacy of the vaccine was further improved by utilizing the layer-by-layer (LBL) nanoparticle that incorporates PAM_3Cys-T1BT* on the surface of LBL microparticles. The formulation included three repeats of CS-T1 region and five repeats of B-cell epitope. Immunized mice exhibited high titer of anti-repeat antibody responses against CS peptides and efficient opsonization of the particle provoking DC activation [88]. The detailed information regarding these formulations is recently reviewed where covalent incorporation of designed *Plasmodium* polypeptides elicited an immune response against *P. berghei*, resulting in higher antibody titer and IFN-γ levels than the positive control. The higher Th2 response in comparison with Th1 proved to be highly efficacious [89]. Thus, the incorporation of TLR2 agonist augmented innate response and favored antigen-specific antibody production. Several lipopeptide-based synthetic TLR2 agonists are currently available [71], and first-generation SAR studies on the PAM_2CS series of compounds [90] led to a simplified second-generation monoacyl lipopeptide PAMCS (**1**) in which the spacing between the ester-linked acyl group and the thioether played a crucial role in determining activity [91]. Few recently discovered small-molecule TLR2 agonists (diprovocims and dihydropyridine–quinolone

Table 14.3 Synthetic TLR adjuvant-based approaches for enhanced immunogenicity of malaria vaccines.

Synthetic TLR adjuvants	Malarial antigen as a vaccine candidate	Immune responses	Ref.
Pam3Cys (TLR2 agonist)	*PfCSP*-T1BT*K20	Enhanced DC activation, higher sporozoite-specific neutralizing antibody titer and IFN-γ levels, better production of effector T cells and Th2 response than Th1 response	[71]
3D-MPL (TLR4 agonist)	*PfCSP*	Improved CD4+ Th1 response, higher anti-CSP antibody titer	[72]
3D-MPL (TLR4 agonist)	*PfCelTOS*	Higher *PfCelTOS*-specific and sporozoite-neutralizing antibodies increased IFNγ producing splenocytes	[73]
GLA (TLR4 agonist)	*PfCelTOS*	Higher IgG2a antibody and IFNγ production, eliciting Th1 response, increased secretion of long-lived plasma cells	[74]
GLA-SE (TLR4 agonist)	*PfCelTOS*	A higher level of plasma IgG2a antibody titers, increased production of IFNγ, activating long-lived antibody-secreting plasma cells	[75]
GLA-SE (TLR4 agonist)	*PfGLURP* and *PfMSP3* (GMZ2)	Higher cytophilic antibody IgG2a in comparison with IgG1 increased production of IFNγ, Th1-based T-cell response	[76]
Flagellin (TLR5 agonist)	*PfCSP*	Higher IgG1 antibody favoring Th2 response increased level of sporozoite-neutralizing antibodies	[77]
Flagellin (TLR5 agonist)	*PfMSP1*	Higher cytophilic antibody IgG1 and IgG2b, Th2 adaptive response	[78]
Imiquimod (TLR7 agonist)	*PfCSP*-T1BT*	High levels of sporozoite-neutralizing antibodies, higher Th1-type IgG2 and Th2-type IgG1 antibody production	[79]
AddaVax (TLR7/8 and TLR 9 agonist)	*PfCSP*-T1BT*	Improved anti-CS-repeat antibodies and IgG2c production, higher sporozoite-neutralizing antibody	[79]
CpG-ODNs (TLR9 agonist)	*PfCSP*	An increased anti-CSP antibody titer, induction of Th1 responses, and specific memory B cells	[80]
CpG-ODNs (TLR9 agonist)	*PfSERA5*	Improved activation of CD4+ T cells, effector memory cells, and higher Th1/Th2 response	[81]

carboxamides) are shown in Figure 14.3 that might induce potential antimalarial efficacy in malaria vaccines [92, 93].

14.4.2 TLR4

Being the most explored member of the TLR family, TLR4 interacts chiefly with the lipid A portion of the lipopolysaccharide (LPS), activating host inflammatory

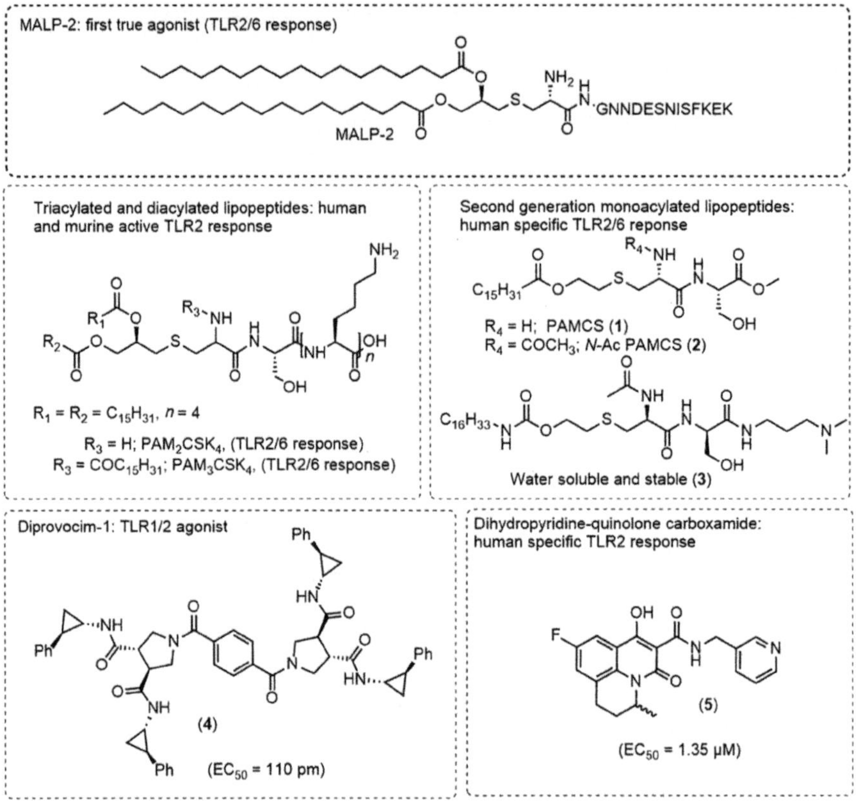

Figure 14.4 TLR2 agonistic lipopeptides: MALP-2 to second-generation lipopeptides (**1**–**3**) and new classes of TLR2 agonists such as diprovocims (**4**) and dihydropyridine–quinolone carboxamides (**5**).

pathways. All LPS-like and non-lipid-like TLR4 activators (Figure 14.5) have demonstrated qualitative antibody responses; however, 3D-MPL (3-*O*-deacylated monophosphoryl lipid A) [94, 95] and GLA [96] have been explored as a potent malarial vaccine adjuvant. Glucopyranosyl lipid adjuvant (GLA)-based formulations activate the TLR4 receptor molecules, switching a Th1 bias response, inducing a high level of IgG2a antibody titer. GLA-based emulsion adjuvants were utilized for improving the immunogenicity of *PfCelTOS* (*Plasmodium falciparum* cell traversal protein for ookinetes and sporozoites). The immunological significance of *PfCelTOS* suggested that antibodies against *PfCelTOS* may block sporozoite infection in the hepatocytes and inhibit their passage through the mosquito midgut [73]. *In vivo* studies in mice and rodents indicated that *PfCelTOS* elicited protective immunity with antigen-specific monoclonal antibody generation, impairing sporozoite infectivity and parasite development both in humans and mosquito vector [74]. However, to be utilized as a subunit vaccine induction of sterile or long-living protection is pivotal. To improve its protective efficacy, recombinant *PfCelTOS* was formulated with synthetic TLR4 ligand GLA-SE (squalene-based stable emulsion). The inclusion of GLA-SE in the vaccine formulation resulted

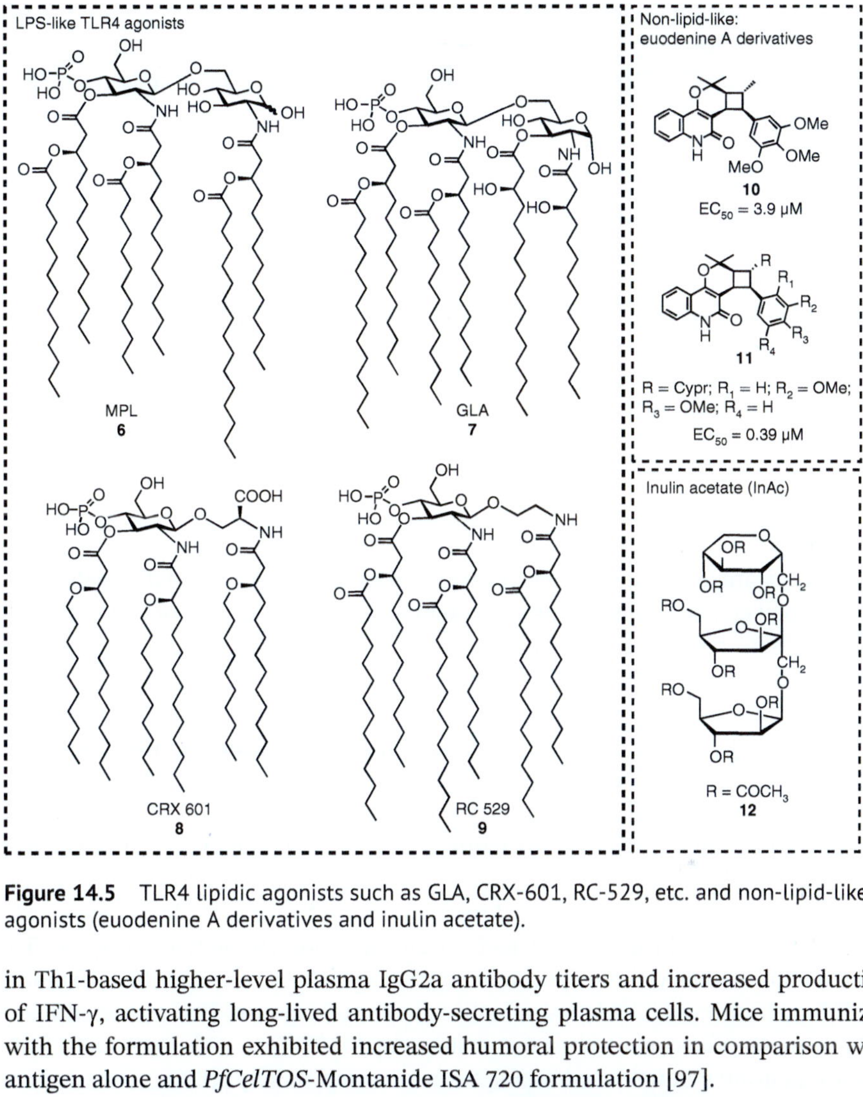

Figure 14.5 TLR4 lipidic agonists such as GLA, CRX-601, RC-529, etc. and non-lipid-like agonists (euodenine A derivatives and inulin acetate).

in Th1-based higher-level plasma IgG2a antibody titers and increased production of IFN-γ, activating long-lived antibody-secreting plasma cells. Mice immunized with the formulation exhibited increased humoral protection in comparison with antigen alone and *PfCelTOS*-Montanide ISA 720 formulation [97].

Another leading *P. falciparum* vaccine candidate is GMZ2, a hybrid protein of GLURP and MSP3, both associated with a higher titer of human IgG antibodies [75, 98]. GMZ2 includes conserved epitope sequences of GLURP at the 5′ end in frame with conserved B-cell epitope sequences of MSP3 at the 3′ end. Immuno-epidemiological studies indicated that cytophilic antibodies specific for these proteins have been associated with reduced malarial risk [99, 100]. Immunization of mice with the hybrid protein generated strong and specific antibody titer mainly of IgG1 and IgG2 isotype. The immunogenicity of the hybrid was also profound in the clinically immune African adults who produced hybrid-specific naturally occurring IgG antibodies [101]. To confer a long-term immunity, synthetic TLR-based adjuvants were formulated to enhance the humoral immunity for GMZ2. TLR4 agonist GLA in stable emulsion upon formulation with GMZ2 elevated the cytophilic isotype IgG2a in comparison with IgG1 antibody. Infected mice models exhibited GLURP- and MSP3-specific long-lasting cytophilic antibodies with an increased ratio of IgG2a/IgG1, suggesting class switching of B cells from IgG1 to IgG2a isotype. Additionally, GLA-SE-GMZ2 promoted increased production of IFN-γ and decreased production of IL-5, indicating induction of Th1-based T-cell response compared with Th2 type. Thus, adjuvantation of GMZ2 with synthetic TLR4 agonist GLA-SE resulted in improved production of antigen-specific long-lasting cytophilic antibodies by plasma cells, generating a humoral response. The efficiently produced cytophilic antibodies trigger antibody-dependent cellular inhibition (ADCI), providing protection against re-infection [102]. Very recently few novel structural classes of compounds (euodenine A derivatives, **10–11**, and inulin acetate, **12**) have demonstrated TLR4 activation that might show the potential application in malaria [76, 103].

14.4.3 TLR5

Even though TLR5 agonists are the least explored in malarial immunity, their use as an adjuvant for *Plasmodium* proteins seems possible. Bacterial flagellin, the subunit of flagellar filament, acts as a potent human TLR5 agonist provoking strong inflammatory responses [104]. Several murine and primate studies have shown the utilization of flagellin (FliC), especially from *Salmonella* species, in several viral and Flu vaccines for enhanced immunogenicity [105]. Binding of FliC to the extracellular region of TLR5 expressed on APCs mediates MyD88-dependent Th2 responses. The ability of FliC to reduce IL-10 production and boost adaptive immunity was utilized for improving the immunogenicity of MSP1 and CSP vaccine candidates against *P. falciparum*. A study by Bargeiri et al. evidenced the use of *Salmonella* FliC flagellin (a TLR5 agonist) as an adjuvant for malarial antigen MSP1. *Plasmodium*-infected mice immunized with FliC-His6-tagged MSP1 formulation elicited higher IgG1 and IgG2b cytophilic antibody than IgG2c. The formulation exhibited limited induced of splenocytes to secrete a moderate amount of IFN-γ, favoring a Th2-based adaptive immune response. The strong immune response was elicited upon co-formulation of MSP1-FliC with CpG ODN 1826 (TLR9 adjuvant)/Quil-A, modulating better immunogenicity [106].

A similar approach was made for enhancing the protective efficacy of *P. falciparum* circumsporozoite protein (CSP). Efficacy and potency enhancement was monitored by fusion of CSP-T1BT* triepitope peptide with STF (Salmonella enterica *Typhimurium* FliC). Both the full length (STF2) and the truncated flagellin protein (STF2Δ) were fused with CSP [107]. Immunization of infected mice with either formulation provided similar protection against infection. The formulation triggered predominantly IgG1 response, with minimal IFN-γ production, favoring Th2 response. Interaction of FliC with TLR5 receptor activates TLR5 downstream cascade producing inflammatory cytokines such as IL-5, IL-6, and minimal IFN-γ. This enabled switching of T cells toward Th2 response. Immunization with the formulation also elicited a high level of sporozoite-neutralizing antibody, thereby reducing the pre-erythrocytic parasite burden within the hepatocytes. Thus, the use of adjuvants with malarial antigens may provide an ideal formulation to improve the potency and protection by the malarial vaccine.

14.4.4 TLR7/8

The ability of TLR7 to recognize pathogen-specific RNA and trigger an immune response to bridge the gap between innate and adaptive response is already known. Being an endosomally localized TLR, the agonists of TLR7 may function effectively as an adjuvant enhancing the efficacy of subunit malaria vaccines. Imiquimod and gardiquimod, a synthetic small molecule of the imidazoquinoline series, an analog of ssRNA ligand, are recognized by TLR7, promoting CD4+ and CD8+ T-cell responses against virally infected cells, basal and squamous cell carcinomas, leishmaniasis, etc. [77, 78, 108, 109]. Being structurally and phylogenetically related, these receptors respond differently to certain ligands, for instance, imiquimod selectively activates TLR7, whereas few non-polymeric agonists such as CL097, 14 (Figure 14.6), induce mixed TLR7/8 response. The relevant application of the TLR7 agonist, imiquimod, has been shown by a study involving incorporation of imiquimod along with *P. falciparum* CS peptide T1BT* [110]. The topical application of FDA-approved imiquimod on the skin of murine models after immunization with CS peptide elicited high anti-CSP antibody titer. Immunization

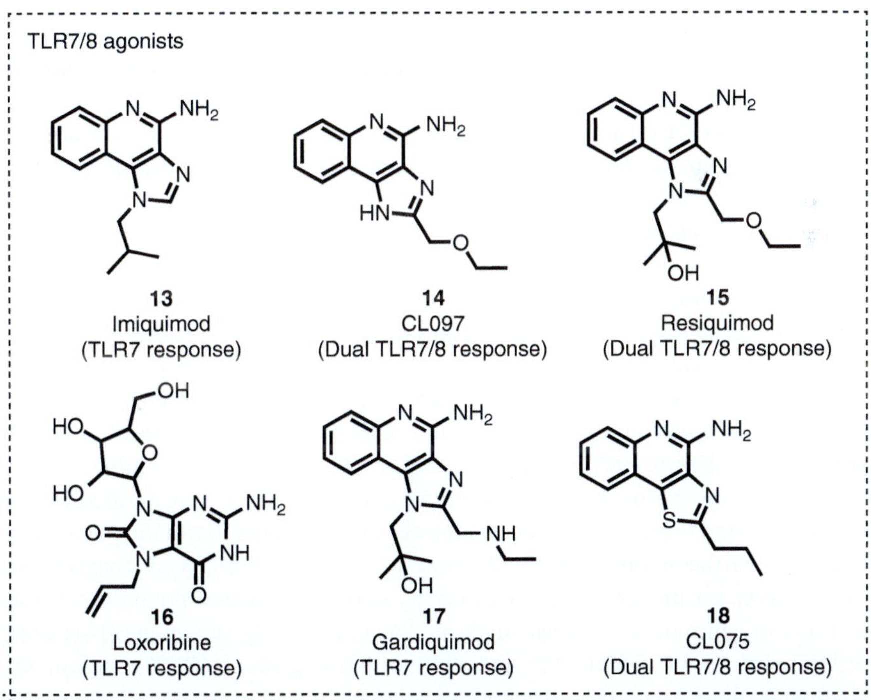

Figure 14.6 TLR7/8 agonists in malaria vaccines such as imiquimod (**13**), CL097 (**14**), and resiquimod (**15**) and other potential TLR7/8 agonists not explored in malaria vaccines (**16–18**).

with the peptide-adjuvant formulation promoted a mixed Th1/Th2 response, chiefly including Th1-type IgG2a/IgG2c antibodies along with IgG1 isotype. The peptides plus topical imiquimod (**13**) immunization induced high levels of sporozoite-neutralising CS-specific antibodies inhibiting the infection caused by mosquito-injected sporozoite *in vivo*. Moreover, a few applications of imiquimod with CS peptide resulted in high-level production of Th1-type IgG2 and Th2-type IgG1 antibodies in infected and immunized mice in comparison with immunization with peptide alone. Application of topical adjuvant retains the sporozoites at the site of infection for prolong period, capable of eliciting stronger immunity by extended antigen presentation. This approach of topical application of an adjuvant at the site of vaccine immunization on the skin may thus provide an outlook for obtaining sterile immunity in humans.

Skin plays a vital role in the malarial pathogenesis, the site of inoculation, and initiation of the parasite life cycle in the human host and a reservoir for several host immune cells such as dendritic cells, Langerhans cells, and γδ T cells inducing effector immune responses. The presence of several antigens presenting cells in the dermis layer stimulates antibody secretion, arresting the sporozoite migration to the hepatocytes and further blood-stage infection. Vaccine candidates eliciting such first line of defense are of prime focus against malaria, and the use of adjuvants that enhance such immune responses is also pivotal. The previous study utilized topical application of synthetic TLR7 imiquimod, while some studies utilized the ability of damage-associated molecular patterns (DAMPs) to promote an immune response [110, 111]. Skin scarification results in the damage to the dermal layer, along with the better presentation of PAMPs, initiating tissue damage-mediated antibody responses. Studies that represent colocalization of CS peptide with imiquimod (Aldara) at the site of SS elicited higher peak of Th1/Th2 response with IgG1 and IgG2c opsonizing antibody isotypes. Activation of TLR7 with Aldara promotes the synthesis of CS-specific T cells secreting IFN-γ and sporozoite-neutralising antibodies that block sporozoite invasion and egress-inhibiting infection of hepatocytes and blood cells. Immunization with CSP-Aldara protects the mice models against challenge by *Plasmodium*-infected mosquitoes. However, these vaccine adjuvants often associated with repeated dosage result in higher expenditure. Co-formulation of different TLRs may seem promising providing enhanced immunogenicity and protection at a lesser dosage. AddaVax, a creme formulation of TLR7/8 agonist resiquimod (**15**, Figure 14.5) and TLR 9 agonist CpG along with CS peptide (T1BT*) via SS, enhanced the protection by improving the anti-CS-repeat antibodies and IgG2c production. Improved protection may be conferred predominantly by phagocytosis due to the increase in the opsonizing antibody. Enhanced phagocytosis and release of serum sporozoite-neutralizing antibody together potently promote the humoral immunity against malaria. Several highly active TLR7-specific (gardiquimod **16**, loxoribine **17**) and dual TLR7/8 agonists (CL075, **18**) of the imidazoquinoline and other structural classes are recently reported and are not explored in malaria vaccines [79, 112].

14.4.5 TLR9

This intracellular receptor is known to be expressed by B cells, macrophages, and plasmacytoid DCs. TLR9 recognizes DNA from the viral and bacterial origin and self-DNA while forming immune complexes [113] but has been shown to get activated by (Figure 14.6) hemozoin-associated DNA [114]. Within the RBCs, parasite metabolizes hemoglobin and releases porphyrin molecules that are toxic to the parasite; thus it polymerizes them into hemozoin crystals within the food vacuole. When phagocytized by the APCs, these crystals along with *Plasmodium*-bound DNA interact with TLR9 ligand-binding domain and activate the MyD88-dependent IRF5/7 pathway. This activates different MyD88-dependent PRRs such as inflammasomes and TLR9 and triggers the production of cytokines such as TNFα, IL-6, IL-12, and IL-1β (Figure 14.7). Akira et al. have devised a method where hemozoin, a non-self-DNA TLR9 ligand, has been utilized in the detection and measurement of malaria infection having the capacity to screen malaria vaccines and therapeutic medicines [115].

The criteria for recognition of non-self-DNA involve unmethylated CpG motifs from nucleotide sequences [116]. Hemmi et al. included that CpG-ODN in a cell initiates the binding with TLR-9 and ultimately triggers signal transduction. Following binding with CpG-ODN, the TIR domain of TLR 9 engages itself with MyD88 adaptor protein and stimulates immune responses to include induction of pro-inflammatory and Th1 cytokines (IL-6, IL-1, TNF-α, IFN-γ, and IL-12) [117]. CpG–ODNs are similar to native CpGs and have strong CD8+ T-cell responses.

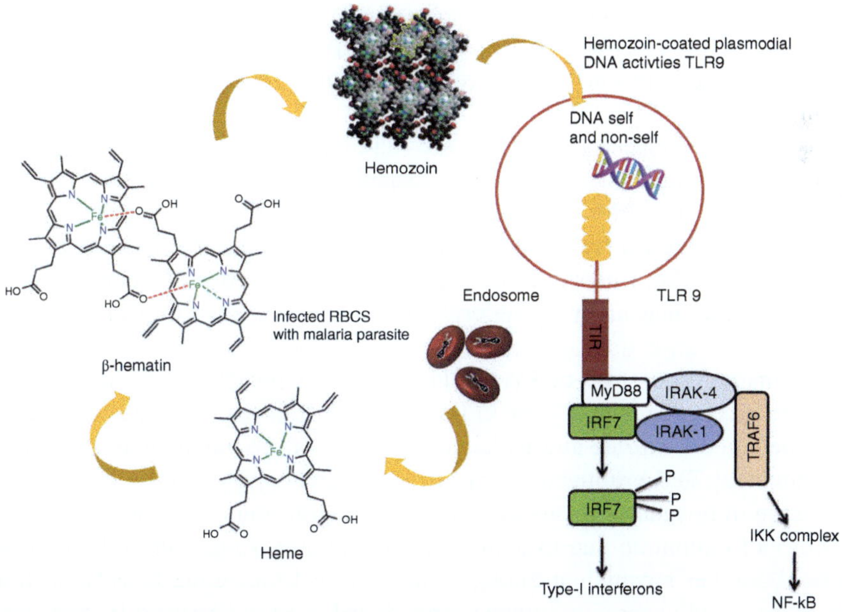

Figure 14.7 Hemozoin formation and TLR9 signaling pathway.

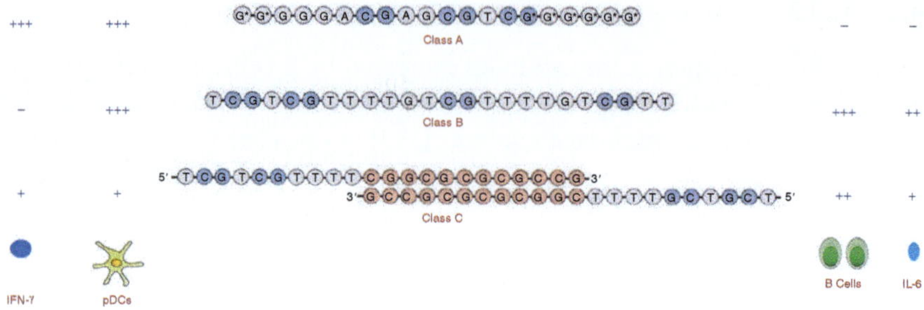

Figure 14.8 ODN classes of TLR9 agonists and their immune responses: Class A ODNs activate pDCs cells and induce highest IFN-γ levels compared with other classes, Class B ODNs activate B-cells and pDCs cells with IL-6 induction, and Class C ODNs show the moderate response for IFN-γ and IL-6 induction.

To date, four classes of ODNs with different structures have been characterized (Figure 14.8). Class A consists of mixed phosphodiester and phosphorothioate sequence, contains polyG motifs, and forms large structures. They activate pDCs to induce high levels of IFN-α with a lower level of NFκB stimulation. Class B ODNs contain one or more CpG motifs with purely phosphorothioate backbone and activate B cells and induce a higher level of IL-6 secretion. Class C ODNs exhibit intermediate stimulatory properties as they form palindromic motifs and contain only a phosphorothioate backbone. The phosphodiester backbone of ODNs can easily undergo degradation by nucleases, while a phosphorothioate backbone can bind non-specifically to proteins in serum causing unwanted side effects. Efforts are made to develop CpG–ODNs exclusively with a phosphodiester backbone, providing resistance to nuclease activity with immune-stimulatory properties of naturally occurring ODNs [118].

It has been investigated that vaccines containing TLR9 agonist CpG result in prolong and premature development of malaria protein-specific memory B-cell responses in malaria-naive individuals [119]. Similarly, an immunogenic hybrid fusion protein generated from CSP of *Plasmodium* vivax and/or *P. falciparum* and surface antigen S from hepatitis B virus supplemented with CpG TLR9 agonist boosted the immunogenicity of the protein by increasing the anti-CSP antibody titer [114].

Symptomatic blood stage of *Plasmodium* possesses several potent antigens as a probable vaccine candidate. One of the potential antigens is SERA5, expressed during the late trophozoite and schizont stages. Literature reports that utilization of recombinant SERA antigen (SE47) in non-human primates conferred protective immunity against *Plasmodium* [120]. However, the challenge remains in terms of its formulation due to its hydrophobic nature. Tougan et al. [121] thus generated another recombinant antigen SE36 (lacked the serine repeats) with a hydrogel-based adjuvant aluminium hydroxide gel (AHG). Observed in primates, SE36/AHG demonstrated that a higher anti-SE36 titer that retained in plasma more than a year, however, induced lower titer amounts upon clinical trials. This elevated the prerequisite for immune-stimulation of immune-responsive cells against the antigen SE36. Synthetic CpG adjuvants (K3 ODNs) containing unmethylated cytosine–guanosine dinucleotides were employed with Se36/AHG. The formulation aggravated the role of effector CD4+ T cells augmenting mixed Th1/Th2 response in non-human primates, eliciting effector memory cells. Such studies thus reveal the effectiveness of synthetic TLR adjuvants in improvising vaccine development to combat malaria [121].

14.5 Conclusion

Exploring novel antigens is a never-ending path in terms of vaccination. However, for malarial vaccines, antigenic polymorphism and reduced antigen-specific immune-stimulation have been a major setback. Despite the use of several adjuvants for enhanced vaccine immunogenicity, the major hindrance pertaining to long-lasting vaccination is inadequate production of T- and B-cell responses. It is vital for an adjuvant to evoke cellular and humoral responses effectively. The new research in synthetic adjuvants may emerge as a promising measure to accelerate malaria vaccine development. The hitch may be untangled by expanding the plethora of cytokine storm and enhancing protective immunity by providing enormous opsonizing, neutralizing, and cytophilic antibody. Insights into the MyD88-dependent PRRs and their differential expression and divergent mode of action during a complicated and uncomplicated state of malaria may prove benefactor. Moreover, each antigen may animate variable immune responses, augmenting discrete TLR-based signaling. Furthermore, co-stimulation of TLRs with different antigens and conjugation of vaccine antigen with synthetic TLR adjuvants may provide a synergistic approach to fight malaria.

Abbreviations

3D-MPL	3-*O*-deacylated monophosphoryl lipid A
ADCI	antibody-dependent cellular inhibition
AMA1	apical membrane protein 1
CFA	complete Freund's adjuvant
CLRs	C-type lectin receptors
CRP	C-reactive protein
CSP	circumsporozoite protein
CTLs	cytotoxic T lymphocytes
DC	dendritic cell
EBA-175	erythrocyte binding protein
GLA	glucopyranosyl lipid adjuvant
GlcN	glucosamine
GPI	glycosyl phosphatidylinositol
Hz	hemozoin
IFN	interferons

IL	interleukins
Ino	inositol
iRBCs	infected red blood cells
ISCOMs	immunostimulating complexes
LBL	layer by layer
LPS	lipopolysaccharide
Man	mannose sugar residues
MCP-1	monocyte chemoattractant protein-1
MHC	major histocompatibility complex
MIP-1a	macrophage inflammatory protein-1a
MSP1	merozoite surface protein 1
NLRs	nod-like receptors
NO	nitric oxide
PAMPs	pathogen-associated molecular patterns
pDC	plasmacytoid dendritic cells
PE	phosphoethanolamine
PfCelTOS	*Plasmodium falciparum* cell traversal protein for ookinetes and sporozoites
PRRs	pattern recognition receptors
QS-21	saponin
STF2	*Salmonella enterica Typhimurium* FliC
STF2Δ	truncated *Salmonella enterica Typhimurium* FliC
TBV	transmission blocking vaccines
Tfh	T-follicular helper cells
TLR	toll-like receptor
TNF	tumor necrosis factor
Tregs	T-regulatory cells
μMT mice	B-cell knockout mice

References

1 Fauci, A.S. and Morens, D.M. (2012). The perpetual challenge of infectious diseases. *New England Journal of Medicine* 366 (5): 454–461.

2 Oakes, R.S. and Jewell, C.M. (2018 Dec). A plug-and-play approach for malaria vaccination. *Nature Nanotechnology* 13 (12): 1096.

3 Rts, S.C. (2015). Efficacy and safety of RTS, S/AS01 malaria vaccine with or without a booster dose in infants and children in Africa: final results of a phase 3, individually randomised, controlled trial. *The Lancet* 386 (9988): 31–45.

4 World Health Organization (2018). Malaria vaccine: WHO position paper, January 2016–recommendations. *Vaccine* 36 (25): 3576–3577.

5 Regules, J.A., Cicatelli, S.B., Bennett, J.W. et al. (2016). Fractional third and fourth dose of RTS, S/AS01 malaria candidate vaccine: a phase 2a controlled human malaria parasite infection and immunogenicity study. *The Journal of Infectious Diseases* 214 (5): 762–771.

6 Oyen, D., Torres, J.L., Wille-Reece, U. et al. (2017). Structural basis for antibody recognition of the NANP repeats in *Plasmodium falciparum* circumsporozoite protein. *Proceedings of the National Academy of Sciences of the United Stated of America* 114 (48): E10438–E10445.

7 Kusi, K.A., Faber, B.W., Thomas, A.W., and Remarque, E.J. (2009). Humoral immune response to mixed *Pf* AMA1 alleles; multivalent *Pf* AMA1 vaccines induce broad specificity. *PLoS One* 4 (12): e8110.

8 Ouattara, A., Mu, J., Takala-Harrison, S. et al. (2010). Lack of allele-specific efficacy of a bivalent AMA1 malaria vaccine. *Malaria Journal* 9 (1): 1–3.

9 Campeotto, I., Goldenzweig, A., Davey, J. et al. (2017). One-step design of a stable variant of the malaria invasion protein RH5 for use as a vaccine immunogen. *Proceedings of the National Academy of Sciences of the United States of America* 114 (5): 998–1002.

10 Utami, R.A. (2018). Association between antibody responses to blood stage parasitic antigens and protection from *Plasmodium falciparum* and *Plasmodium vivax* Malaria in Timika, Indonesia.

11 Douglas, A.D., Williams, A.R., Illingworth, J.J. et al. (2011). The blood-stage malaria antigen *Pf*RH5 is susceptible to vaccine-inducible cross-strain neutralizing antibody. *Nature Communications* 2 (1): 1–9.

12 Foquet, L., Schafer, C., Minkah, N.K. et al. (2018). *Plasmodium falciparum* liver stage infection and transition to stable blood stage infection in liver-humanized and blood-humanized FRGN KO mice enables testing of blood stage inhibitory antibodies (reticulocyte-binding protein homolog 5) in vivo. *Frontiers in Immunology* 9: 524.

13 Bustamante, L.Y., Powell, G.T., Lin, Y.C. et al. (2017). Synergistic malaria vaccine combinations identified by systematic antigen screening. *Proceedings of the National Academy of Sciences of the United States of America* 114 (45): 12045–12050.

14 Chen, L., Xu, Y., Wong, W. et al. (2017). Structural basis for inhibition of erythrocyte invasion by antibodies to *Plasmodium falciparum* protein CyRPA. *eLife* 6: e21347.

15 Volz, J.C., Yap, A., Sisquella, X. et al. (2016). Essential role of the PfRh5/PfRipr/CyRPA complex during *Plasmodium falciparum* invasion of erythrocytes. *Cell Host & Microbe* 20 (1): 60–71.

16 Talaat, K.R., Ellis, R.D., Hurd, J. et al. (2016). Safety and immunogenicity of Pfs25-EPA/Alhydrogel®, a transmission blocking vaccine against *Plasmodium falciparum*: an open label study in malaria naïve adults. *PLoS One* 11 (10): e0163144.

17 Huang, W.C., Deng, B., Lin, C. et al. (2018). A malaria vaccine adjuvant based on recombinant antigen binding to liposomes. *Nature Nanotechnology* 13 (12): 1174.

18 Menon, V., Kapulu, M.C., Taylor, I. et al. (2018). Assessment of antibodies induced by multivalent transmission-blocking malaria vaccines. *Frontiers in Immunology* 8: 1998.

19 Singh, S.K., Roeffen, W., Mistarz, U.H. et al. (2017). Construct design, production, and characterization of *Plasmodium falciparum* 48/45 R0.6C subunit protein produced in *Lactococcus lactis* as candidate vaccine. *Microbial Cell Factories* 16 (1): 97.

20 Singh, S.K., Thrane, S., Chourasia, B.K. et al. (2019). Pfs230 and Pfs48/45 fusion proteins elicit strong transmission-blocking antibody responses against *Plasmodium falciparum*. *Frontiers in Immunology* 10: 1256.

21 Overstreet, M.G., Chen, Y.C., Cockburn, I.A. et al. (2011). CD4+ T cells modulate expansion and survival but not functional properties of effector and memory CD8+ T cells induced by malaria sporozoites. *PLoS One* 6 (1): e15948.

22 Carvalho, L.H., Sano, G.I., Hafalla, J.C. et al. (2002). IL-4-secreting CD4+ T cells are crucial to the development of CD8+ T-cell responses against malaria liver stages. *Nature Medicine* 8 (2): 166.

23 Nardin, E.H. and Nussenzweig, R.S. (1993). T cell responses to pre-erythrocytic stages of malaria: role in protection and vaccine development against pre-erythrocytic stages. *Annual Review of Immunology* 11 (1): 687–727.

24 Pied, S.Y., Nussler, A., Pontent, M. et al. (1989). C-reactive protein protects against pre-erythrocytic stages of malaria. *Infection and Immunity* 57 (1): 278–282.

25 Franklin, B.S., Parroche, P., Ataíde, M.A. et al. (2009). Malaria primes the innate immune response due to interferon-γ induced enhancement of toll-like receptor expression and function. *Proceedings of the National Academy of Sciences of the United Stated of America* 106 (14): 5789–5794.

26 Taylor-Robinson, A.W. and Smith, E.C. (1999). A dichotomous role for nitric oxide in protection against blood stage malaria infection. *Immunology Letters* 67 (1): 1–9.

27 Roetynck, S., Baratin, M., Vivier, É., and Ugolini, S. (2006). NK cells and innate immunity to malaria. *Medecine Sciences: M/S.* 22 (8, 9): 739–744.

28 Pied, S., Roland, J., Louise, A. et al. (2000). Liver CD4− CD8− NK1. 1+ TCRαβ intermediate cells increase during experimental malaria infection and are able to exhibit inhibitory activity against the parasite liver stage in vitro. *The Journal of Immunology* 164 (3): 1463–1469.

29 Su, Z. and Stevenson, M.M. (2002). IL-12 is required for antibody-mediated protective immunity against blood-stage *Plasmodium chabaudi* AS malaria infection in mice. *The Journal of Immunology* 168 (3): 1348–1355.

30 Stevenson, M.M., Tam, M.F., Wolf, S.F., and Sher, A. (1995). IL-12-induced protection against blood-stage *Plasmodium chabaudi AS* requires IFN-gamma and TNF-alpha and occurs via a nitric oxide-dependent mechanism. *The Journal of Immunology* 155 (5): 2545–2556.

31 Stevenson, M.M. and Riley, E.M. (2004). Innate immunity to malaria. *Nature Reviews. Immunology* 4 (3): 169.

32 von der Weid, T., Honarvar, N., and Langhorne, J. (1996). Gene-targeted mice lacking B cells are unable to eliminate a blood stage malaria infection. *The Journal of Immunology* 156 (7): 2510–2516.

33 Langhorne, J., Cross, C., Seixas, E. et al. (1998). A role for B cells in the development of T cell helper function in a malaria infection in mice. *Proceedings of the National Academy of Sciences of the United Stated of America* 95 (4): 1730–1734.

34 Urban, B.C., Ing, R., and Stevenson, M.M. (2005). *Early Interactions Between Blood-Stage Plasmodium Parasites and the Immune System in Immunology and Immune-Pathogenesis of Malaria*, 25–70. Berlin, Heidelberg: Springer.

35 Bouharoun-Tayoun, H., Oeuvray, C., Lunel, F., and Druilhe, P. (1995). Mechanisms underlying the monocyte-mediated antibody-dependent killing of *Plasmodium falciparum* asexual blood stages. *Journal of Experimental Medicine* 182 (2): 409–418.

36 Stevenson, M.M. and Tam, M.F. (1993). Differential induction of helper T cell subsets during blood-stage *Plasmodium chabaudi* AS infection in resistant and susceptible mice. *Clinical and Experimental Immunology* 92 (1): 77–83.

37 Linke, A., Kühn, R., Müller, W. et al. (1996). *Plasmodium chabaudi*: differential susceptibility of gene-targeted mice deficient in IL-10 to an erythrocytic-stage infection. *Experimental Parasitology* 84 (2): 253–263.

38 Aribot, G., Rogier, C., Sarthou, J.L. et al. (1996). Pattern of immunoglobulin isotype response to *Plasmodium falciparum* blood-stage antigens in individuals living in a holo endemic area of Senegal (Dielmo, West Africa). *The American Journal of Tropical Medicine and Hygiene* 54 (5): 449–457.

39 Matsumoto, S., Yukitake, H., Kanbara, H. et al. (2000). *Mycobacterium bovis* bacillus calmette-guerin induces protective immunity against infection by *Plasmodium yoelii* at blood-stage depending on shifting immunity toward Th1 type and inducing protective IgG2a after the parasite infection. *Vaccine* 19 (7, 8): 779–787.

40 Taylor-Robinson, A.W. and Phillips, R.S. (1994). B cells are required for the switch from Th1-to Th2-regulated immune responses to *Plasmodium chabaudi* infection. *Infection and Immunity* 62 (6): 2490–2498.

41 Perlmann, H., Helmby, H., Hagstedt, M. et al. (1994). IgE elevation and IgE anti-malarial antibodies in *Plasmodium falciparum* malaria; association of high IgE levels with cerebral malaria. *Clinical and Experimental Immunology* 97 (2): 284–292.

42 Perlmann, P.E., Perlmann, H.E., Looareesuwan, S.O. et al. (2000). Contrasting functions of IgG and IgE antimalarial antibodies in uncomplicated and severe *Plasmodium falciparum* malaria. *The American Journal of Tropical Medicine and Hygiene* 62 (3): 373–377.

43 Vukovic, P., Hogarth, P.M., Barnes, N. et al. (2000). Immunoglobulin G3 antibodies specific for the 19-kilodalton carboxyl-terminal fragment of *Plasmodium yoelii* merozoite surface protein 1 transfer protection to mice deficient in Fc-γRI receptors. *Infection and Immunity* 68 (5): 3019–3022.

44 Majarian, W.R., Daly, T.M., Weidanz, W.P., and Long, C.A. (1984). Passive immunization against murine malaria with an IgG3 monoclonal antibody. *The Journal of Immunology* 132 (6): 3131–3137.

45 Obeng-Adjei, N., Portugal, S., Tran, T.M. et al. (2015). Circulating Th1-cell-type Tfh cells that exhibit impaired B cell help are preferentially activated during acute malaria in children. *Cell Reports* 13 (2): 425–439.

46 Hisaeda, H., Maekawa, Y., Iwakawa, D. et al. (2004). Escape of malaria parasites from host immunity requires CD4+ CD25+ regulatory T cells. *Nature Medicine* 10 (1): 29.

47 Minigo, G., Woodberry, T., Piera, K.A. et al. (2009). Parasite-dependent expansion of TNF receptor II–positive regulatory T cells with enhanced suppressive activity in adults with severe malaria. *PLoS Pathogens* 5 (4): e1000402.

48 Engwerda, C.R. and Good, M.F. (2005). Interactions between malaria parasites and the host immune system. *Current Opinion in Immunology* 17 (4): 381–387.

49 Hviid, L. (2005). Naturally acquired immunity to *Plasmodium falciparum* malaria in Africa. *Acta Tropica* 95 (3): 270–275.

50 Gazzinelli, R.T. and Denkers, E.Y. (2006). Protozoan encounters with toll-like receptor signalling pathways: implications for host parasitism. *Nature Reviews. Immunology* 6 (12): 895.

51 Kawai, T. and Akira, S. (2011). Toll-like receptors and their crosstalk with other innate receptors in infection and immunity. *Immunity* 34 (5): 637–650.

52 Coban, C., Ishii, K.J., Kawai, T. et al. (2005). Toll-like receptor 9 mediates innate immune activation by the malaria pigment hemozoin. *Journal of Experimental Medicine* 201 (1): 19–25.

53 Parroche, P., Lauw, F.N., Goutagny, N. et al. (2007). Malaria hemozoin is immunologically inert but radically enhances innate responses by presenting malaria DNA to toll-like receptor 9. *Proceedings of the National Academy of Sciences of the United Stated of America* 104 (6): 1919–1924.

54 Krishnegowda, G., Hajjar, A.M., Zhu, J. et al. (2005). Induction of proinflammatory responses in macrophages by the glycosyl phosphatidyl inositols of *Plasmodium falciparum* cell signaling receptors, glycosyl phosphatidyl inositol (GPI) structural requirement, and regulation of GPI activity. *Journal of Biological Chemistry* 280 (9): 8606–8616.

55 Nebl, T., De Veer, M.J., and Schofield, L. (2005). Stimulation of innate immune responses by malarial glycosyl phosphatidyl inositol via pattern recognition receptors. *Parasitology* 130 (S1): S45–S62.

56 Dostert, C., Guarda, G., Romero, J.F. et al. (2009). Malarial hemozoin is a Nalp3 inflammasome activating danger signal. *PLoS One* 4 (8): e6510.

57 Griffith, J.W., Sun, T., McIntosh, M.T., and Bucala, R. (2009). Pure hemozoin is inflammatory in vivo and activates the NALP3 inflammasome via release of uric acid. *The Journal of Immunology* 183 (8): 5208–5220.

58 Naik, R.S., Branch, O.H., Woods, A.S. et al. (2000). Glycosyl phosphatidyl inositol anchors of *Plasmodium falciparum*: molecular characterization and naturally elicited antibody response that may provide immunity to malaria pathogenesis. *Journal of Experimental Medicine* 192 (11): 1563–1576.

59 Durai, P., Govindaraj, R.G., and Choi, S. (2013). Structure and dynamic behavior of T oll-like receptor 2 subfamily triggered by malarial glycosyl phosphatidyl inositols of *Plasmodium falciparum*. *The FEBS Journal* 280 (23): 6196–6212.

60 Gowda, D.C. (2007). TLR-mediated cell signaling by malaria GPIs. *Trends in Parasitology* 23 (12): 596–604.

61 Baccarella, A., Fontana, M.F., Chen, E.C., and Kim, C.C. (2013). Toll-like receptor 7 mediates early innate immune responses to malaria. *Infection and Immunity* 81 (12): 4431–4442.

62 Kim, C.C., Nelson, C.S., Wilson, E.B. et al. (2012). Splenic red pulp macrophages produce type I interferons as early sentinels of malaria infection but are dispensable for control. *PLoS One* 7 (10): e48126.

63 Haque, A., Best, S.E., Ammerdorffer, A. et al. (2011). Type I interferons suppress CD4+ T-cell-dependent parasite control during blood-stage *Plasmodium* infection. *European Journal of Immunology* 41 (9): 2688–2698.

64 Hunt, N.H. and Grau, G.E. (2003). Cytokines: accelerators and brakes in the pathogenesis of cerebral malaria. *Trends in Immunology* 24 (9): 491–499.

65 de Kossodo, S. and Grau, G.E. (1993). Profiles of cytokine production in relation with susceptibility to cerebral malaria. *The Journal of Immunology* 151 (9): 4811–4820.

66 Baccarella, A., Huang, B.W., Fontana, M.F., and Kim, C.C. (2014). Loss of toll-like receptor 7 alters cytokine production and protects against experimental cerebral malaria. *Malaria Journal* 13 (1): 354.

67 Olivier, M., Van Den Ham, K., Shio, M.T. et al. (2014). Malarial pigment hemozoin and the innate inflammatory response. *Frontiers in Immunology* 5: 25.

68 Coban, C., Igari, Y., Yagi, M. et al. (2010). Immunogenicity of whole-parasite vaccines against *Plasmodium falciparum* involves malarial hemozoin and host TLR9. *Cell Host & Microbe* 7 (1): 50–61.

69 Giribaldi, G., Prato, M., Ulliers, D. et al. (2010). Involvement of inflammatory chemokines in survival of human monocytes fed with malarial pigment. *Infection and Immunity* 78 (11): 4912–4921.

70 Shio, M.T., Eisenbarth, S.C., Savaria, M. et al. (2009). Malarial hemozoin activates the NLRP3 inflammasome through Lyn and Syk kinases. *PLoS Pathogens* 5 (8): e1000559.

71 Kaur, A., Patil, M.T., Mehta, S.K., and Salunke, D.B. (2018). An efficient and scalable synthesis of potent TLR2 agonistic PAM2CSK4. *RSC Advances* 8 (18): 9587–9596.

72 Dutta, S., Inventor; US Secretary of Army, Assignee. (2018). Soluble recombinant plasmodium falciparum circumsporozoite protein, use in vaccines, methods of making and uses thereof. United States patent US 9,919,040, filed 14 July 2015.

73 Kariu, T., Ishino, T., Yano, K. et al. (2006). CelTOS, a novel malarial protein that mediates transmission to mosquito and vertebrate hosts. *Molecular Microbiology* 59 (5): 1369–1379.

74 Espinosa, D.A., Vega-Rodriguez, J., Flores-Garcia, Y. et al. (2017). The *Plasmodium falciparum* cell-traversal protein for ookinetes and sporozoites as a candidate for pre-erythrocytic and transmission-blocking vaccines. *Infection and Immunity* 85 (2): e00498–e00416.

75 Dodoo, D., Theisen, M., Kurtzhals, J.A. et al. (2000). Naturally acquired antibodies to the glutamate-rich protein are associated with protection against *Plasmodium falciparum* malaria. *The Journal of Infectious Diseases* 181 (3): 1202–1205.

76 Kumar, S., Kesharwani, S.S., Kuppast, B. et al. (2016). Discovery of inulin acetate as a novel immune-active polymer and vaccine adjuvant: synthesis, material characterization, and biological evaluation as a toll-like receptor-4 agonist. *Journal of Materials Chemistry B* 4 (48): 7950–7960.

77 Zhang, W.W. and Matlashewski, G. (2008). Immunization with a toll-like receptor 7 and/or 8 agonist vaccine adjuvant increases protective immunity against *Leishmania major* in BALB/c mice. *Infection and Immunity* 76 (8): 3777–3783.

78 Itoh, T. and Celis, E. (2005). Transcutaneous immunization with cytotoxic T-cell peptide epitopes provides effective antitumor immunity in mice. *Journal of Immunotherapy (Hagerstown, Md.: 1997)* 28 (5): 430.

79 Yoo, E., Salunke, D.B., Sil, D. et al. (2014). Determinants of activity at human toll-like receptors 7 and 8: quantitative structure–activity relationship (QSAR) of diverse heterocyclic scaffolds. *Journal of Medicinal Chemistry* 57 (19): 7955–7970.

80 Mata, E., Salvador, A., Igartua, M. et al. (2013). Malaria vaccine adjuvants: latest update and challenges in preclinical and clinical research. *BioMed Research International* 2013: 282913.

81 Ezoe, S., Palacpac, N.M., Tetsutani, K. et al. (2020). First-in-human randomised trial and follow-up study of *Plasmodium falciparum* blood-stage malaria vaccine BK-SE36 with CpG-ODN (K3). *Vaccine* 38, 2 (46): 7246–7257.

82 Salunke, D.B., Shukla, N.M., Yoo, E. et al. (2012). Structure–activity relationships in human toll-like receptor 2-specific monoacyl lipopeptides. *Journal of Medicinal Chemistry* 55 (7): 3353–3363.

83 Salunke, D.B., Connelly, S.W., Shukla, N.M. et al. (2013). Design and development of stable, water-soluble, human toll-like receptor 2 specific monoacyl lipopeptides as candidate vaccine adjuvants. *Journal of Medicinal Chemistry* 56 (14): 5885–5900.

84 Cohen, J., Marchand, M., Ockenhouse, C.F., and Yadav, A. (2008). Vaccines for malaria. WO2008009652 A1, filed 16 July 2007.

85 Powell, T.J. (2013). Microparticle vaccine against malaria. WO2013148426 A1, filed 20 March 2013.

86 Powell, T.J. and Boyd, J.G. (2013). Antigenic compositions and methods. WO2013148427 A1, filed 20 March 2013.

87 Nardin, E.H., Calvo-Calle, J.M., Oliveira, G.A. et al. (2001). A totally synthetic polyoxime malaria vaccine containing *Plasmodium falciparum* B cell and universal T cell epitopes elicits immune responses in volunteers of diverse HLA types. *The Journal of Immunology* 166 (1): 481–489.

88 Powell, T.J., Tang, J., DeRome, M.E. et al. (2013). *Plasmodium falciparum* synthetic LbL microparticle vaccine elicits protective neutralizing antibody and parasite-specific cellular immune responses. *Vaccine* 31 (15): 1898–1904.

89 Kaur, A., Kannan, D., Mehta, S.K. et al. (2018). Synthetic toll-like receptor agonists for the development of powerful malaria vaccines: a patent review. *Expert Opinion on Therapeutic Patents* 28 (11): 837–847.

90 Wu, W., Li, R., Malladi, S.S. et al. (2010). Structure–activity relationships in toll-like receptor-2 agonistic diacyl thioglycerol lipopeptides. *Journal of Medicinal Chemistry* 53 (8): 3198–3213.

91 Agnihotri, G., Crall, B.M., Lewis, T.C. et al. (2011). Structure–activity relationships in toll-like receptor 2-agonists leading to simplified monoacyl lipopeptides. *Journal of Medicinal Chemistry* 54 (23): 8148–8160.

92 Morin, M.D., Wang, Y., Jones, B.T. et al. (2018). Diprovocims: a new and exceptionally potent class of toll-like receptor agonists. *Journal of the American Chemical Society* 140 (43): 14440–14454.

93 Hu, Z., Banothu, J., Beesu, M. et al. (2018). Identification of human toll-like receptor 2-agonistic activity in dihydropyridine–quinolone carboxamides. *ACS Medicinal Chemistry Letters* 10 (1): 132–136.

94 Ballou, W.R.J., Diderlaurent, A.M., and Van der Most, R.G. (2015). Novel methods for inducing an immune response. WO2015150568, filed 02 April 2015.

95 Angov, E., Bergmann-Leitner, E.S., and Ockenhouse, C.F. (2015). Novel malaria vaccines. WO2015091734, filed 18 December 2014.

96 Fox, C., Reed, S.G., Baldwinj, S., and Vedvick, T. (2013). Improved adjuvant formulations comprising TLR4 agonists and methods of using the same. WO2013119856, filed 07 February 2013.

97 Fox, C.B., Baldwin, S.L., Vedvick, T.S. et al. (2012). Effects on immunogenicity by formulations of emulsion-based adjuvants for malaria vaccines. *Clinical and Vaccine Immunology* 19 (10): 1633–1640.

98 Oeuvray, C., Bouharoun-Tayoun, H., Gras-Masse, H. et al. (1994). Merozoite surface protein-3: a malaria protein inducing antibodies that promote *Plasmodium falciparum* killing by cooperation with blood monocytes. *Blood* 84 (5): 1594–1602.

99 Theisen, M., Soe, S., Jessing, S.G. et al. (2000). Identification of a major B-cell epitope of the *Plasmodium falciparum* glutamate-rich protein (GLURP), targeted by human antibodies mediating parasite killing. *Vaccine* 19 (2, 3): 204–212.

100 Oeuvray, C., Theisen, M., Rogier, C. et al. (2000). Cytophilic immunoglobulin responses to *Plasmodium falciparum* glutamate-rich protein are correlated with protection against clinical malaria in Dielmo. *Senegal. Infection and Immunity* 68 (5): 2617–2620.

101 Theisen, M., Soe, S., Brunstedt, K. et al. (2004). A *Plasmodium falciparum* GLURP–MSP3 chimeric protein; expression in Lactococcus lactis, immunogenicity and induction of biologically active antibodies. *Vaccine* 22 (9, 10): 1188–1198.

102 Lousada-Dietrich, S., Jogdand, P.S., Jepsen, S. et al. (2011). A synthetic TLR4 agonist formulated in an emulsion enhances humoral and Type 1 cellular immune responses against GMZ2–A GLURP–MSP3 fusion protein malaria vaccine candidate. *Vaccine* 29 (17): 3284–3292.

103 Neve, J.E., Wijesekera, H.P., Duffy, S. et al. (2014). Euodenine A: a small-molecule agonist of human TLR4. *Journal of Medicinal Chemistry* 57 (4): 1252–1275.

104 Smith, K.D., Andersen-Nissen, E., Hayashi, F. et al. (2003). Toll-like receptor 5 recognizes a conserved site on flagellin required for protofilament formation and bacterial motility. *Nature Immunology* 4 (12): 1247.

105 Taylor, D.N., Treanor, J.J., Strout, C. et al. (2011). Induction of a potent immune response in the elderly using the TLR-5 agonist, flagellin, with a recombinant hemagglutinin influenza–flagellin fusion vaccine (VAX125, STF2. HA1 SI). *Vaccine* 29 (31): 4897–4902.

106 Bargieri, D.Y., Leite, J.A., Lopes, S.C. et al. (2010). Immunogenic properties of a recombinant fusion protein containing the C-terminal 19 kDa of *Plasmodium falciparum* merozoite surface protein-1 and the innate immunity agonist FliC flagellin of *Salmonella typhimurium*. *Vaccine* 28 (16): 2818–2826.

107 Carapau, D., Mitchell, R., Nacer, A. et al. (2013). Protective humoral immunity elicited by a needle-free malaria vaccine comprised of a chimeric *Plasmodium falciparum* circumsporozoite protein and a toll-like receptor 5 agonist, flagellin. *Infection and Immunity* 81 (12): 4350–4362.

108 Zuber, A.K., Bråve, A., Engström, G. et al. (2004). Topical delivery of imiquimod to a mouse model as a novel adjuvant for human immunodeficiency virus (HIV) DNA. *Vaccine* 22 (13, 14): 1791–1798.

109 Hung, I.F., Zhang, A.J., To, K.K. et al. (2016). Topical imiquimod before intradermal trivalent influenza vaccine for protection against heterologous non-vaccine and antigenically drifted viruses: a single-centre, double-blind, randomised, and controlled phase 2b/3 trial. *The Lancet Infectious Diseases.* 16 (2): 209–218.

110 Othoro, C., Johnston, D., Lee, R. et al. (2009). Enhanced immunogenicity of *Plasmodium falciparum* peptide vaccines using a topical adjuvant containing a potent synthetic toll-like receptor 7 agonist, imiquimod. *Infection and Immunity* 77 (2): 739–748.

111 Nace, G., Evankovich, J., Eid, R., and Tsung, A. (2012). Dendritic cells and damage-associated molecular patterns: endogenous danger signals linking innate and adaptive immunity. *Journal of Innate Immunity* 4 (1): 6–15.

112 Salunke, D.B., Yoo, E., Shukla, N.M. et al. (2012). Structure–activity relationships in human toll-like receptor 8-active 2,3-diamino-furo[2,3-*c*] pyridines. *Journal of Medicinal Chemistry* 55 (18): 8137–8151.

113 Krieg, A.M., Yi, A.K., Matson, S. et al. (1995). CpG motifs in bacterial DNA trigger direct B-cell activation. *Nature* 374 (6522): 546.

114 Coronado, L.M., Nadovich, C.T., and Spadafora, C. (2014). Malarial hemozoin: from target to tool. *Biochimica et Biophysica Acta (BBA) – General Subjects* 1840 (6): 2032–2041.

115 Akira, S., Ishii, K.J., and Coban, C. (2006). Detection/Measurement of malaria infection disease utilizing natural immunity by hemozoin, screening of preventive of therapeutic medicine for malaria infection disease and regulation of natural immunity induction. WO200606195, filed 23 December 2005.

116 Hemmi, H., Takeuchi, O., Kawai, T. et al. (2000). A toll-like receptor recognizes bacterial DNA. *Nature* 408 (6813): 740.

117 Latz, E., Verma, A., Visintin, A. et al. (2007). Ligand-induced conformational changes allosterically activate toll-like receptor 9. *Nature Immunology* 8 (7): 772.

118 Meng, W., Yamazaki, T., Nishida, Y., and Hanagata, N. (2011). Nuclease-resistant immunostimulatory phosphodiester CpG oligodeoxynucleotides as human toll-like receptor 9 agonists. *BMC Biotechnology* 11 (1): 88.

119 Crompton, P.D., Mircetic, M., Weiss, G. et al. (2009). The TLR9 ligand CpG promotes the acquisition of *Plasmodium falciparum*-specific memory B cells in malaria-naive individuals. *The Journal of Immunology* 182 (5): 3318–3326.

120 Suzue, K., Ito, M., Matsumoto, Y. et al. (1997). Protective immunity induced in squirrel monkeys with recombinant serine repeat antigen (SERA) of *Plasmodium falciparum*. *Parasitology International* 46 (1): 17–25.

121 Tougan, T., Aoshi, T., Coban, C. et al. (2013). TLR9 adjuvants enhance immunogenicity and protective efficacy of the SE36/AHG malaria vaccine in nonhuman primate models. *Human Vaccines & Immunotherapeutics* 9 (2): 283–290.

15

Pure TLR7 Agonistic BBIQ is a Potential Adjuvant Against *Plasmodium berghei* ANKA Challenge *In Vivo*

Ruchika Saroa[1], Deepender Kaushik[2], Aruna Rakha[3], Upma Bagai[4,†], Sukhbir Kaur[1], and Deepak B. Salunke[2,4]

[1] *Panjab University, Department of Zoology, Chandigarh 160014, India*
[2] *Panjab University, Department of Chemistry and Centre of Advanced Studies in Chemistry, Chandigarh 160014, India*
[3] *Post Graduate Institute of Medical Education & Research, Department of Translational and Regenerative Medicines, Chandigarh 160012, India*
[4] *Panjab University, National Interdisciplinary Centre of Vaccine, Immunotherapeutics and Antimicrobials, Chandigarh 160014, India*

15.1 Introduction

Malaria is one of the oldest diseases known to humans for millennia, and *Plasmodium falciparum* is the causative agent responsible for millions of deaths worldwide. It is the only species that directly affects the central nervous system causing neurological deficits and cognitive sequelae. The evolvement of an effective vaccine against malaria is the best hope to control this hazard [1]. Several models are developed to represent human malaria and the *Plasmodium berghei* ANKA (PbA) infection in CBA or C57BL/6 mice is the most widely used model. PbA is the main source of cerebral syndrome in rodents having various similarities to the human cerebral malaria. During PbA infection, infected erythrocytes are sequestered into various organs resulting in the congestion of blood vessels leading to death of the host [2].

Pattern-recognition receptors (PRRs) such as toll-like receptors (TLRs), nucleotide binding oligomerization domain like receptor-like receptors (NLRs), and RIG-I-like receptors are being targeted to discover new small molecule immune modulators as well as vaccine adjuvants. Several antigens when combined with TLR agonists are known to provide long-lasting and protective immunity to host by stimulating the expansion of naïve T cells towards a T helper 1 (Th1) phenotype [3]. The TLR ligands also aid in promoting the differentiation and maturation of dendritic cells (DCs) [4]. TLR1, TLR2, TLR4, TLR5, TLR6, and TLR11 are expressed on the cell

† Deceased (8 September 2018).

Drug Development for Malaria: Novel Approaches for Prevention and Treatment, First Edition. Edited by Pravin Kendrekar.

surface, whereas TLR3, TLR7, TLR8, and TLR9 are expressed in intracellular vesicles such as endosome and endoplasmic reticulum [5]. TLR7/8 agonists activate antigen presenting cells (APCs) and enhance both humoral and cellular immune responses and have demonstrated potential as vaccine adjuvants [6].

Resiquimod, a synthetic small molecule activating both TLR7 and TLR8, when given parenterally produces anti-viral effects through the induction of pro-inflammatory cytokines and was shown to have potential to act as an adjuvant [7]. Imiquimod, a pure TLR7 agonist, has been studied as a topical vaccine adjuvant to co-injected protein, topically co-applied peptides and subcutaneously injected dendritic cells and DNA vaccines [8]. Topically applied resiquimod-induced pro-inflammatory cytokines and improved antibody responses to subcutaneously administered antigen and also proved to be an effective topical adjuvant for promoting cytotoxic T lymphocyte (CTL) responses [7].

TLR7 agonists are more potent than TLR8 agonists at inducing (interferon) IFN-α and IFN-regulated chemokines such as IFN-inducible protein and IFN-inducible T cell α chemo attractant [9]. By contrast, TLR8 agonists are more potent at inducing pro-inflammatory cytokines and chemokines, such as TNF-α, IL-12, and MIP-1α, via activation of p38 MAPK and NF-κB pathways [10].

However, potent induction of pro-inflammatory cytokines such as TNF-α by TLR8 agonists may lead to excess toxicity [11]. In light of this, the present study was designed to evaluate the immune response generated in rodent host post-immunised with 10 000 g fraction formulated with highly potent pure TLR7 agonistic 1-benzyl-2-butyl-1*H*-imidazo[4,5-*c*]quinolin-4-amine (BBIQ) [12] against *P. berghei* ANKA challenge.

Immunisation of mice with 10 000 g fraction emulsified in Freund complete adjuvant/Freund incomplete adjuvant (FCA/FIA) showed an activation of an effective cell mediated as well as humoral immune responses against lethal rodent malaria parasite proving that this fraction has a great potential to act as a vaccine when combined with an effective adjuvant [13]. Mice immunised with parasite constituents formulated in FCA/FIA against lethal *P. berghei* NK-65 have also been reported to exhibit significant increase in CD4 and CD8 T cells in spleen leading to the complete clearance of parasite from the system [14].

Recently, the efficacy of pure TLR7 agonistic BBIQ in combination with a suboptimal dose of chloroquine against PbA *in vivo* was investigated wherein a strong but short-lived Th1 mediated immune response was observed [15]. The present study was designed to evaluate the adjuvant capability of BBIQ in combination with blood stage fraction of PbA against its challenge.

15.2 Material and Methods

15.2.1 Experimental Animals

Outbred (LACA) mice five to six weeks old of both sexes were purchased from Central Animal House of Panjab University, Chandigarh. Mice were kept in plastic cages with water and food *ad libitum*. The care as well as sacrifice of the animals was done by following the guidelines approved by the Institutional Animal Ethics Committee.

15.2.2 Ethical Clearance

Ethical clearance was obtained from Panjab University, Chandigarh (PU/IAEC/S/16/132).

15.2.3 Parasite Infection

ANKA strain of *P. berghei* (PbA) was initially procured from National Institute of Malaria Research (NIMR), New Delhi and used in the present study. PbA was maintained *in vivo* by intra-peritoneal (i.p.) inoculation of 10^6 infected red blood cells (iRBCs) from infected to normal mice. Giemsa-stained thin blood smears were made to check the course of infection by the following formula.

$$\frac{\text{Number of infected RBCs/reticulocytes}}{\text{Total number of RBCs/reticulocytes}} \times 100$$

15.2.4 Isolation of Blood Stage Fraction

Cell free parasite was isolated from PbA-infected mice blood by the method of Bagai and Pawar [13]. Grey-coloured parasite pellet was suspended in 0.25 M sucrose in phosphate-buffered saline (PBS [pH 7.2]), homogenised and subjected to subcellular fractionation to isolate 10 000 g [16]. The concentration of protein in fraction was estimated by method of Lowry et al. using bovine serum albumin (BSA) as standard and was found to be 16.56 mg/ml [17]. 100 μg/dose of 10 000 g fraction was used for the immunisation studies.

15.2.5 Adjuvant

Synthetic imidazoquinolines are the first generation TLR7/8 agonists and 1-benzyl-2-butyl-1*H*-imidazo[4,5-*c*]quinolin-4-amine (BBIQ, Figure 15.1) is one of the most active TLR7 agonists [18] which has not been explored as an adjuvant with different *Plasmodium* antigens.

Synthesis of BBIQ was achieved from 2,4-quinolinediol in six steps using the procedures as reported by Shukla et al. [18] with minor modifications [15]. Recently, the process for the production of BBIQ on large scale was also optimised from inexpensive phthalimide and was confirmed to be a pure TLR7 agonist with no TLR8 agonist ability. The manner in which BBIQ binds and activates human TLR7 was also characterised using *in silico* molecular modelling studies [12].

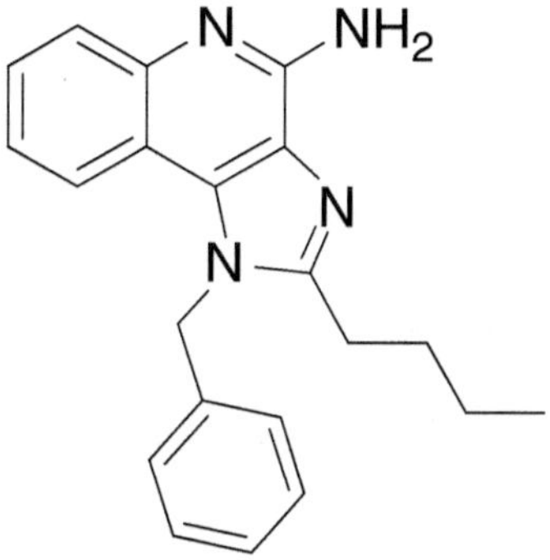

Figure 15.1 Structure of 1-benzyl-2-butyl-1*H*-imidazo[4,5-*c*] quinolin-4-amine (BBIQ), a synthetic small molecule TLR7 agonist used as an adjuvant.

15.3 Immunisation Protocol and Post-challenge Regime

A schematic representation detailing about the overall immunization schedule and post challenge regime is shown in Figure 15.2. In particular, five groups (GP-I to GP-V) having 30 mice each were employed in the study. GP-I was kept as normal control. GP-II was administered with PBS (subcutaneously [s.c.]) on D0, D14, and D28.

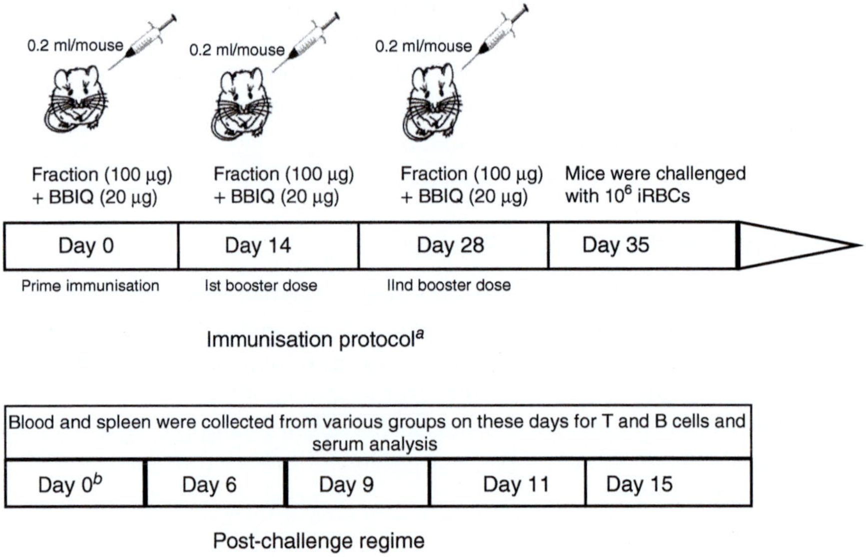

[a] Total 30 mice were included for immunisation
[b] Five mice were sacrificed on D35 of immunisation. This day was considered as D0 post-challenge

Figure 15.2 A schematic diagram showing the immunisation protocol and post-challenge regime of mice immunised with fraction along with adjuvant (GP-III).

Table 15.1 Immunisation protocol.[a)]

Immunisation/Challenge	Group-II	Group-III	Group-IV	Group-V
Prime immunisation; D0 (Dose/mouse) (s.c.)	PBS 0.2 ml	10 000 g fraction (100 μg) + BBIQ (20 μg)	BBIQ (20 μg)	10 000 g (100 μg)
Ist booster; D14 (Dose/mouse) (s.c.)	PBS 0.2 ml	10 000 g fraction (100 μg) + BBIQ (20 μg)	BBIQ (20 μg)	10 000 g (100 μg)
IInd booster; D28 (Dose/mouse) (s.c.)	PBS 0.2 ml	10 000 g fraction (100 μg) + BBIQ (20 μg)	BBIQ (20 μg)	10 000 g (100 μg)
Inoculated/ Challenge; D35 (i.p.)	10^6 iRBCs	10^6 iRBCs	10^6 iRBCs	10^6 iRBCs

a) Five mice from GP-III, GP-IV, and GP-V were sacrificed before challenge.

These mice were inoculated with 10^6 iRBCs (i.p.) on D35. Mice of GP-III, GP-IV, and GP-V were immunised according to Table 15.1 and challenged with 10^6 iRBCs (i.p.) on D35.

15.4 Study Design

Course of parasitaemia post-infection and post-immunisation was monitored in GP-II and GP-III, GP-IV, and GP-V, respectively, by preparing Giemsa stained thin blood smears till death of the mouse or clearance of the parasite from the blood. Percent infection was calculated by the formula explained earlier.

Five mice from each group were sacrificed on D0, D6, D9, D11, and D15 for splenic T cell analysis (CD3, CD4, CD8 and CD4, CD25, FoxP3), splenic B cell analysis (CD19), detection of antibody level (IgG1 and IgG2a) and cytokine analysis (IFN-γ, TNF-α, IL-12, IL-10, and IL-27) in serum samples.

15.5 Isolation of Splenic Lymphocytes from Mice

Spleen from mice of various groups as explained above was dissected out and teased it into a single cell suspension. Cell suspension was washed with cold fluorescence activating cell sorter buffer (FACS) (1 M PBS + 2% FCS + 2 mM ethylene diamine tetra acetic acid [EDTA] pH-7.2) buffer. Red blood cells were lysed using lysis buffer (0.8% ammonium chloride in PBS [pH-7.2]) followed by incubation on ice for 15 minutes. Lymphocytes were collected after washing thrice with FACS buffer [19] and then counted using Neubauer's chamber. 0.5×10^6 lymphocytes were subjected to cell surface and intracellular staining as well [14].

15.6 FACS Analysis of Isolated Lymphocytes

Lymphocytes were stained with anti-mouse CD3-fluorescein isothiocyanate (FITC), anti-mouse CD4-PE, anti-mouse CD8-APC, and anti-mouse CD19-brilliant violet [14]. They were subjected to surface staining using anti-mouse CD4-FITC and anti-mouse CD25-APC followed by intracellular staining with anti-mouse FoxP3-PE. Samples were then analysed on FACS Calibur (BD) and results were analysed using BD FACS DIVA 8.2 software.

15.7 IgG1 and IgG2a Antibody Response

The presence of parasite specific antibodies was monitored in sera samples collected from various groups by enzyme-linked immunosorbent assay (ELISA) [20]. Serum samples were obtained by centrifuging blood at 200 g for 10 minutes. Twofold dilutions were made of each serum sample for the detection of IgG1 and IgG2a antibodies [13]. Optical density of each well was determined by ELISA reader (BioTek, USA) at 490 nm.

15.8 Estimation of Various Cytokines

Levels of IFN-γ, TNF-α, IL-12, IL-10, and IL-27 in serum samples of various groups were measured by sandwich ELISA [21]. Cytokine analysis was performed as per manufacturer's protocol (Qayee-Bio and Diaclone, France). 500 μl of serum was collected from each animal and stored at −20 °C for further use. Serum samples of GP-I and GP-II were diluted in 1 : 4 ratio, whereas GP-IV, GP-V, and GP-VI in 1 : 8 ratio with standard diluent (provided in kits). The absorbance of each well was read on a spectrophotometer at 450 nm. The quantitative estimation was done using standard curve obtained for individual cytokine as mentioned in the respective protocol.

15.9 Statistical Analysis

Student's *t*-test was used for statistical analysis; results with $p < 0.05$ were considered to be statistically significant.

15.10 Results and Discussion

15.10.1 Course of Infection

GP-I was not infected with 10^6 iRBCs, so smears were clear of any infection on all days. Mice of GP-II showed an increase in parasitaemia from D2 to D15 post-infection. On D4, 3.05 ± 0.94% infection was recorded on D4 and all mice of GP-II died on D15 (Figure 15.3). In GP-III, highest infection was found to be 2.9 ± 0.34% on D6 which was cleared by D9. After this, no parasite was observed in GP-III and all mice were clear of infection as seen till D21, whereas parasite appeared late in GP-IV by D6 and all the mice of this group died by D15. In GP-V, on D2, 2.54 ± 0.67% infection was observed. It increased to 4.89 ± 2.88% on D4. Mice of GP-V showed similar course of infection as observed in GP-II and all mice in this group died on D15 (Figure 15.3).

15.10.2 Flow Cytometric Analysis of Splenic T Cells and T reg Cells

T cells are known to provide protective immunity to host against infection; however, both humoral and cell-mediated immune responses are required for providing complete protection to the host against *Plasmodium*. The balance between Th1 and Th2 immune response is necessary for the effective clearance of parasite from the system as well as protecting mice from neurological symptoms [22].

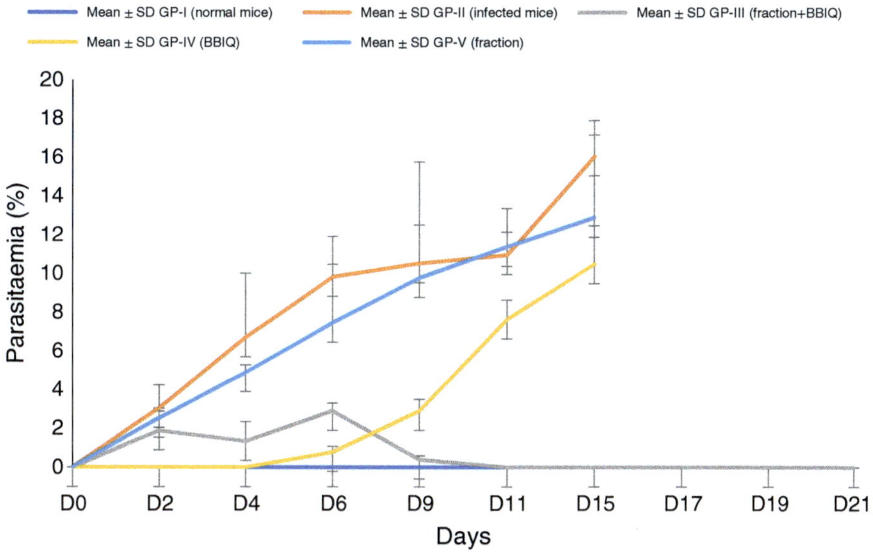

Figure 15.3 Line graph showing the parasitaemia in GP-II (infected control), GP-III (mice immunised with fraction + BBIQ), GP-IV (mice immunised with BBIQ), and GP-V (mice immunised with fraction). The parasitaemia was determined by examining Giemsa-stained thin blood smears. Parasitaemia (mean ± S.D.) of the infected and immunised mice is plotted vs days.

In the present study, the percentage of splenic CD3 T cells was found to be higher (D0 and D11) in mice post-immunisation with fraction + BBIQ in comparison to infected controls. This increase in percentage of CD3 T cells depicted the activation of higher number of T cells against the challenge upon immunisation, whereas their percentage was found to be declined on these similar days in mice immunised with BBIQ alone (Figure 15.4a). Splenic CD3 T cells were further gated for splenic CD4 and CD8 T cells and an increase was observed in splenic CD4 and CD8 T cells in mice post-immunised with fraction emulsified in adjuvant on D6, D11, and D15 (Figure 15.4b,c). This increase in CD4 and CD8 T cells predicted the genesis of effective T cell-mediated responses in host against the challenge as all mice in this group cleared the parasite by D11.

However, mice immunised with fraction alone exhibited an increase in percentages of splenic CD3 (D11), CD4 (D6 and D11), and CD8 (D6, D11 and D15) T cells as compared to infected controls, though CD3, CD4, and CD8 T cells were higher in mice but they were not capable to clear the parasite from blood. Hence, all mice post-immunised with fraction died of challenge by D15 (Figure 15.4a–c).

T reg cells are suppressor T cells which carry out their suppressive activities through secretion of IL-10, TGF-β, and IL-35. They control the inflammation caused by excessive proliferation of T cells [21]. Percentage of splenic T reg cells was found to be higher on various days of experiment suggesting their role in suppressing the inflammatory action of T cells in host post-immunisation (fraction + adjuvant) (Figure 15.4d). Percentage of T reg cells was also higher in mice immunised with

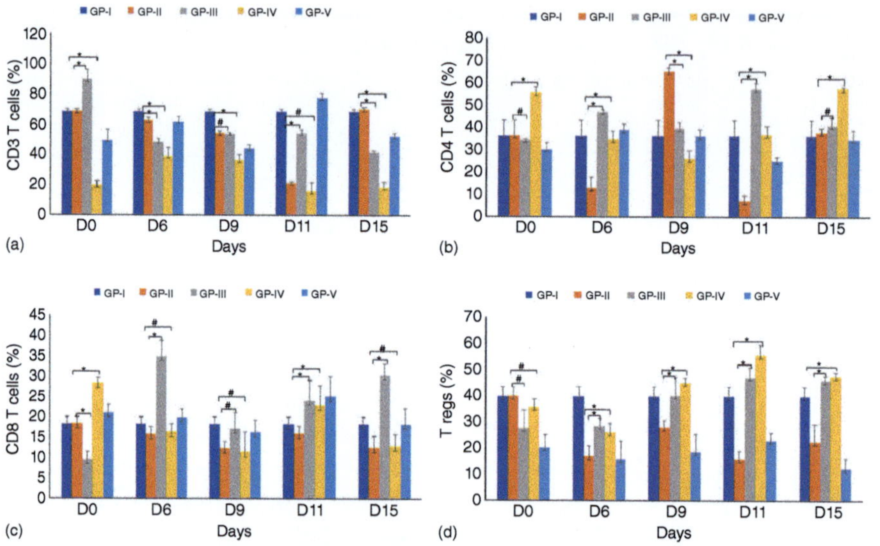

Figure 15.4 Histograms showing the percentages of splenic CD3, CD4, CD8 T, and T regulatory cells of various groups of animals. CD3 (a), CD4 (b), CD8 (c), and T reg cells (d) in GP-I (normal control), GP-II (infected control), GP-III (mice immunised with fraction + BBIQ), GP-IV (mice immunised with BBIQ), and GP-V (mice immunised with fraction) on D0, D6, D9, D11, and D15. Data expressed are the mean ± S.D. *: $p < 0.05$; significant, #: $p > 0.05$; non-significant. GP-II vs GP-III, GP-II vs GP-IV, and GP-II vs GP-V.

adjuvant alone (D6, D9, D11, and D15) and fraction alone (D11), but no survival was observed in both groups. This may point towards the inhibition of effective T cell responses by T reg cells in these mice and aided in parasite growth.

15.10.3 Cytokine Profiling

IFN-γ is a defining cytokine of Th1 cells required for inhibiting the asexual stages of parasite and provides partial protection against *Plasmodium chabaudi* infection. $CD8^+$ T cells also provide protection against liver stages through the secretion of IFN-γ. Complete protection against liver stages of *P. yoelii* is known to be mediated through IFN-γ secretion by CD8 T cells [23].

IL-12 is known to provide protection against the blood stage of *P. chabaudi* through IFN-γ production and $CD4^+$ T cells expansion [24]. The concentration of IFN-γ and IL-12 was higher in mice post-immunised with fraction + BBIQ on D9 and D11 signifying the generation of substantial Th1 response in host. Due to this, all mice in this group were cleared of infection and survived the challenge (Figure 15.5a,c).

IL-10 was reported to be a key immunoregulator during *Plasmodium* infection. The proliferation of CD4 and CD8 T cells and production of TNF-α and IFN-γ were mitigated by IL-10 and limit the immunopathology associated with the disease [25]. Lower level of TNF-α on D9 and D11 post immunization specify no inflammation in mice post immunization with fraction and adjuvant. In addition, higher levels of IL-10 on similar days also authenticate the suppression of inflammation in mice

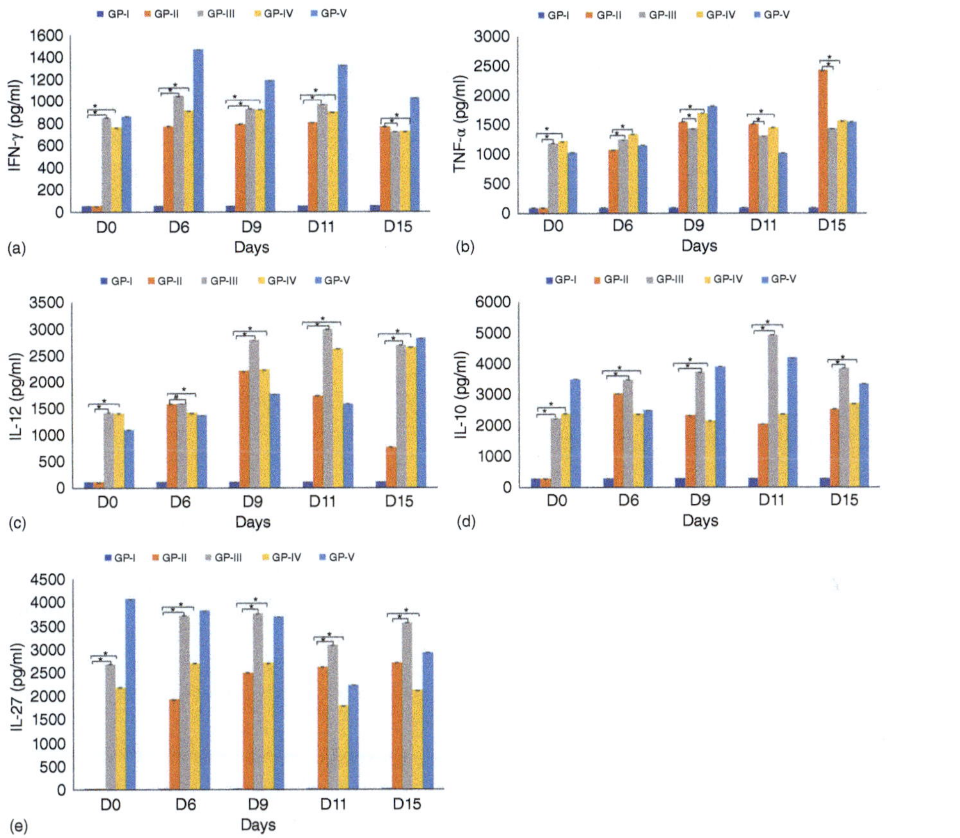

Figure 15.5 Level of various cytokines in GP-I (normal controls), GP-II (infected controls), GP-III (mice immunised with fraction + BBIQ), GP-IV (mice immunised with BBIQ), and GP-V (mice immunised with fraction). Sera sample was analysed for the presence of IFN-γ (a), TNF-α (b), IL-12 (c), IL-10 (d), and IL-27 (e) by sandwich ELISA. Data expressed are the mean ± S.D. of the cytokine concentrations from two different assays. *: $p < 0.05$; significant, #: $p > 0.05$; non-significant. GP-II vs GP-III, GP-II vs GP-IV, and GP-II vs GP-V.

(Figure 15.5b). Increased IL-10 on experimental days in these mice may play a key role in inhibiting the Th1-mediated inflammation. Contrarily, a reverse trend was observed in the level of TNF-α in mice administered with BBIQ alone. On D6 and D9, TNF-α was higher in mice administered with BBIQ alone pointing to the inflammation in host. On similar days, TNF-α was higher in mice post-immunised with fraction alone which may aid in immune-mediated inflammation in host (Figure 15.5b).

IL-27 suppresses the development of Th17-mediated inflammation and stimulates $CD4^+$ T cells to produce IL-10. It has a regulatory role in limiting the immunopathology during infection [26]. Increased level of IL-27 on D6, D9, D11, and D15 post-immunisation with fraction + BBIQ may assist in putting down the Th1 and Th17-mediated inflammation in mice (Figure 15.5e), whereas lower level of IL-27 in mice immunised with adjuvant alone (D11 and D15) points towards the immune-mediated pathology inside the host (Figure 15.5e).

15.10.4 Flow Cytometric Analysis of Splenic B Cells

Complete clearance can be achieved by the activation of various cells such as macrophages and B cells. CD4 T cells helped B cells to produce antimalarial antibodies-specific IgG responses against *P. chabaudi* infection [27]. In the present study, mice immunised with fraction along with adjuvant showed elevated levels of CD4 T cells and B cells on D6 and D11. This increase in CD19 B cells might have helped in clearance of parasite in host via secreting anti-parasitic antibodies, whereas they were found to be lower in mice post-immunised with adjuvant alone and fraction alone on D9 and D11. This may signify that antibodies secreted from B cells may mediate the complete clearance of parasite in mice post-immunisation (fraction + BBIQ) (Figure 15.6).

15.10.5 IgG1 and IgG2a Response

Sera levels of IgG1 and IgG2a were also higher on D6, D9, and D15 in mice post-immunisation with fraction along with adjuvant confirming that CD4 T cells, CD19 B cells and IgG1 and IgG2a together mediated complete clearance of parasite in these mice. After parasite clearance, level of IgG1 was declined in these mice sustaining Th1 response inside the host (Figure 15.7a,b).

A decline in B cells and IgG2a on D6, D9, and D11 in mice immunised with BBIQ alone was observed (Figure 15.7a). Due to their lower levels, all mice post-immunisation with adjuvant alone died after challenge because of the insufficient secretion of anti-parasitic antibodies. Elevated levels of only IgG1 (D0, D6, and D9) post-immunisation of mice with adjuvant alone in comparison to infected controls indicate the generation of Th2 immune responses inside the host. But this was not sustainable and capable as well to control the parasite growth thereby,

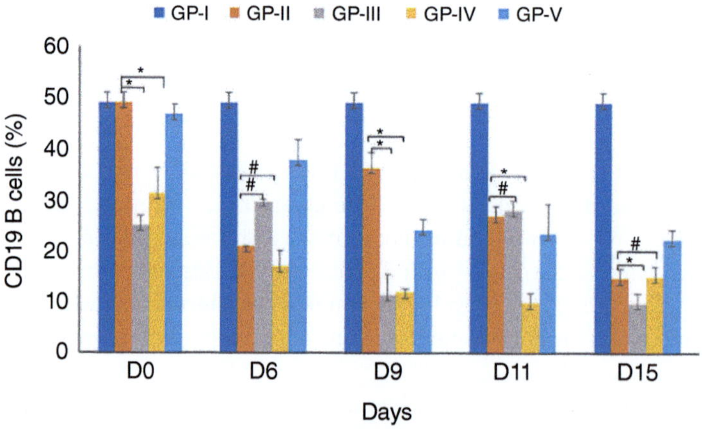

Figure 15.6 Histogram showing the percentage of splenic CD19+ B cells of various groups. GP-I (normal controls), GP-II (infected controls), GP-III (mice immunised with fraction + BBIQ), GP-IV (mice immunised with BBIQ), and GP-V (mice immunised with fraction) on D0, D6, D9, D11, and D15. Data expressed are the mean ± S.D. *: $p < 0.05$; significant, #: $p > 0.05$; non-significant. GP-II vs GP-III, GP-II vs GP-IV, and GP-II vs GP-V.

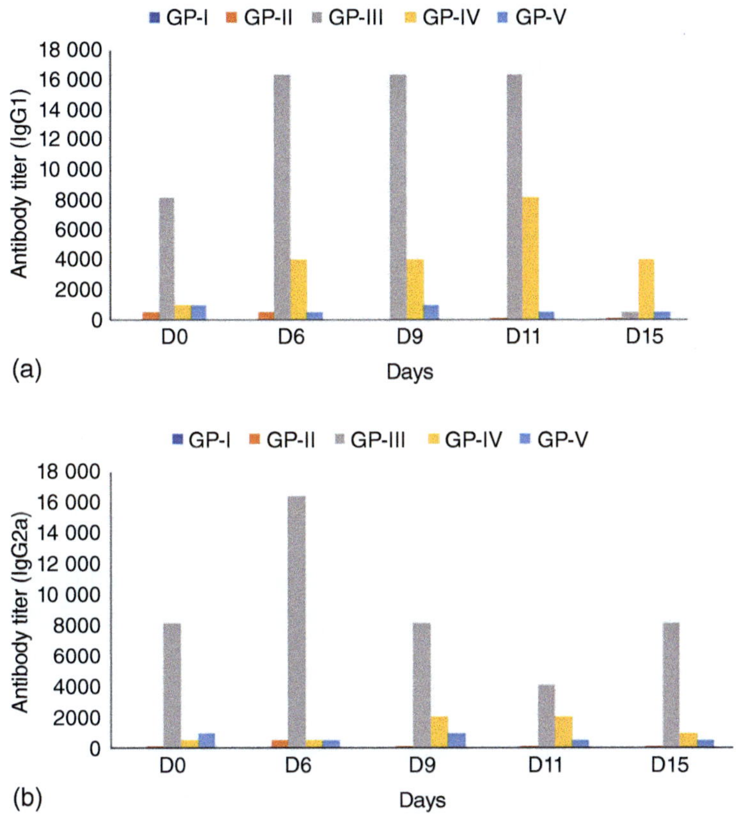

Figure 15.7 Histograms showing IgG1 (a) and IgG2a (b) response in GP-I (normal controls [not detected]), GP-II (infected controls), GP-III (mice immunised with fraction + BBIQ), GP-IV (mice immunised with BBIQ), and GP-V (mice immunised with fraction). Serum IgG antibodies to blood-stage PbA antigen were measured by ELISA on D0, D6, D9, D11, and D15.

parasite appeared on D9 and all mice died in this group by D15 (Figure 15.7a). However, mice post-immunised with fraction alone exhibited a constant decline in IgG1 and IgG2a aiding parasite growth inside the host (Figure 15.7a,b).

Later, leftover mice from GP-III with complete clearance of parasite were reinjected with 10^6 iRBCs (i.p.) after one month of immunisation. They showed regular course of infection as in infected controls and died on D8 post-infection with 10.4% parasitaemia. It can also be seen that on D15, frequency of CD3, CD4, and IgG1 was lower depicting the protection for shorter duration.

15.11 Conclusion

A blood stage fraction along with TLR7 agonist (BBIQ) displayed complete but interim protection against the challenge in mice. The duration of protection may increase by adding one booster dose in immunisation protocol. The further efficacy studies with variable immunisation protocol and possible application of pure TLR8 agonists as well as dual TLR7/8 agonists with blood stage fraction are currently ongoing to achieve complete and long-lasting protection against *Plasmodium* challenge. To the best of our knowledge, this is the first study to demonstrate the use of pure TLR7 agonist as an adjuvant with blood stage fraction of *P. berghei* ANKA against its challenge. A better and complete understanding of TLR agonists as an adjuvant with various antigens of *Plasmodium* will prove helpful in the designing of effective vaccine against the cerebral malaria in humans.

Conflict of Interests

The authors declare no conflict of interest.

Funding

The authors are indebted to University Grant Commission (UGC), New Delhi for the award of Junior Research Fellowship. The Special Assistance Programme of UGC [F.4-28/2015(CAS-II) (SAP-II)] and Fund for Improvement of S&T Infrastructure of DST [SR/FST/LSI-545/2012(C)] are gratefully acknowledged.

Acknowledgment

Ruchika Saroa performed the research and drafted the manuscript. Late Prof Upma Bagai and Dr Deepak B. Salunke designed the research study and helped in analysing the results. Prof. Sukhbir Kaur helped in designing and writing the manuscript. Dr Aruna Rakha helped in flow cytometry work, Deepender Kaushik synthesised the TLR7 agonist. It is a pleasure to acknowledge the technical work of CSIF for immunophenotyping by flow cytometer (B.D. FACS Calibur) at PGIMER, Chandigarh.

References

1 Mungala-Odera, V., Snow, R.W., and Newton, C.R. (2004). The burden of the neurocognitive impairment associated with *Plasmodium falciparum* malaria in sub-Saharan Africa. *The American Journal of Tropical Medicine and Hygiene* 71: 64–70.

2 Engwerda, C.R., Mynott, L.T., Sawhney, S. et al. (2002). Locally up-regulated lymphotoxin α not systemic tumor necrosis factor α is the principle mediator of murine cerebral malaria. *The Journal of Experimental Medicine* 195: 1371–1377.

3 Maisonneuve, C., Bertholet, S., Philpott, D.J., and Gregorio, D.E. (2014). Unleashing the potential of NOD- and toll-like agonist as vaccine adjuvants. *PNAS* 111: 12294–12299.

4 Tomai, M.A. and Vasilakos, J.P. (2012). TLR agonists as vaccine adjuvants. In: *Innovation in Vaccinology* (ed. S. Baschieri), 205–228. Dordrecht: Springer.

5 Kumar, H., Kawai, T., and Akira, S. (2009). Toll-like receptors and innate immunity. *Biochemical and Biophysical Research Communications* 388: 621–625.

6 Dowling, J.D. (2018). Recent advances in the discovery and delivery of TLR7/8 agonists as vaccine adjuvants. *Immunohorizons* 2: 185–197.

7 Chang, A.B., Cross, L.J., Najar, M.H., and Dutz, J.P. (2009). Topical resiquimod promotes priming of CTL to parenteral antigens. *Vaccine* 27: 5791–5799.

8 Othoro, C., Johnston, D., Lee, R. et al. (2009). Enhanced immunogenicity of *Plasmodium falciparum* peptide vaccines using a topical adjuvant containing a potent synthetic toll-like receptor 7 agonist, Imiquimod. *Infection and Immunity* 77: 739–748.

9 Gorden, K.B., Gorski, K.S., Gibson, S.J. et al. (2005). Synthetic TLR agonists reveal functional differences between human TLR7 and TLR8. *Journal of Immunology* 174: 1259–1268.

10 Levy, O., Suter, E.E., Miller, R.L., and Wessels, M.R. (2006). Unique efficacy of toll-like receptor 8 agonists in activating human neonatal antigen-presenting cells. *Blood* 108: 1284–1290.

11 Warshakoon, H.J., Hood, J.D., Kimbrell, M.R. et al. (2009). Potential adjuvantic properties of innate immune stimuli. *Human Vaccines* 5: 381–394.

12 Kaushik, D., Dhingra, S., Patil, M.T. et al. (2020). BBIQ, a pure TLR7 agonist, is an effective influenza vaccine adjuvant. *Human Vaccines* 16: 1989–1996, https://doi.org/10.1080/21645515.2019.1710409.

13 Bagai, U. and Pawar, A. (2013). A blood stage fraction of *Plasmodium berghei* induces protective and long lasting immune response in BALB/c mice. *Parasitology International* 62: 329–336.

14 Kumar, V., Rakha, A., Saroa, R., and Bagai, U. (2015). $CD4^+$ T cells expansion in *P. berghei* (NK-65) infected and immunized BALB/C mice. *Journal of Clinical and Experimental Pathology* 5: 229–234.

15 Saroa, R., Kaushik, D., Bagai, U. et al. (2019). Efficacy of TLR7 agonistic imidazoquinoline as immunochemotherapeutic agent against *P. berghei* ANKA infected rodent host. *Bioorganic and Medicinal Chemistry Letters* 29: 1099–1105.

16 Banyal, H.S., Pandey, V.C., and Dutta, G.P. (1979). Subcellular fractionation and localization of marker enzymes of erythrocytic stages of *Plasmodium knowlesi*. *Indian Journal of Parasitology* 3: 9–14.

17 Lowry, O.H., Rasebrough, N.J., Farr, A.L., and Randall, R.J. (1951). Protein measurement with phenol reagent. *The Journal of Biological Chemistry* 193: 265–275.

18 Shukla, N.M., Malladi, S.S., Mutz, C.A. et al. (2010). Structure-activity relationships in human toll-like receptor 7-active imidazoquinoline analogues. *Journal of Medicinal Chemistry* 53: 4450–4465.

19 Czuprynski, C.J. and Brown, J.F. (1999). *In vitro* analysis, isolation and preparation of lymphocytes from infected animals. In: *Immunology of Infection* (ed. S.H.E. Kaufmann and D. Kabelitz), 189–194. New York.

20 Lee, H.D., Chu, B.K., Kang, J.H. et al. (2019). Previous infection with *Plasmodium berghei* confers resistance to *Toxoplasma gondii* infection in mice. *The Korean Journal of Parasitology* 57: 93–99.

21 Kaur, S., Kaur, T., and Joshi, J. (2016). Immunogenicity and protective efficacy of DNA vaccine against visceral leishmaniasis in BALB/c mice. *Journal of Biomedical Research* 30: 304–313.

22 Podoba, J.E. and Stevenson, M.M. (1991). $CD4^+$ and $CD8^+$ T lymphocytes both contribute to acquired immunity to blood-stage *Plasmodium chabaudi* AS. *Infection and Immunity* 59: 51–58.

23 Nie, C.Q., Bernard, N.J., Schofield, L., and Hansen, D.S. (2007). $CD4^+$ $CD25^+$ regulatory T cells suppress $CD4^+$ T-cell function and inhibit the development of *Plasmodium berghei*-specific TH1 responses involved in cerebral malaria pathogenesis. *Infection and Immunity* 75: 2275–2282.

24 Su, Z. and Stevenson, M.M. (2002). IL-12 is required for antibody-mediated protective immunity against blood-stage *Plasmodium chabaudi* AS malaria infection in mice. *Journal of Immunology* 168: 1348–1355.

25 Perez-Mazliah, D. and Langhorne, J. (2015). CD4 T-cell subsets in malaria: TH1/TH2 revisited. *Frontiers in Immunology* 5: 671–674.

26 Kimura, D., Miyakoda, M., Kimura, K. et al. (2016). Interleukin-27-producing $CD4^+$ T cells regulate protective immunity during malaria parasite Infection. *Immunity* 44: 672–682.

27 Langhorne, J., Meding, S.J., Eichmann, K., and Gillard, S.S. (1989). The response of $CD4^+$ T cells to *Plasmodium chabaudi chabaudi*. *Immunological Reviews* 112: 71–94.

Index

Drug Development for Malaria: Novel Approaches for Prevention and Treatment, First Edition.
Edited by Pravin Kendrekar.

c

d

k

l

n

o

p

q